Limb Salvage Surgery in Bone Tumors

This book brings together a wide spectrum of surgical techniques for tumor excision and limb reconstruction, with special emphasis on practical biological options often used in developing countries. A unique section on pelvic tumors explores reconstruction strategies beyond megaprostheses. Unlike most books on musculoskeletal neoplasms that focus primarily on tumor pathology and outcomes, this volume emphasizes reconstruction techniques and presents the wide range of available options. It bridges a critical gap in surgical oncology literature, making it a valuable reference that deserves a place on every oncologist's shelf.

Key Features:

- Explains complex surgical concepts with clarity, supported by high-quality full-color illustrations
- Engaging and practical resource for orthopedic surgeons, oncologists, residents, trainees, and fellows
- Blends evidence with step-by-step guidance to serve as a trusted companion for young surgeons

Love Kapoor MS (orthopedics), Fellowship in Musculoskeletal Oncology (AIIMS, New Delhi). *Assistant Professor, Department of Orthopedics, National Cancer Institute, All India Institute of Medical Sciences, New Delhi, India*

Venkatesan Sampath Kumar MS (orthopedics), DNB (orthopedics), MRCS (Glasgow), MNAMS, FRCS (trauma and orthopedics, Glasgow). *Additional Professor, Department of Orthopaedics, All India Institute of Medical Sciences, New Delhi, India*

Shah Alam Khan MS (Orthopaedics), DNB (Orthopaedics), MRCS (Edinburgh), M.Ch Orth (Liverpool), FRCS (Glasgow). *Professor, Department of Orthopaedics, All India Institute of Medical Sciences, New Delhi, India*

Limb Salvage Surgery in Bone Tumors

Love Kapoor
Venkatesan Sampath Kumar
Shah Alam Khan

CRC Press
Taylor & Francis Group
Boca Raton London New York

CRC Press is an imprint of the
Taylor & Francis Group, an **informa** business

Designed cover image: Love Kapoor, Venkatesan Sampath Kumar, and Shah Alam Khan

First edition published 2026
by CRC Press
2385 NW Executive Center Drive, Suite 320, Boca Raton FL 33431

and by CRC Press
4 Park Square, Milton Park, Abingdon, Oxon, OX14 4RN

CRC Press is an imprint of Taylor & Francis Group, LLC

ISBN: 978-0-367-42130-4 (hbk)
ISBN: 978-1-041-25150-7 (pbk)
ISBN: 978-0-367-82200-2 (ebk)

DOI: 10.1201/9780367822002

Typeset in Times
by SPi Technologies India Pvt Ltd (Straive)

This Book is Dedicated

To our **Patients**,
who, with extraordinary resilience, place their trust in us as surgeons.
Their journeys remind us that limb salvage is not only a technical achievement but also a profound human endeavor—one that restores mobility, dignity, and hope in the face of life-altering disease;

To our **Mentors**,
who guided us with wisdom and instilled in us the pursuit of excellence;

And to our **Families**,
whose unwavering support and sacrifices made this work possible.

Contents

Author Biographies ... ix
Preface ... xi
Acknowledgment ... xii

SECTION I General Principles

Chapter 1 Clinical Presentation, Classification, and Staging of Bone Tumors ... 3
Chapter 2 Imaging of Bone Tumors ... 8
Chapter 3 Biopsy of Bone Tumors ... 22
Chapter 4 Fundamentals of Surgical Management of Bone Tumors ... 31

SECTION II Upper Extremity

Chapter 5 Proximal Humerus Resection and Reconstruction ... 43
Chapter 6 Scapular Resection and Reconstruction ... 55
Chapter 7 Distal Humerus Resection and Reconstruction ... 62
Chapter 8 Resections and Reconstructions around the Wrist ... 71

SECTION III Lower Extremity

Chapter 9 Proximal Femur Resection and Reconstruction ... 83
Chapter 10 Distal Femur Resection and Reconstruction ... 93
Chapter 11 Proximal Tibia Resection and Reconstruction ... 105
Chapter 12 Distal Tibia Resection and Reconstruction ... 118
Chapter 13 Fibular Resections ... 126

SECTION IV Pelvic and Sacral Resections

Chapter 14 Pelvic Resections and Reconstructions ... 137
Chapter 15 Sacral Resection and Reconstruction ... 151

SECTION V Miscellaneous

Chapter 16 Resections and Reconstructions in Skeletally Immature ... 165
Chapter 17 Intercalary Resection and Reconstruction ... 176

Chapter 18 Partial Limb Salvage in Extensive Extremity Sarcomas 188
Chapter 19 Limb Salvage in Benign Bone Tumors 196
Chapter 20 Management of Appendicular Skeletal Metastasis 207
Chapter 21 Bone Grafting, Allograft, and Tissue Processing 218
Chapter 22 Recent Advances in Limb Salvage Surgery 223

Index 230

Author Biographies

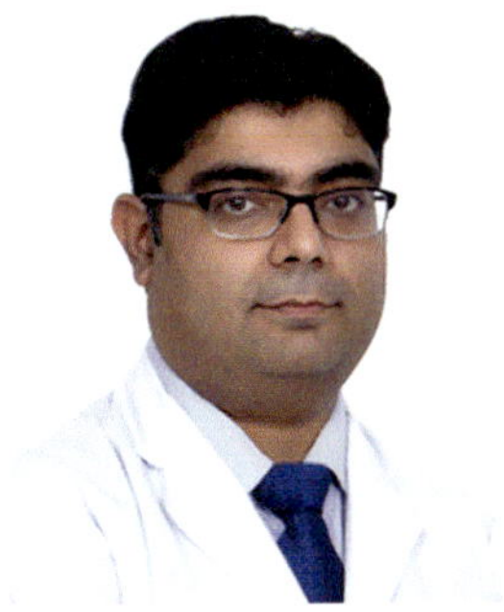

Dr. Love Kapoor

Love Kapoor is an Assistant Professor in the Department of Orthopedics at the National Cancer Institute, All India Institute of Medical Sciences (AIIMS), New Delhi, with a focused expertise in musculoskeletal oncology. After completing his MBBS and MS (Orthopedics) from Government Medical College and Hospital, Chandigarh, he pursued a fellowship in Musculoskeletal Oncology at AIIMS, New Delhi, where he honed his skills in complex limb salvage procedures and multidisciplinary cancer care.

An enthusiastic academic and researcher, Dr. Kapoor has authored more than 18 PubMed-indexed publications in reputed international journals, with contributions on biological reconstructions, endoprosthetic replacements, pelvic resections, and novel techniques in limb salvage surgery. His scholarly work has appeared in leading journals such as *Journal of Surgical Oncology, International Orthopedics, Journal of Hand Surgery*, and *JSES International*. He has also contributed to book chapters in the field of orthopedic oncology.

Deeply passionate about oncology, Dr. Kapoor is committed to combining clinical practice with academic advancement. He is actively involved in teaching and mentoring young orthopedic surgeons, fostering a culture of inquiry and innovation. His research orientation is aimed at improving functional outcomes, enhancing reconstructive techniques, and ensuring oncological safety for patients undergoing limb salvage surgery.

Dr. Kapoor embodies the new generation of surgeon-scientists, dedicated to advancing musculoskeletal oncology through patient-centered care, academic excellence, and innovative research.

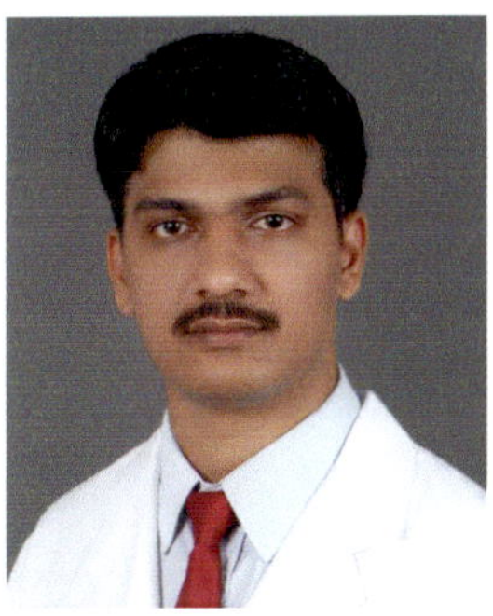

Dr. Venkatesan Sampath Kumar

Dr. Venkatesan Sampath Kumar is an Additional Professor in the Department of Orthopedics at the AIIMS, New Delhi, with specialized expertise in orthopedic oncology. He completed his MBBS from Madras Medical College, followed by MS (orthopedics) from AIIMS, New Delhi. He holds additional qualifications, including DNB (orthopedics), MRCS (Glasgow), MNAMS, and FRCS (trauma and orthopedics, Glasgow).

Dr. Kumar further trained internationally through prestigious fellowships, including a Commonwealth Fellowship in Orthopedic Oncology at the Robert Jones and Agnes Hunt Hospital, Oswestry (UK), a fellowship in Lower Limb Surgery at Wrightington Hospital (UK), and a fellowship in Orthopedic Oncology at Memorial Sloan Kettering Cancer Center (USA).

He has authored numerous publications in indexed international journals, spanning clinical research in orthopedic oncology, pediatric orthopedics, and trauma, with contributions to leading journals such as the *Journal of Surgical Oncology, International Orthopedics, The Bone & Joint Journal*, and *Journal of Hand Surgery*. He has also contributed chapters to international reference texts, including *Sarcoma: A Multidisciplinary Approach to Treatment* and *Turek's Orthopedics*.

Dr. Kumar is an active member of multiple professional societies, including the Indian Orthopedic Association, International Society of Limb Salvage (ISOLS), and Indian Musculoskeletal Oncology Society (IMSOS). His clinical practice and academic work focus on advancing musculoskeletal oncology, improving outcomes of limb salvage surgery, and contributing to collaborative global research.

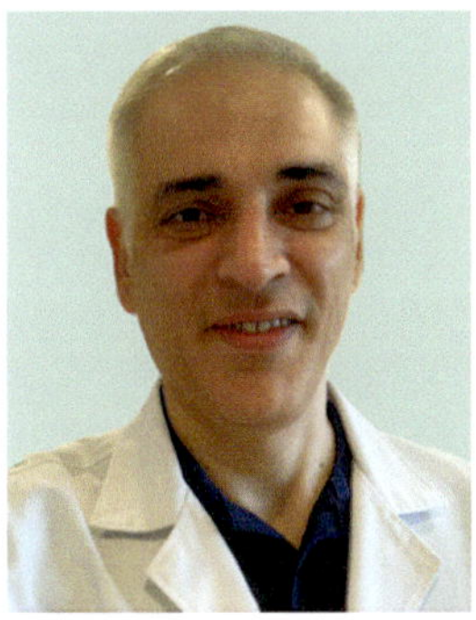

Prof. Shah Alam Khan

Prof. Shah Alam Khan is Professor in the Department of Orthopedics at the AIIMS, New Delhi, and is among the leading figures in the field of musculoskeletal oncology. He completed his MS (orthopedics) from Jawaharlal Nehru Medical College, Aligarh, Uttar Pradesh, and holds additional qualifications, including DNB (orthopedics), MRCS (Edinburgh), M.Ch. orthopedics (Liverpool), and FRCS (Glasgow).

Prof. Khan has more than two decades of academic, clinical, and research experience, with significant contributions to orthopedic oncology, musculoskeletal trauma, and reconstructive surgery. He has authored a large number of publications in reputed international and national journals such as the *Journal of Surgical Oncology, Journal of Bone and Joint Surgery* (American), *International Orthopedics, Pediatric Blood Cancer, Clinical Oncology*, and others. His work has shaped contemporary approaches to osteosarcoma, Ewing sarcoma, and giant cell tumors, as well as innovative reconstructive methods, particularly in resource-constrained environments.

He has contributed chapters to multiple textbooks and has authored numerous books. Prof. Khan has also been recognized with several academic awards and gold medals throughout his career, reflecting his excellence in both undergraduate and postgraduate training.

As a senior academic and clinician, Prof. Khan has been a mentor to generations of orthopedic surgeons and oncologists, fostering academic rigor, innovation, and patient-centered care. His leadership at AIIMS has significantly advanced the discipline of orthopedic oncology in India and abroad.

Preface

The field of musculoskeletal oncology has witnessed a remarkable transformation over the past few decades, shifting from amputation as the default mode of treatment for malignant bone tumors to the era of sophisticated limb salvage procedures that prioritize both oncological clearance and functional preservation. This paradigm shift has been made possible by parallel advances in oncological imaging, histopathology, neoadjuvant chemotherapy, surgical techniques, biomaterials, and reconstructive strategies. Today, limb salvage is not only a feasible option in the majority of patients with bone tumors, but in many centers, it is the standard of care.

Limb Salvage in Bone Tumors has been conceptualized to provide a comprehensive, detailed, and practical overview of this evolving discipline. While the literature is replete with individual studies, review articles, and technical notes, the need for a consolidated resource that brings together surgical principles, operative nuances, reconstructive options, complication management, and outcome analysis remains pressing—especially for surgeons and trainees working in high-volume centers and those in the formative stages of their careers. This volume seeks to address that gap by presenting the subject in a structured, evidence-based, and clinically oriented manner.

The intention behind this book is not merely to catalog techniques but to offer a thoughtful discussion of decision-making in bone tumor surgery. Limb salvage is not a "one-size-fits-all" concept. The choice of procedure is guided by several factors: tumor biology, anatomical location, patient age and expectations, availability of reconstruction methods, and institutional expertise. Equally important are the multidisciplinary inputs from medical oncologists, radiation oncologists, radiologists, and rehabilitation specialists, all of whom contribute to optimizing patient outcomes. By highlighting these interconnections, the book underscores the importance of a team-based approach in musculoskeletal oncology.

Each chapter has been designed with a dual purpose—first, to present the fundamental principles of a specific anatomical resection or reconstruction, and second, to delve into the operative details, supported by illustrative cases, diagrams, and clinical images. The contributors have drawn on their own clinical experience and institutional data, ensuring that the discussions remain grounded in real-world practice. This emphasis on practical applicability is expected to benefit readers who may be confronted with similar surgical challenges in their own practices.

The scope of the book extends beyond the purely surgical domain. Chapters also address perioperative care, rehabilitation, functional outcome assessment, and long-term follow-up. The discussion of complications—whether related to infection, implant failure, or tumor recurrence—is candid, reflecting the reality that limb salvage is not without risks. Yet, the very act of acknowledging these challenges equips surgeons with foresight and strategies to mitigate them. A section has also been devoted to newer frontiers in limb salvage, including 3D bioprinting, patient-specific implants, and biological reconstructions, which offer a glimpse into the future of musculoskeletal oncology.

As editors and contributors, we are acutely aware of the diversity of contexts in which limb salvage is practiced worldwide. Resource-rich centers may employ custom endoprostheses and navigation-assisted resections, whereas surgeons in low-resource settings may rely on innovative biological methods such as recycled autografts or allograft-prosthetic composites. By presenting a spectrum of reconstructive strategies, this book attempts to be inclusive and relevant across varied health-care environments. The underlying principle remains the same—providing the best possible functional and oncological outcome within the given constraints.

The book also emphasizes the importance of long-term oncological surveillance. A successful limb salvage procedure is measured not only by the immediate functional result but also by the durability of reconstruction, the ability to detect and treat recurrence, and the quality of life that patients regain over years of survivorship. By integrating long-term perspectives, we hope to remind readers that limb salvage is a journey that extends well beyond the operating room.

This work is the result of collective efforts by a group of surgeons, oncologists, and academicians who share a common passion for musculoskeletal oncology. Their willingness to contribute chapters, share cases, and distill years of experience into accessible writing has been invaluable. We are equally indebted to our mentors, colleagues, and students, whose discussions and queries have shaped our understanding of the subject and underscored the need for such a resource.

We hope that *Limb Salvage in Bone Tumors* will serve as a valuable reference for orthopedic surgeons, oncologists, residents, and allied specialists. Whether used as a guide in the operating theater, a resource for academic preparation, or a foundation for further research, this book aims to inspire thoughtful practice and continuous learning in the service of patients with bone tumors.

Shah Alam Khan
Venkatesan Sampath Kumar
Love Kapoor

Acknowledgment

We gratefully acknowledge all those whose support has made this book possible. We are indebted to our mentors and teachers in the field of musculoskeletal oncology, whose guidance and encouragement laid the foundation for our academic and clinical journey.

We extend our sincere thanks to our colleagues in the Departments of Orthopedics, Medical Oncology, Pathology, Radiodiagnosis, Radiation Oncology, Nuclear Medicine, and Anesthesiology at the AIIMS, New Delhi, India. Their collaboration, expertise, and multidisciplinary commitment have been invaluable in advancing the care of patients with bone tumors, significantly enriching the perspective of this work.

We are also thankful to our students and residents, whose curiosity and enthusiasm constantly inspire us to refine our knowledge and practice. Our heartfelt gratitude goes to our families, whose patience, understanding, and unwavering support sustained us through the long hours of writing and editing.

Above all, we express our deepest appreciation to our patients. Their strength and resilience in the face of illness continue to be our greatest motivation and the true inspiration behind this book.

Section I

General Principles

1 Clinical Presentation, Classification, and Staging of Bone Tumors

INTRODUCTION

Bone tumors represent a diverse group of neoplastic conditions arising from osseous or cartilaginous tissue, with biological behavior ranging from indolent benign lesions to highly aggressive malignancies. Although rare, accounting for less than 1% of all adult malignancies and approximately 15% of pediatric cancers, primary bone tumors pose significant diagnostic and therapeutic challenges due to their potential for local destruction, systemic spread, and the functional implications of their treatment.

Over the last two decades, there has been a significant enhancement in both survival outcomes and quality of life for patients with bone sarcomas, largely owing to progress in multimodal therapeutic strategies. The integration of limb salvage surgical techniques with systemic chemotherapy and, in select cases, radiotherapy has enabled curative treatment in a substantial proportion of patients with bone and soft tissue sarcomas. Presently, limb-sparing resections have supplanted amputations in over 90% of cases. These multidisciplinary advances have contributed to a notable rise in five-year survival rates among adolescents, improving from around 50% in the 1970s to approximately 75%–80% in recent years [1]. A thorough understanding of the underlying biology and pathology of bone and soft tissue neoplasms remains critical for devising effective treatment plans.

This chapter aims to provide a comprehensive overview of the clinical manifestations, classification paradigms, and staging systems pertinent to bone tumors. It underscores the importance of a systematic approach to clinical evaluation, integration of imaging and histologic data, and application of established staging frameworks in the diagnosis and multidisciplinary management of patients with bone tumors.

CLINICAL EVALUATION OF BONE TUMORS

A thorough clinical evaluation is the cornerstone of the diagnostic workup of bone tumors. Given the overlapping features between benign and malignant lesions, a meticulous history, physical examination, and appropriate use of initial imaging are essential to formulate a differential diagnosis and guide further investigations or referral to a musculoskeletal oncologist.

HISTORY

The clinical presentation of bone tumors varies widely, from incidental findings on radiographs to severe pain and functional impairment. Pain is the most common symptom and should be carefully characterized. Benign lesions often cause mild, activity-related discomfort that is responsive to analgesics. In contrast, malignant tumors typically produce pain that is progressive, persistent at rest, and often more pronounced at night. A history of trauma may occasionally unmask an underlying lesion but should not be assumed to be causal. Patient age at presentation is an important variable that can help guide the diagnosis (Table 1.1).

Systemic symptoms such as fever, malaise, and weight loss may suggest malignancy or infection. A detailed personal and family history is crucial, particularly in individuals with known genetic syndromes (e.g., Li-Fraumeni, hereditary retinoblastoma, Rothmund-Thomson syndrome), prior radiation exposure, Paget's disease, or predisposing bone conditions such as multiple enchondromatosis or osteochondromas.

PHYSICAL EXAMINATION

The physical examination should begin with an inspection and palpation of the affected region, assessing for swelling, tenderness, changes in the overlying skin, local warmth, or the presence of a palpable mass. Malignant tumors often present with a firm, fixed mass, sometimes with associated neurovascular compromise or regional lymphadenopathy. Joint involvement may manifest with decreased range of motion or joint effusion (Figure 1.1 and Table 1.2).

Neurovascular examination is critical to evaluate for deficits suggestive of compression or invasion. Assessment of limb function, gait, and load-bearing capacity provides

TABLE 1.1
Common Diagnoses by Age

Age	Benign	Malignant
0–5 years	Histiocytosis	Metastatic neuroblastoma
5–20 years	Nonossifying fibroma Aneurysmal bone cyst Simple bone cyst Osteoid osteoma Osteochondroma	Osteosarcoma Ewing sarcoma
20–40 years	Giant cell tumor Fibrous dysplasia Enchondroma	Lymphoma Ewing sarcoma
>40 years	Enchondroma Bone infarct Infection	Metastatic carcinoma Lymphoma Multiple myeloma Chondrosarcoma

DOI: 10.1201/9780367822002-2

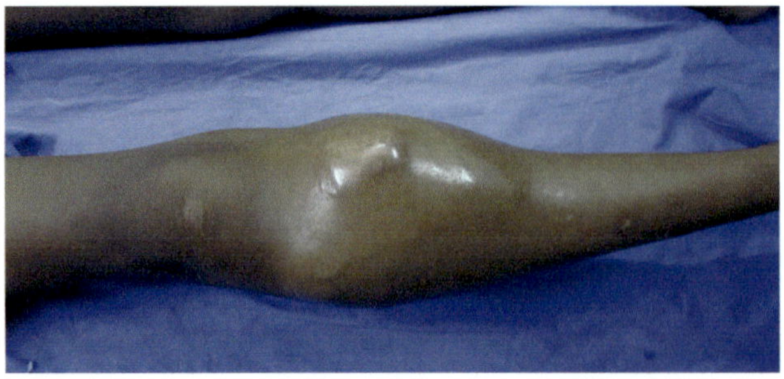

FIGURE 1.1 Clinical photograph of a young adolescent male presenting with a progressively enlarging swelling around the knee joint of three months' duration. The overlying skin appears shiny and stretched, with prominence of superficial veins. Malignant bone tumors typically present with persistent pain (often worsening at night or at rest), swelling, functional limitation, and occasionally constitutional symptoms. On physical examination, such swellings are usually firm to hard in consistency, ill-defined with indistinct margins merging into surrounding tissues, tender on deep palpation, adherent to underlying structures, and associated with raised local temperature.

TABLE 1.2

Comparison of Clinical Presentation of Benign vs. Malignant Bone Tumors

Clinical Feature	Benign Bone Tumors	Malignant Bone Tumors
History	Often incidental; history of minor trauma or found during evaluation for unrelated symptoms. Pain is usually mild, intermittent, and mechanical.	Progressive pain, worsening at night or rest; may include systemic symptoms such as fever, weight loss. Often no history of trauma.
Chief Complaints	Mild pain, swelling, deformity, or incidental finding on imaging. Usually nondisabling.	Persistent pain, swelling, functional limitation, or mass. May include constitutional symptoms and reduced limb function.
Physical Examination		
Overlying Skin	Normal appearance; no dilated veins; freely mobile over the lesion.	Shiny with dilated veins; may have surgical (biopsy) scar; adherent to underlying tissues.
Consistency of Swelling	Soft to firm; fluctuant or well-circumscribed.	Firm to hard; solid and often fixed.
Margins of Swelling	Well-defined; clearly demarcated from surrounding tissues.	Ill-defined; imperceptibly merges into surrounding tissues.
Tenderness on Palpation	Non-tender or mildly tender.	Tender on deep palpation.
Local Temperature	Normal.	Raised local temperature.

insight into the lesion's functional impact. In older adults, suspicion should remain high for metastatic disease, multiple myeloma, or lymphoma, necessitating a focused examination, including breast and prostate.

CLASSIFICATION OF BONE TUMORS

Bone tumors exhibit a wide range of morphological characteristics and biological behaviors. Significant progress has been made in understanding their molecular biology, classification, and clinical management since the release of the fourth edition of the World Health Organization (WHO) classification of soft tissue and bone tumors in 2013 [2]. Building upon these developments, the fifth edition of the WHO classification, introduced in April 2020, incorporated refined diagnostic categories and updated molecular insights to enhance prognostication and treatment strategies for bone tumors (Table 1.3) [3, 4].

STAGING OF BONE TUMORS

Bone tumor staging provides a framework for patient evaluation, helps direct treatment, and stratifies risk or prognosis. The Enneking staging system, introduced in 1980, was the first structured approach developed for musculoskeletal tumors and has since been endorsed by the Musculoskeletal Tumor Society (MSTS) [5–7]. Variables used to assign a stage to malignant bone tumors include tumor grade based on histology, extent of tumor, and presence or absence of metastatic disease based on appropriate imaging studies. Despite its age, this system remains widely utilized, especially among orthopedic oncologists, due to its anatomical focus, straightforward design, and applicability to both bone and soft tissue neoplasms. It integrates anatomical, radiological, and pathological features to stage musculoskeletal tumors (Tables 1.4 and 1.5).

Among the various staging frameworks for musculoskeletal malignancies, the most commonly employed today is the American Joint Committee on Cancer (AJCC) staging system, with its latest revision released in 2017. This system follows the TNM classification and incorporates histological grading, which is typically assessed using the Fédération Nationale des Centres de Lutte Contre le Cancer (FNCLCC) grading criteria [8–10] (Table 1.6). The eighth edition of the AJCC system further stratifies bone sarcomas into three distinct anatomical categories based on the tumor's site of origin: the appendicular skeleton, trunk, skull, and facial bones; the spine; and the pelvis.

The AJCC eighth edition staging system uses three grades for bone and soft tissue sarcomas: G1 (well-differentiated low grade), G2 (moderately differentiated high grade), and G3 (poorly differentiated high grade). The AJCC eighth edition revised an earlier four-tiered tumor grading scheme (G1–G4) by eliminating G4. Further, the G2 and G3 designations are now both considered high-grade lesions, resulting in a grade classification that is similar to the two-tiered MSTS staging system.

TABLE 1.3
The 2020 WHO Classification of Bone Tumors

Predominant Tissue	Benign	Intermediate (Locally Aggressive)	Malignant
Osteogenic	Osteoma Osteoid osteoma	Osteoblastoma	Low-grade central osteosarcoma Osteosarcoma NOS Conventional Telangiectatic Small cell Parosteal osteosarcoma Periosteal osteosarcoma High-grade surface osteosarcoma Secondary osteosarcoma
Chondrogenic	Subungual exostosis Bizarre parosteal osteochondromatous proliferation Periosteal chondroma Enchondroma Osteochondroma Chondroblastoma Chondromyxoid fibroma Osteochondromyxoma	Chondromatosis NOS Atypical cartilaginous tumor	Chondrosarcoma grade 1 Chondrosarcoma grade 2 Chondrosarcoma grade 3 Periosteal chondrosarcoma Clear cell chondrosarcoma mesenchymal chondrosarcoma Dedifferentiated chondrosarcoma
Fibrogenic	Fibroma Fibromatosis	Desmoplastic fibroma	Fibrosarcoma
Mixed	Chondromyxoid fibroma		
Osteoclastic giant cell rich tumors	Aneurysmal bone cyst Nonossifying fibroma	Giant cell tumor of bone NOS	Giant cell tumor of bone, malignant
Marrow tumors			Ewing's sarcoma Myeloma
Vascular tissue	Haemangioma	Epithelioid hemangioma	Epithelioid hemangioendothelioma NOS Angiosarcoma
Notochordal tumors	Benign notochordal cell tumor		Chordoma NOS Chondroid chordoma Poorly differentiated chordoma Dedifferentiated chordoma
Other mesenchymal tumors of bone	Chondromesenchymal hamartoma of chest wall Simple bone cyst Fibrous dysplasia Osteofibrous dysplasia Lipoma NOS Hibernoma	Osteofibrous dysplasia-like adamantinoma Mesenchymoma NOS	Adamantinoma of long bones Dedifferentiated adamantinoma Leiomyosarcoma NOS Pleomorphic sarcoma, undifferentiated Bone metastases

Hematopoietic neoplasms of bone: Plasmacytoma of bone
Malignant lymphoma, non-Hodgkin, NOS
Hodgkin disease NOS
Diffuse large B-cell lymphoma NOS
Follicular lymphoma NOS
Marginal zone B-cell lymphoma NOS
T-cell lymphoma NOS
Anaplastic large cell lymphoma NOS
Malignant lymphoma, lymphoblastic, NOS
Burkitt lymphoma NOS
Langerhans cell histiocytosis NOS
Langerhans cell histiocytosis, disseminated
Erdheim-Chester disease
Rosai-Dorfman disease

Abbreviations: NOS; not otherwise specified.

TABLE 1.4
Enneking Staging System for Benign Bone Lesions

Stage	Definition	Behavior	Radiographic Findings	Examples
1	Latent	Remains static or heals spontaneously	Well-defined borders often with sclerotic edges without cortical disruption, permeative growth, and periosteal reaction	Nonossifying fibroma, enchondroma, osteochondroma
2	Active	Progressive growth, limited by natural barriers	Varying amounts of bone destruction or cortical thinning	Osteoid osteoma, chondromyxoid fibroma, unicameral bone cysts
3	Aggressive	Progressive growth, not limited by natural barriers	Expansion of bone with cortical violation and soft tissue extension, causing structural compromise	Giant cell tumor, aneurysmal bone cyst

TABLE 1.5
Enneking Surgical Staging System for Malignant Bone Tumors

Stage	Grade[a]	Site[b]	Distant Metastasis[c]
IA	Low (G1)	Intracompartmental (T1)	None (M0)
IB	Low (G1)	Extracompartmental (T2)	None (M0)
IIA	High (G2)	Intracompartmental (T1)	None (M0)
IIB	High (G2)	Extracompartmental (T2)	None (M0)
III	Any (G)	Any (T)	Regional or distant metastasis (M1)

[a] G1, low grade; G2, high grade.
[b] T1, lesions that remain within an anatomic compartment (intraosseous for bone tumors): T2, lesions extending through or beyond the host cortex.
[c] MO, no distant metastasis; M1, distant metastasis.

TABLE 1.6
AJCC Staging System for Bone Sarcoma

Stage	Primary Tumor (T)[a]	Regional Lymph Nodes (N)[b]	Distant Metastasis (M)[c]	Histologic Grade (G)[d]
IA	T1	N0	M0	G1, GX
IB	T2, T3	N0	M0	G1,GX
IIA	T1	N0	M0	G2, G3
IIB	T2	N0	M0	G2, G3
III	T3	N0	M0	G2, G3
IVA	Any T	N0	M1a	Any G
IVB	Any T	N1	Any M	Any G
	Any T	Any N	M1b	Any G

[a] TX, primary tumor cannot be assessed; TO, no evidence of primary tumor; T1, tumor 8 cm or less in greatest dimension; T2, tumor more than 8 cm in greatest dimension; T3, discontinuous tumors in the primary bone.
[b] NX, regional lymph nodes cannot be assessed; NO, no regional lymph node metastasis; N1, regional lymph node metastasis.
[c] MO, no distant metastasis; M1, distant metastasis; M1a, lung; M1b, metastasis to bone or any other distant sites.
[d] GX, grade cannot be assessed; G1, low histologic grade (well differentiated); G2, high histologic grade (moderately differentiated); G3, high histologic grade (poorly differentiated)

TABLE 1.7
AJCC Definitions of T Categories for Spinal and Pelvic Tumors

Category	Site	Extent of Primary Tumor
TX	Spine	Cannot be assessed
TX	Pelvis	Cannot be assessed
T0	Spine	No evidence of primary tumor
T0	Pelvis	No evidence of primary tumor
T1	Spine	One vertebral segment or two adjacent vertebral segments
T1a	Pelvis	One pelvic segment but no extraosseous extension If greatest dimension $\leq$ 8 cm
T1b	Pelvis	One pelvic segment but no extraosseous extension If greatest dimension > 8 cm
T2	Spine	Three adjacent vertebral segments
T2a	Pelvis	One pelvic segment with extraosseous extension Two segments with extraosseous extension If greatest dimension $\leq$ 8 cm
T2b	Pelvis	One pelvic segment with extraosseous extension Two segments with extraosseous extension If greatest dimension > 8 cm
T3	Spine	At least four adjacent vertebral segments or multiple nonadjacent vertebral segments
T3a	Pelvis	Two pelvic segments with extraosseous extension If greatest dimension $\leq$ 8 cm
T3b	Pelvis	Two pelvic segments with extraosseous extension If greatest dimension > 8 cm
T4	Spine	Extends into spinal canal or great vessels
T4	Pelvis	Spans three pelvic segments or crosses sacroiliac joint
T4a	Spine	Extends into spinal canal
T4a	Pelvis	Involves sacroiliac joint and extends medial to sacral neuroforamen
T4b	Spine	Gross vascular invasion or tumor thrombus in great vessels
T4b	Pelvis	Encases external iliac vessels, or gross tumor thrombus is seen in major pelvic vessels

The AJCC eighth edition also newly defines lesion size (T category), giving unique criteria for osseous lesions in both the pelvis and spine (Table 1.7), which are distinct from criteria in other sites. The regional lymph node

(N category), distant metastases (M category), and histologic (G category) evaluations are the same for lesions in the pelvis and spine as for osseous lesions in other sites. The spine is divided into five segments: the right and left vertebral bodies, the right and left pedicles and transverse processes, and the posterior elements. In the pelvis, the osseous structures are divided into four segments: the sacrum, the iliac wing, the acetabulum and periacetabulum, and the pubic rami, ischium, and symphysis. In the pelvis, similar to the appendicular skeleton, lesion size less than or equal to versus greater than 8 cm is used to differentiate T1a from T2a and T1b from T2b, respectively [1, 4] (Table 1.7). However, both the pelvis and spine T category definitions now reflect involvement of multiple pelvic or vertebral segments, soft tissue extension (e.g., great vessel or spinal canal involvement), and sacroiliac joint transgression (for pelvic lesions; Table 1.7).

SUMMARY

- **Bone tumors often present with nonspecific symptoms**, such as persistent pain or swelling, requiring careful clinical evaluation for timely diagnosis.
- **Benign and malignant bone tumors differ distinctly in clinical and physical examination**, with malignant tumors showing firm, ill-defined masses, tenderness, and raised local temperature.
- **Classification of bone tumors is guided by the WHO system**, incorporating histologic, anatomic, and molecular features to ensure accurate diagnosis and prognostication.
- **The Enneking staging system**, widely used in surgical oncology, categorizes tumors based on grade, anatomical extent, and presence of metastasis.
- **The AJCC eighth edition staging system provides a TNM-based framework**, incorporating tumor size, histological grade, and metastatic spread—tailored for different anatomical sites, including spine and pelvis.

REFERENCES

1. Siegel R, Naishadham D, Jemal A. Cancer statistics, 2013. *CA Cancer J Clin.* 2013;63:11–30.
2. Fletcher CD, Bridges AJ, Hogendoorn CW, et al. *WHO classification of tumours of soft tissue and bone.* 4th ed. Lyon: IARC Press; 2013.
3. The WHO Classification of Tumors Editorial Board. *WHO classification of tumors: soft tissue and bone tumours.* 5th ed. Lyon: IARC Press; 2020.
4. Choi JH, Ro JY. The 2020 WHO classification of tumors of bone: an updated review. *Adv Anat Pathol.* 2021;28(3): 119–138.
5. Enneking WF, Spanier SS, Goodman MA. A system for the surgical staging of musculoskeletal sarcoma. *Clin Orthop Relat Res.* 1980;153:106–120.
6. Jawad MU, Scully SP. Classifications in brief: Enneking classification—benign and malignant tumors of the musculoskeletal system. *Clin Orthop Relat Res.* 2010;468:2000–2002.
7. Musculoskeletal Tumor Society, Enneking WF. Staging of musculoskeletal neoplasms. *Skeletal Radiol.* 1985;13: 183–194.
8. Tanaka K, Ozaki T. New TNM classification (AJCC eighth edition) of bone and soft tissue sarcomas: JCOG Bone and Soft Tissue Tumor Study Group. *Jpn J Clin Oncol.* 2019;49:103–107.
9. Neuville A, Chibon F, Coindre JM. Grading of soft tissue sarcomas: from histological to molecular assessment. *Pathology.* 2014;46:113–120.
10. Lin X, Davion S, Bertsch EC, Omar I, Nayar R, Laskin WB. Federation Nationale des Centers de Lutte Contre le Cancer grading of soft tissue sarcomas on needle core biopsies using surrogate markers. *Hum Pathol.* 2016;56:147–154.

2 Imaging of Bone Tumors

INTRODUCTION

The accurate diagnosis and effective management of bone tumors are critically dependent on comprehensive imaging evaluation. Although the core imaging modalities—plain radiography, ultrasonography, computed tomography (CT), magnetic resonance imaging (MRI), and nuclear scintigraphy—have remained consistent over the years, their clinical application has evolved significantly. Traditionally employed for anatomical and morphological assessment, imaging now plays an essential role in tissue characterization, staging, treatment response evaluation, and long-term surveillance.

Technological advancements, particularly in MRI, CT, and nuclear medicine, have enhanced the sensitivity and specificity of imaging in musculoskeletal oncology. These improvements have not only allowed for more precise lesion localization and definition at initial presentation but have also facilitated more accurate monitoring of disease progression and therapeutic outcomes. Importantly, these benefits have been achieved with markedly reduced radiation exposure, a critical consideration, especially in younger patient populations.

Emerging imaging techniques such as high-field-strength MRI, diffusion-weighted imaging (DWI), dynamic contrast–enhanced (DCE) MRI, whole-body MRI, and hybrid PET-CT systems have expanded the diagnostic horizon. These modalities enable earlier detection of subtle pathological changes, improved delineation of tumor margins, and reliable assessment of tumor viability and necrosis, thereby supporting more informed clinical decisions.

This chapter provides an overview of the role of imaging in the management of bone tumors, detailing the indications, advantages, and limitations of each modality in the contemporary diagnostic and therapeutic landscape. Soft tissue tumors are excluded from this discussion to maintain a focused approach on osseous neoplasms.

IMAGING ASSESSMENT AT DIAGNOSIS

Radiographic Evaluation of Bone Tumors

Conventional radiography remains the cornerstone in the initial evaluation of suspected bone tumors, providing essential information about the lesion's anatomical location, biological behavior, and aggressiveness. Despite the availability of advanced imaging techniques, plain radiographs often offer the first clues toward a differential diagnosis and guide subsequent imaging [1]. A systematic and structured radiographic analysis facilitates differentiation between benign and malignant bone tumors.

This analysis includes the evaluation of several key parameters:

- **Age of the Patient**: Skeletally immature patients are more likely to harbor benign lesions such as simple bone cysts or aneurysmal bone cysts, whereas primary malignant tumors such as osteosarcoma or Ewing sarcoma are more frequent in adolescents and young adults. In older adults (>40 years), metastatic bone disease becomes a more common consideration.
- **Location and Part of the Bone Involved**: Long bones are commonly affected in both benign and malignant tumors, while flat bones are more frequently associated with malignant lesions such as chondrosarcoma. Specific regions within bones also provide diagnostic clues: epiphyseal lesions often indicate giant cell tumor or chondroblastoma, metaphyseal lesions may suggest osteochondroma or osteosarcoma, and diaphyseal involvement is characteristic of Ewing sarcoma or adamantinoma (Table 2.1, Figure 2.1).
- **Common Matrix Types and Associated Tumors** (Figure 2.2)
    - **Osteoid matrix**: Osteoid osteoma, osteosarcoma
    - **Chondroid matrix**: Enchondroma, chondrosarcoma, osteochondroma
    - **No matrix**: Giant cell tumor, Fibrous dysplasia, eosinophilic granuloma

Key distinguishing features between benign and malignant bone lesions are summarized in Table 2.2. These radiological parameters not only help establish a diagnosis but also act as a medical triage system to guide further investigations (Figures 2.3–2.5).

TABLE 2.1
Common Diagnoses by Location of Lesion in Long Bones

Site	Benign	Malignant
Long Bones		
Epiphyseal	Chondroblastoma	Clear cell
	Giant cell tumor	chondrosarcoma
Metaphyseal	Nonossifying fibroma	Osteosarcoma
	Aneurysmal bone cyst	Chondrosarcoma
	Simple/unicameral bone cyst	Metastatic bone disease
	Enchondroma	
	Osteochondroma	
Diaphyseal	Fibrous dysplasia	Ewing sarcoma
	Histiocytosis	Adamantinoma
	Osteoid osteoma	Lymphoma
		Metastatic bone disease

DOI: 10.1201/9780367822002-3

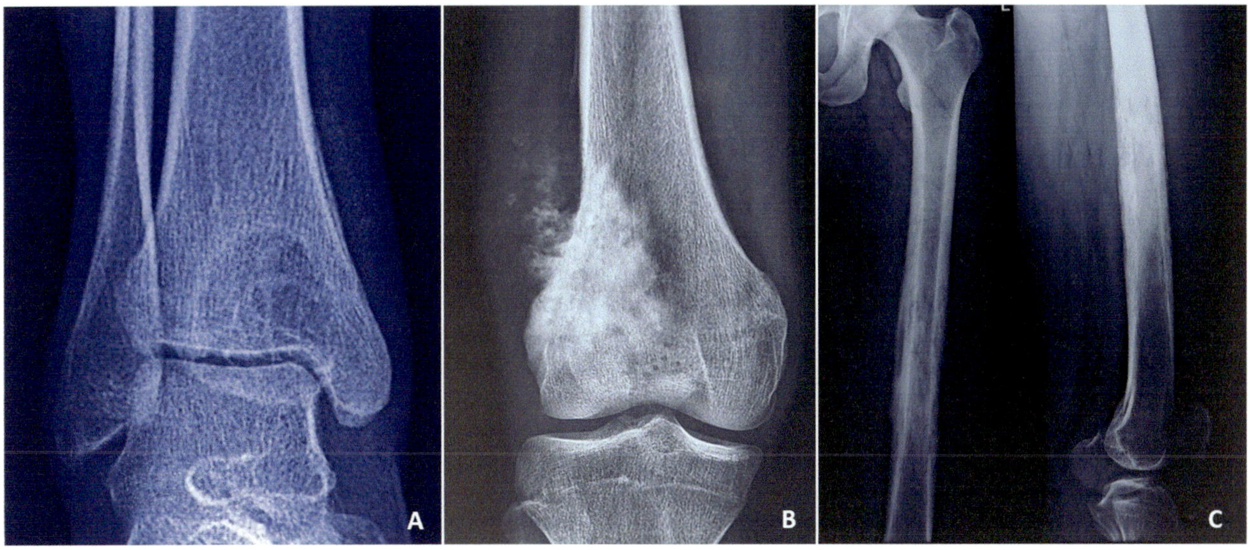

FIGURE 2.1 Lesions in the specific regions within bones provide diagnostic clues. (A) Epiphyseal lesions often indicate giant cell tumor or chondroblastoma, (B) metaphyseal lesions may suggest osteochondroma or osteosarcoma, and (C) diaphyseal involvement is characteristic of Ewing sarcoma or adamantinoma.

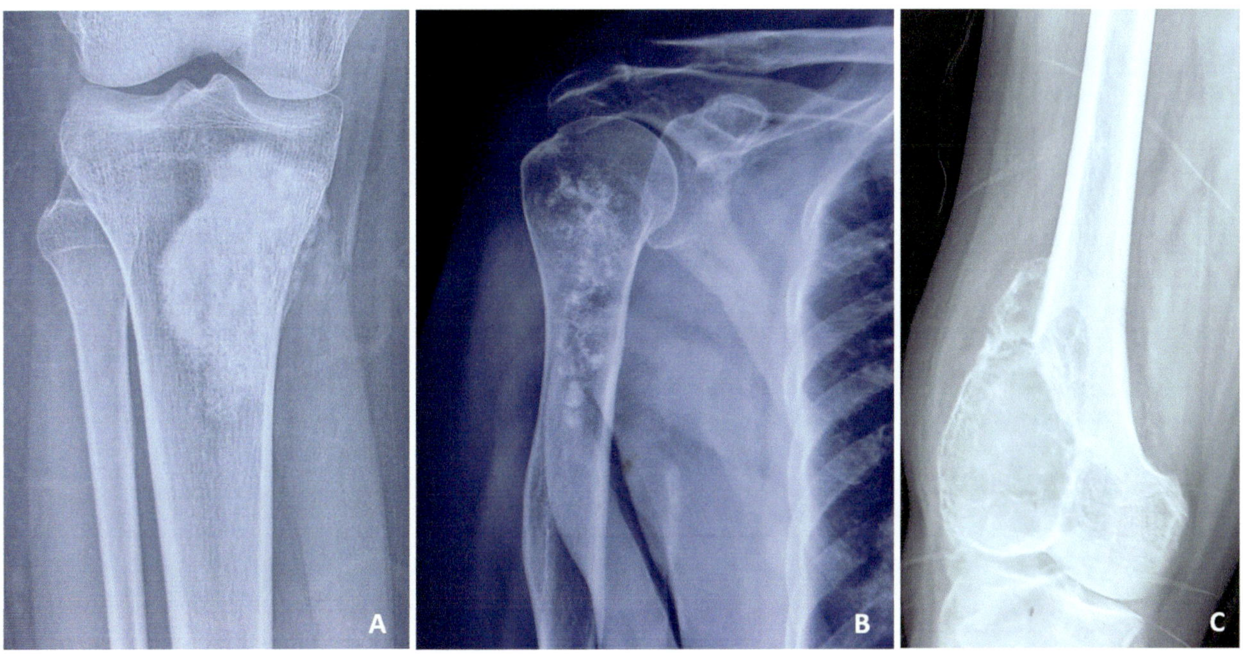

FIGURE 2.2 Common matrix types in bone tumors. (A) Osteoid matrix in Osteosarcoma. (B) Chondroid matrix in Enchondroma. (C) No matrix in Giant cell tumor.

The application of radiographic pattern recognition can substantially enhance diagnostic accuracy. For instance, a metaphyseal osteolytic lesion with a narrow zone of transition and absent periosteal reaction in a young patient may suggest a benign pathology such as a simple bone cyst or nonossifying fibroma. In contrast, an ill-defined mixed-density lesion with cortical destruction and a spiculated periosteal reaction in an adolescent strongly favors a diagnosis of osteosarcoma. The structured assessment of plain radiographs remains an indispensable tool for the initial evaluation of bone tumors. Its judicious application aids in early diagnosis, helps prevent misdiagnosis, and avoids inappropriate surgical interventions, enabling timely referrals for appropriate oncologic management.

TABLE 2.2
Radiological Features Differentiating Benign and Malignant Bone Tumors

Feature	Suggestive of Benign Lesion	Suggestive of Malignant Lesion
Age	Skeletally immature (e.g., ABC, SBC)	>40 years or adolescence (e.g., osteosarcoma)
Bone Involved	Long/Flat bone	Flat bones are more commonly involved in malignancy
Part of Bone	Epiphysis (GCT), Metaphysis (Osteochondroma)	Diaphysis (Ewing sarcoma) Metaphysis (osteosarcoma)
Characteristics	Osteolytic/sclerotic, no matrix	Mixed with cortical breach
Matrix Composition	Absent or chondroid	Osteoid or chondroid (suggests malignancy)
Cortical Integrity	Intact cortex	Cortical breach or erosion
Margin/Border	Well-defined	Ill-defined, permeative
Periosteal Reaction (Figure 2.3)	Absent or solid (benign)	Interrupted, lamellated, Codman's triangle
Pathological Fracture (Figure 2.4)	Usually absent	Frequently present in aggressive lesions
Zone of Transition (Figure 2.5)	Narrow (geographic)	Wide (moth-eaten, permeative)

ADVANCED IMAGING

Magnetic Resonance Imaging in Bone Tumor Evaluation

MRI is the modality of choice for the comprehensive evaluation of bone tumors following initial radiographic assessment. It provides unparalleled resolution for assessing the extent of intraosseous tumors, soft tissue involvement, and marrow changes. MRI plays a critical role in staging, surgical planning, biopsy guidance, and evaluation of treatment response (Figures 2.6–2.11).

Conventional MRI sequences include T1-weighted, T2-weighted, and fat-suppressed images. T1-weighted images offer excellent anatomic detail and marrow delineation, whereas T2-weighted and short tau inversion recovery (STIR) sequences highlight edema, necrosis, and soft tissue components. Contrast-enhanced MRI with gadolinium further enhances lesion characterization by differentiating viable tumor from cystic or necrotic areas. Contrast-enhanced MRI is optional and may be influenced by resource availability and the operating surgeon's preference. However, post-contrast sequences can be invaluable in differentiating viable tumor from necrotic or cystic areas.

MRI is the most effective imaging technique for delineating the local extent of the tumor. Importantly, it should always be performed before biopsy to prevent post-biopsy

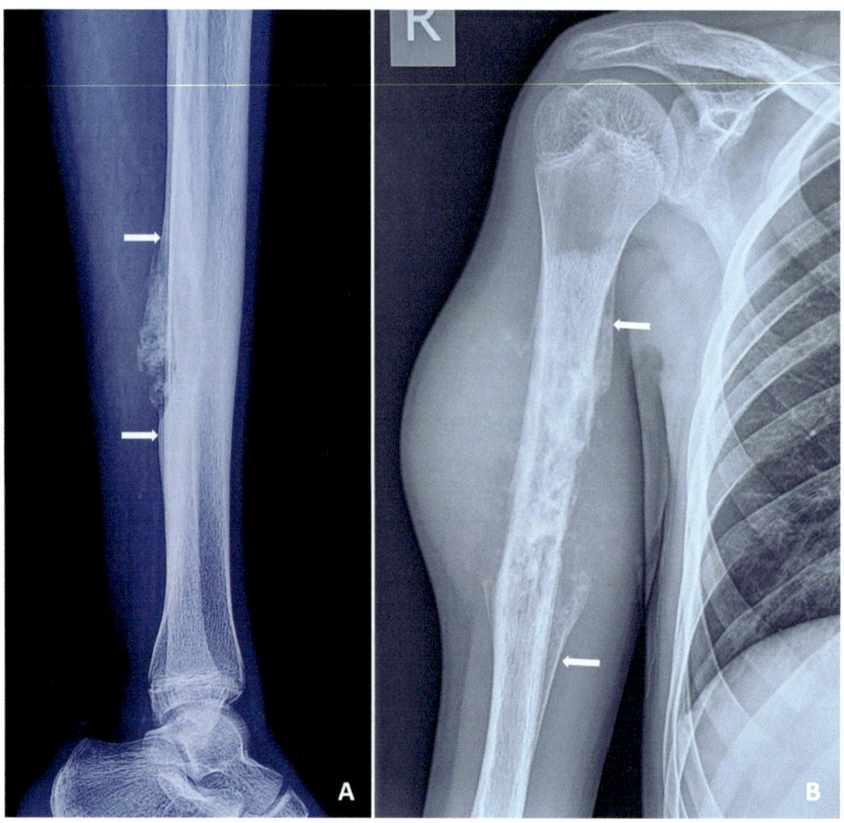

FIGURE 2.3 (A) Lamellated periosteal reaction (white arrows) in an Ewing sarcoma of the tibia. (B) Codman's triangle (white arrows) in Osteosarcoma of the humerus.

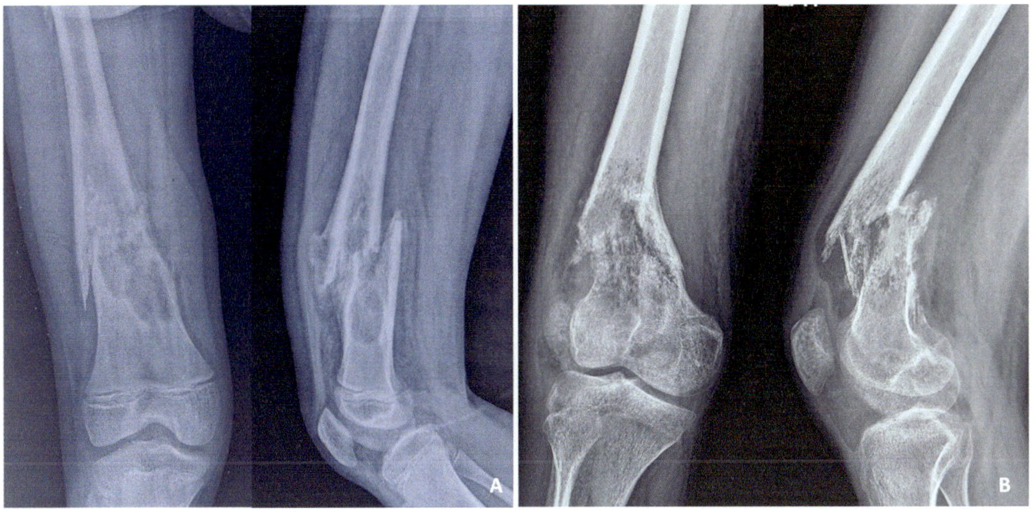

FIGURE 2.4 Pathological fractures are common in malignant bone lesions with extensive bone lysis. (A) Pathological fracture in Ewing sarcoma and (B) osteosarcoma of the femur.

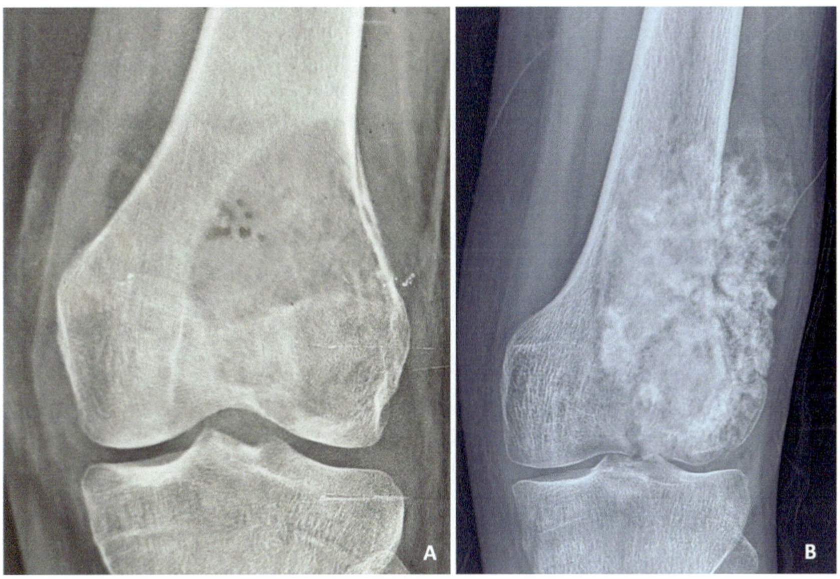

FIGURE 2.5 (A) Benign bone tumors have a narrow zone of transition with a clear demarcation from the normal parent bone, while malignant tumors are typically characterized by a wide zone of transition, with no clear demarcation between the lesion and the parent bone (B).

hemorrhage or edema from obscuring tumor margins. The MRI protocol must include the entire involved bone and adjacent joints to detect possible skip lesions—separate foci of intramedullary tumor without direct continuity with the primary lesion.

MRI should be meticulously evaluated for:

- Intramedullary extent of the tumor
- Extraosseous soft tissue component
- Neurovascular involvement
- Intra-articular extension (Figure 2.12)
- Presence of skip lesions
- Associated bone marrow edema
- Signal characteristics of the lesion

Post-chemotherapy MRI should ideally be performed at least 14 days after the last chemotherapy cycle and within 2 weeks before surgery. A reduction in the size of the soft tissue component is considered indicative of therapeutic response (Figure 2.13).

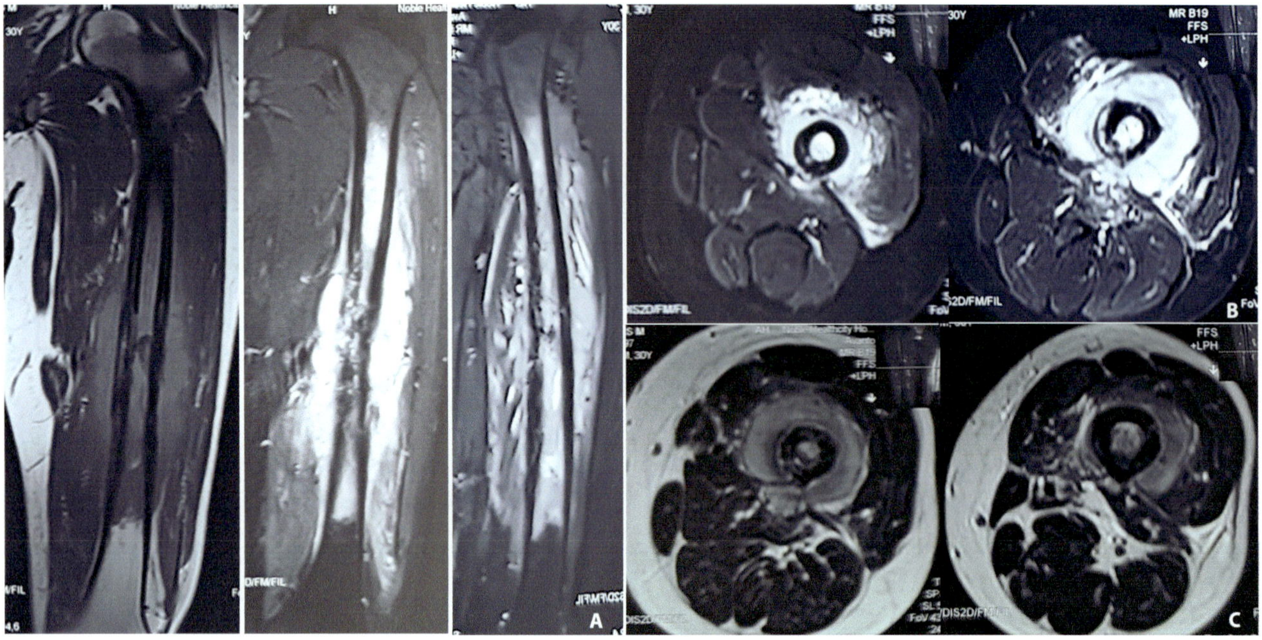

FIGURE 2.6 MRI images of a 19-year-old boy with Ewing sarcoma of the femur. Coronal (A & B) and sagittal (C) images reveal the diaphyseal lesion with cortical destruction and periosteal reaction. Low signal intensity tumor margins are distinguished from the high signal intensity, normal fatty marrow, proximally and distally on T1-weighted images (A). This allows accurate measurements of the entire tumor relative to anatomic landmarks in preparation for limb salvage surgery with an intercalary resection. High signal intensity of tumor margins on T2-weighted images (B & C) indicates an extraosseous soft tissue component.

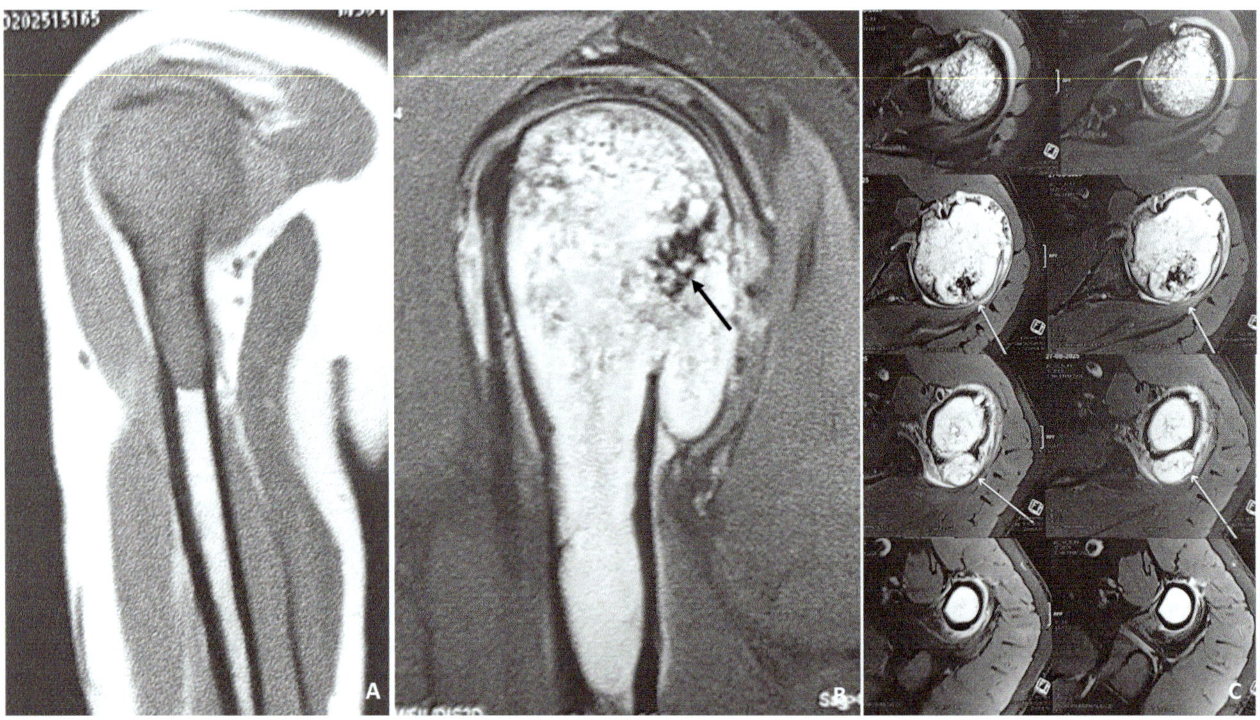

FIGURE 2.7 MRI images of a 36-year-old male with Chondrosarcoma of the proximal humerus reveal a lobulated mass with low to intermediate signal on T1 (A) and high T2 signal (due to the high water content of cartilage), separated by low-intensity septa (B & C). Calcifications are dark on T2 (black arrow).

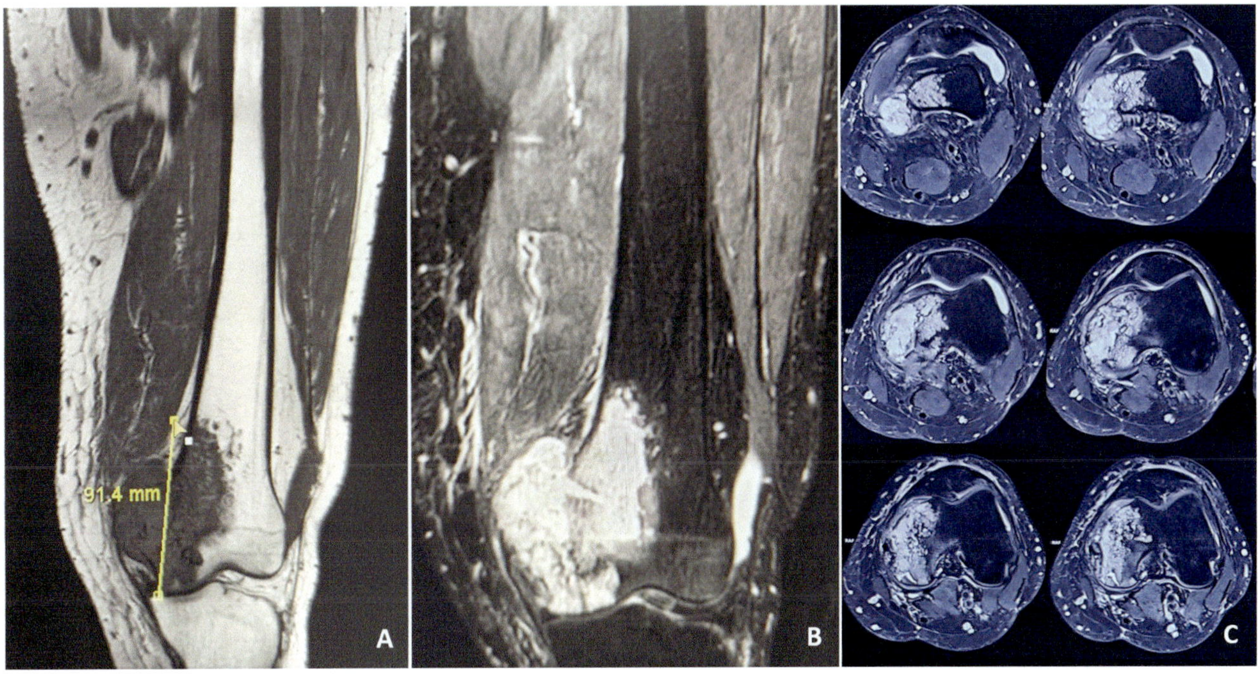

FIGURE 2.8 MRI of a 36-year-old male with chondrosarcoma of the proximal humerus demonstrates a lobulated mass that is hypo- to isointense on T1-weighted sequences, aiding in planning the resection length (A), and hyperintense on T2-weighted images (B), reflecting the high water content characteristic of cartilaginous tumors. Axial sections (C) clearly depict the lesion's proximity to and relationship with the adjacent neurovascular structures.

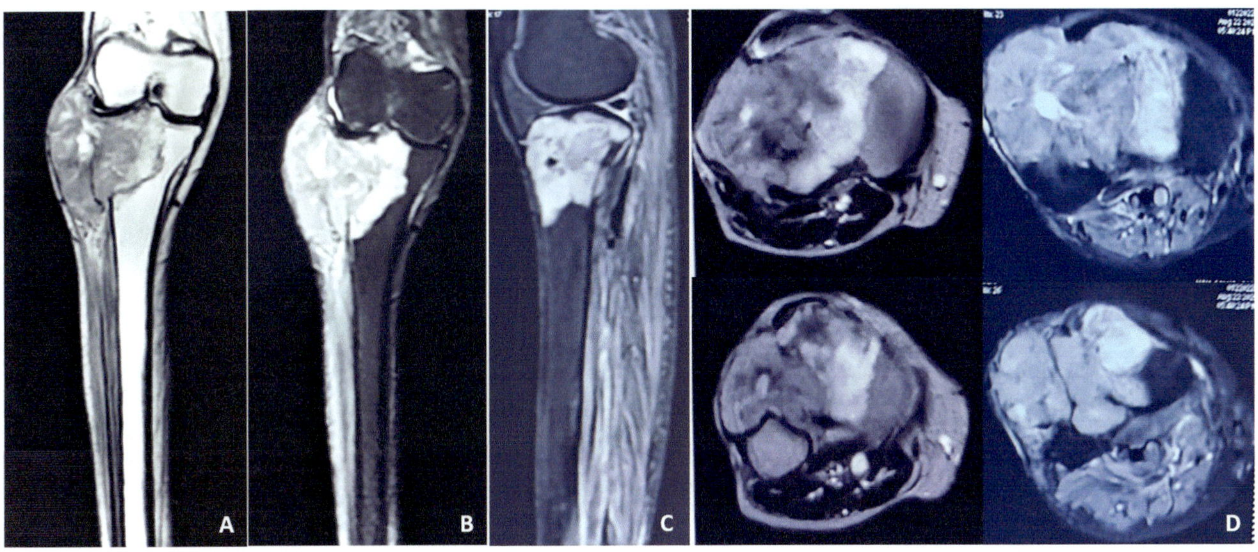

FIGURE 2.9 MRI of a 20-year-old female with distal femoral osteosarcoma. Coronal (A, B) and sagittal (C) images demonstrate a metaphyseal lesion extending up to the articular surface, with lateral cortical breach and extraosseous soft tissue extension. On T1-weighted images (A), the low-signal tumor is clearly demarcated from the high-signal normal fatty marrow, enabling precise measurement of tumor length and relation to anatomic landmarks—essential for planning joint-sacrificing limb salvage resection. T2-weighted images (B, C) reveal hyperintense tumor margins, highlighting the extraosseous component and involvement of the proximal tibiofibular joint. Axial sections (D) delineate the lesion's relationship to adjacent neurovascular structures, critical for surgical planning.

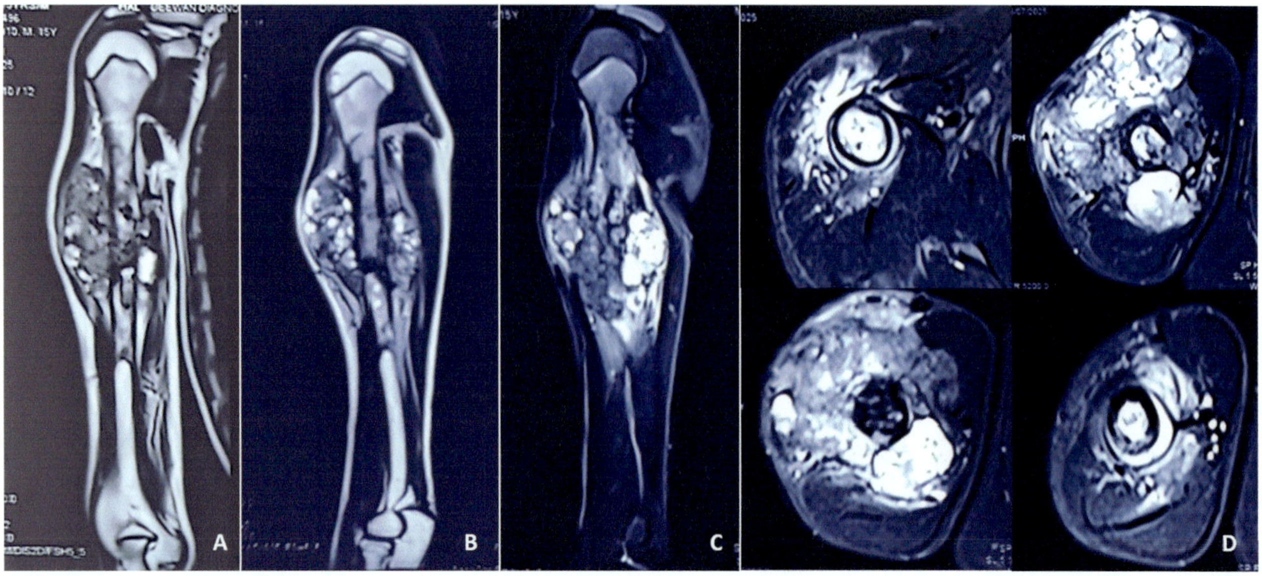

FIGURE 2.10 MRI of a 15-year-old boy with osteosarcoma of the humerus. Coronal and sagittal T1-weighted images (A & B) demonstrate a heterogeneous intramedullary lesion with low signal intensity and cortical destruction. Sagittal T2-weighted image (C) shows a hyperintense tumor with periosteal reaction and extensive soft tissue component. Multiple foci of mineralization appear as signal voids within the mass. Axial sections (D) clearly delineate the circumferential extraosseous extension and its relationship to the surrounding musculature and neurovascular bundle, crucial for surgical planning.

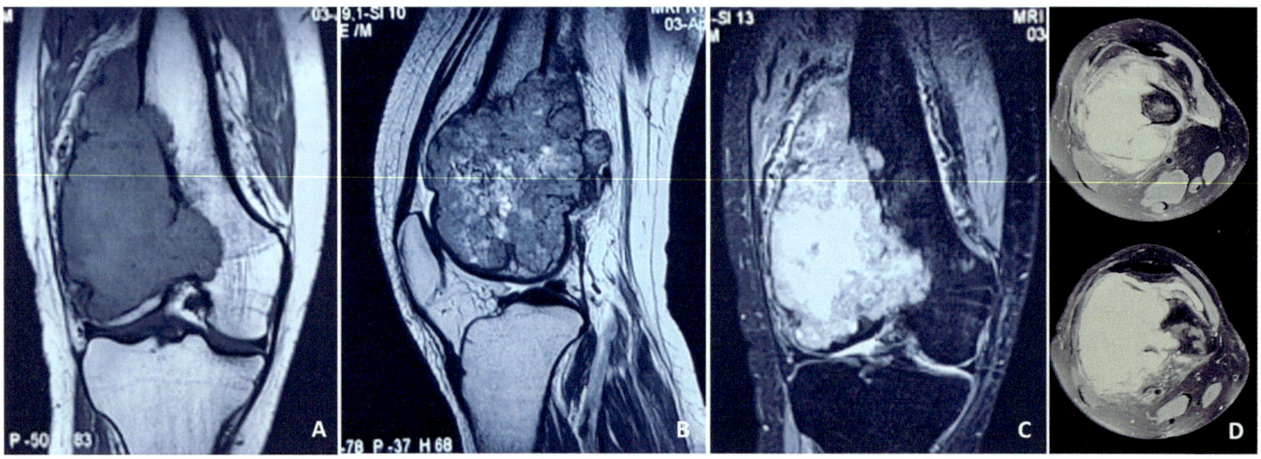

FIGURE 2.11 MRI of a 25-year-old female with a giant cell tumor of the distal femur. Coronal (A & C) and sagittal (B) images demonstrate an expansile, well-defined, lytic lesion involving the epi-metaphyseal region and abutting the subchondral bone plate. The lesion appears dark on T1 (A & B) and bright on T2 (C), showing clear demarcation on the T1 image between fatty marrow and tumor. There is a cortical breach along the anterior, posterior, and lateral cortices with an associated soft tissue component. Axial images (D) delineate the circumferential cortical destruction and the relation of the lesion to surrounding neurovascular structures. MRI not only provides precise mapping of intraosseous and extraosseous extent but also aids in planning the biopsy tract—here favoring a lateral approach—underscoring the importance of obtaining MRI before biopsy to avoid contamination of uninvolved compartments.

Advanced MRI techniques now augment the diagnostic value:

- **DWI**: This sequence reflects tissue cellularity and membrane integrity. Malignant lesions often demonstrate restricted diffusion with corresponding low signal on apparent diffusion coefficient (ADC) maps. Conversely, benign lesions or necrotic regions typically exhibit high ADC values due to increased water mobility [2].
- **Dynamic Contrast–Enhanced (DCE) MRI**: DCE-MRI provides perfusion data by tracking signal intensity changes post-contrast injection over time. Rapid and intense enhancement is more typical of malignant tumors, aiding in differentiation and biopsy planning.

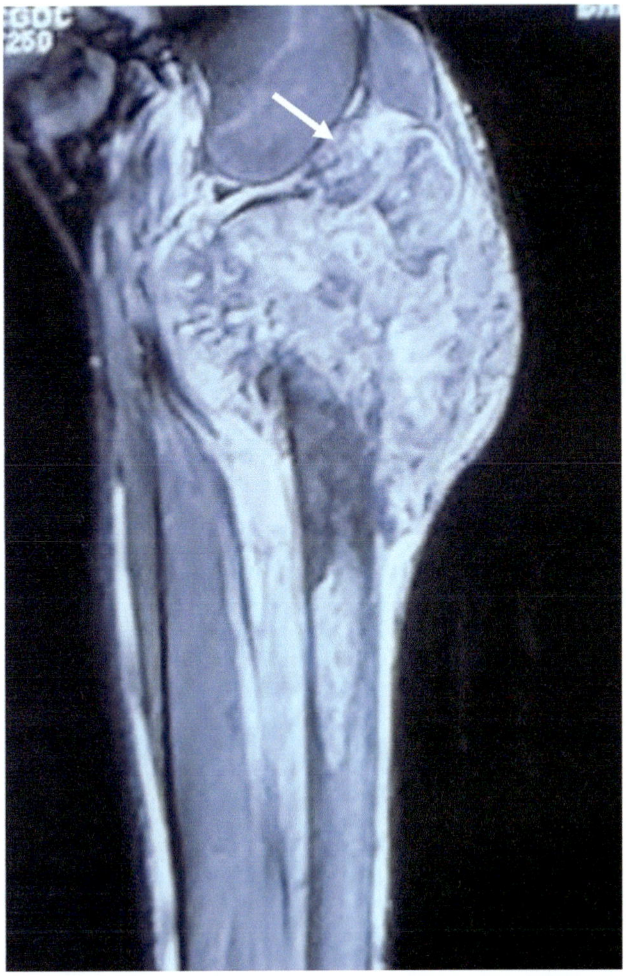

FIGURE 2.12 MRI of a patient with osteosarcoma of the proximal tibia demonstrating intra-articular extension of tumor into the knee joint (white arrow). The lesion shows cortical breach of the tibial plateau with synovial involvement and joint effusion, findings that mandate an extra-articular knee resection to achieve oncologically safe margins. MRI is crucial in such cases as it accurately depicts intra-articular spread, guides the choice between intra- and extra-articular resection, and is indispensable for preoperative surgical planning.

- **High-Field MRI (3T and beyond)**: These systems offer higher signal-to-noise ratios and better spatial resolution, enabling more detailed imaging of complex anatomical regions and small lesions.
- **Magnetic Resonance Angiography (MRA)**: Particularly useful when evaluating tumors near major vessels, MRA facilitates preoperative vascular mapping and planning for limb salvage procedures.

Overall, MRI is indispensable for local staging, evaluating skip lesions, defining anatomical boundaries for resection, and monitoring posttreatment changes, including recurrence. Its multiplanar capability, lack of ionizing radiation, and functional imaging options make it the gold standard for bone tumor imaging beyond radiographs.

Computed Tomography in Bone Tumor Evaluation

CT plays a complementary role in the evaluation of bone tumors, particularly when precise assessment of cortical bone integrity, matrix mineralization, or complex anatomical regions, such as the spine, pelvis, and craniofacial skeleton, is required. While MRI provides superior soft tissue contrast, CT offers unmatched resolution of osseous detail.

Key indications for CT in bone tumor assessment include:

- Evaluation of cortical destruction or breach not clearly delineated on MRI (Figure 2.14)
- Characterization of matrix mineralization patterns (e.g., osteoid, chondroid, or calcific)
- Assessment of anatomical sites that are technically difficult to evaluate with MRI (e.g., pelvis, skull base; Figure 2.15)
- Detection of small pulmonary metastases, particularly in osteosarcoma and Ewing sarcoma
- Surgical planning for resection and reconstruction, particularly in anatomically complex regions

CT is particularly valuable in lesions such as:

- **Osteoid osteoma**, where the nidus and surrounding sclerosis are often best visualized with CT
- **Myositis ossificans**, where zonal ossification patterns can be misleading on MRI but appear clearly on CT
- **Chondroid tumors**, where rings-and-arcs calcification patterns are more easily appreciated. Also, the cortico-medullary continuity of Osteochondroma is clearly defined on CT (Figure 2.16)

When CT is indicated, radiation safety principles must be emphasized. Dose optimization protocols and pediatric-specific settings are especially important given the often young age of patients with primary bone malignancies.

ROLE OF CT ANGIOGRAPHY IN BONE TUMORS

CT Angiography (CTA) plays an important adjunctive role in the preoperative evaluation of bone tumors, particularly those located adjacent to major neurovascular bundles. It provides rapid, high-resolution images of the arterial anatomy and allows assessment of vessel displacement, encasement, or infiltration by the tumor.

Key indications for CTA in bone tumors include:

- Tumors located near large vessels (e.g., proximal femur, pelvis, proximal humerus) (Figure 2.17)
- Planning for limb salvage surgery where vascular preservation is critical
- Evaluation of the feasibility of vascular grafts, vascularized bone transfers, or free flap reconstructions
- Preoperative embolization planning in hypervascular tumors (e.g., ABC, GCT, metastatic RCC)

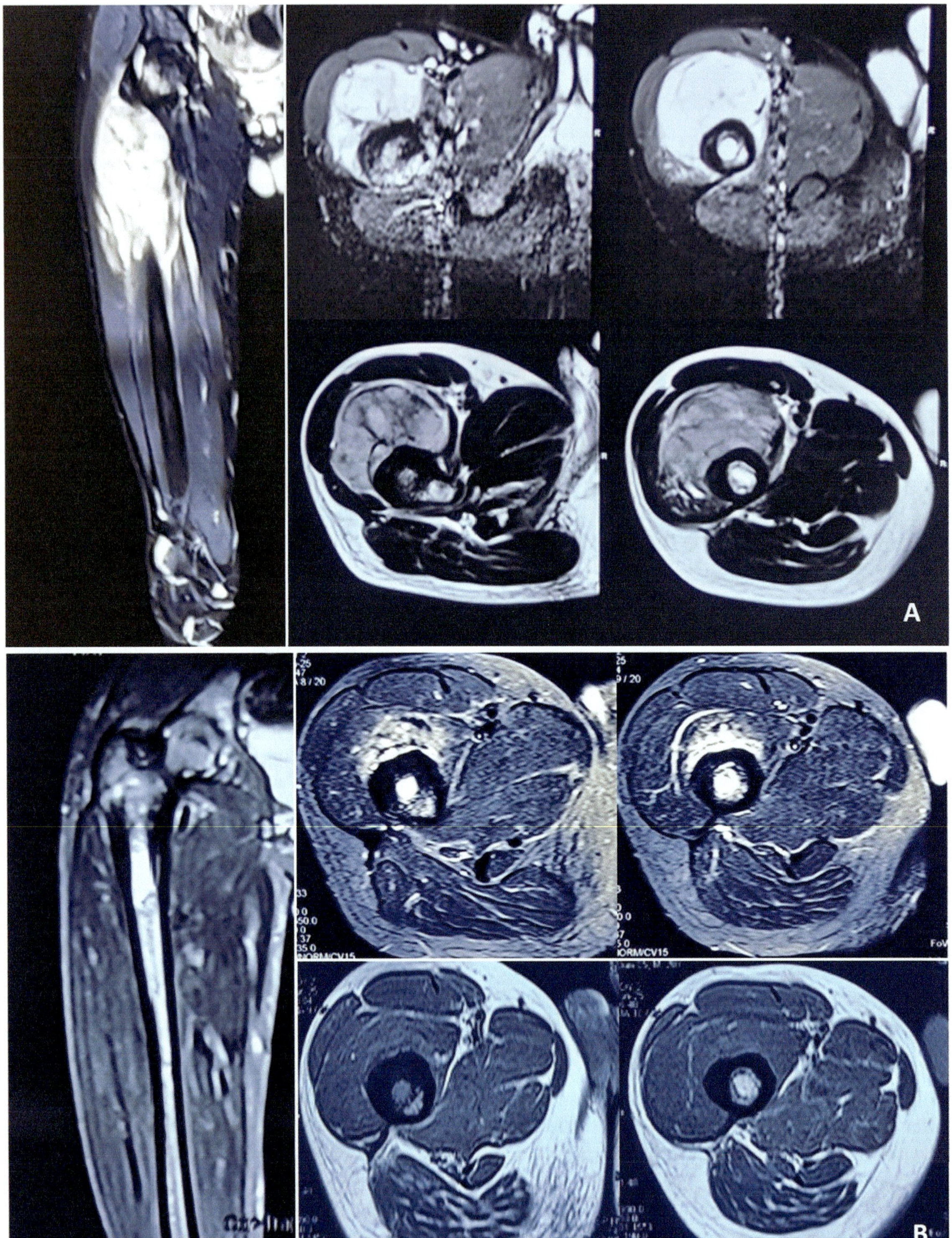

FIGURE 2.13 MRI of a 19-year-old male with Ewing sarcoma of the proximal femur. (A) Pre-chemotherapy images demonstrate a large metaphyseal-diaphyseal lesion with cortical breach and a bulky circumferential soft tissue component. (B) Post-chemotherapy MRI shows marked reduction in the size of the extraosseous soft tissue component and decreased marrow involvement, indicating good therapeutic response. MRI plays a pivotal role in assessing treatment efficacy by allowing precise evaluation of tumor shrinkage, soft tissue resolution, and marrow signal changes. A significant reduction in the soft tissue component, as seen here, is considered a reliable indicator of a favorable response to neoadjuvant chemotherapy and aids in planning definitive surgical resection.

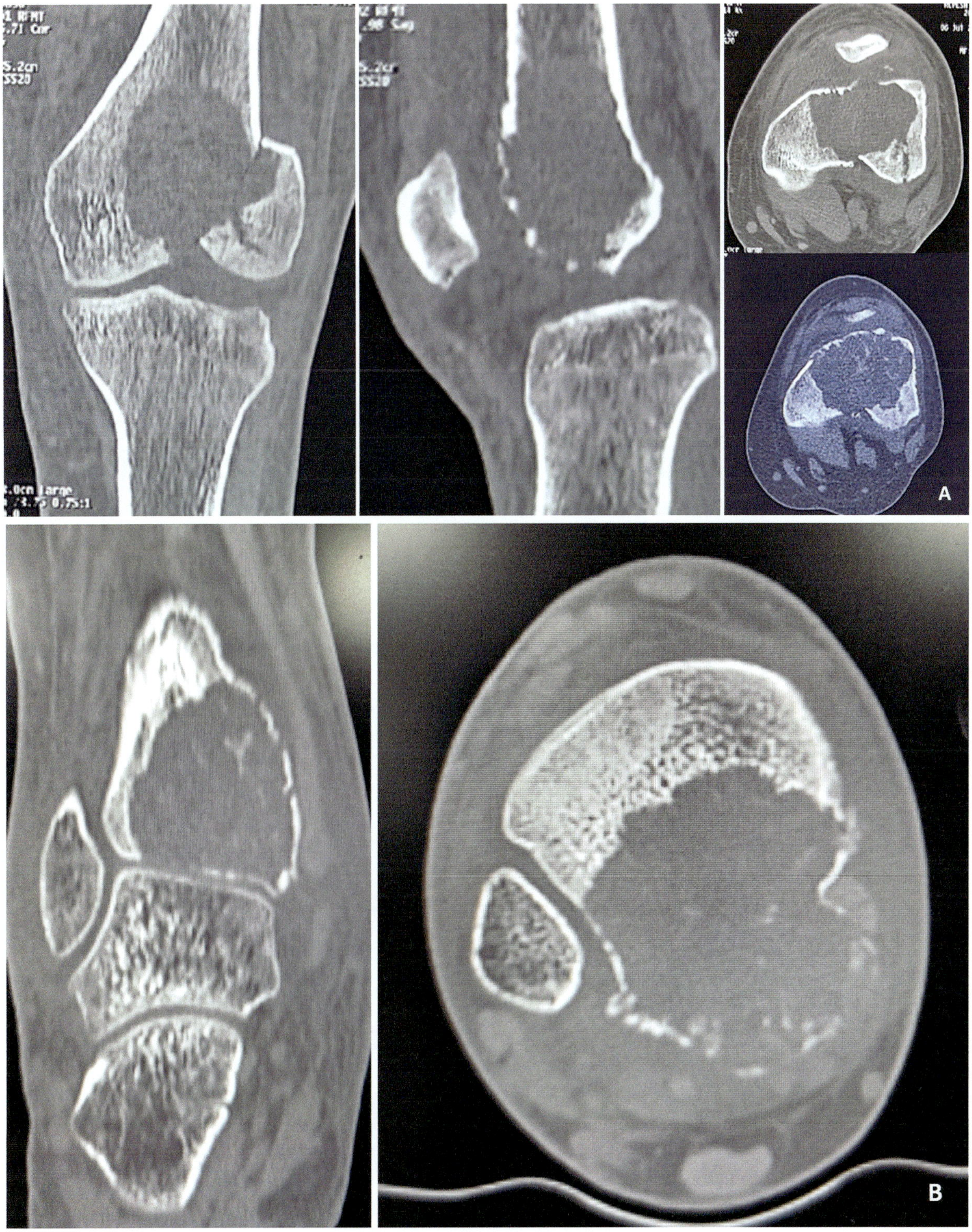

FIGURE 2.14 (A) CT scan images of a giant cell tumor involving the distal femur demonstrating an expansile, lytic lesion with cortical thinning and areas of breach, particularly of the articular cartilage. (B) CT scan of a giant cell tumor of the distal tibia showing cortical destruction with thinning of the anterior cortex and extension close to the articular surface. Subchondral bone involvement is also well delineated. CT imaging is invaluable in assessing cortical integrity and the extent of subchondral bone involvement, which may not be clearly appreciated on MRI. In addition, CT aids surgical planning by identifying the most compromised cortex, thereby guiding the surgical approach for curettage or resection.

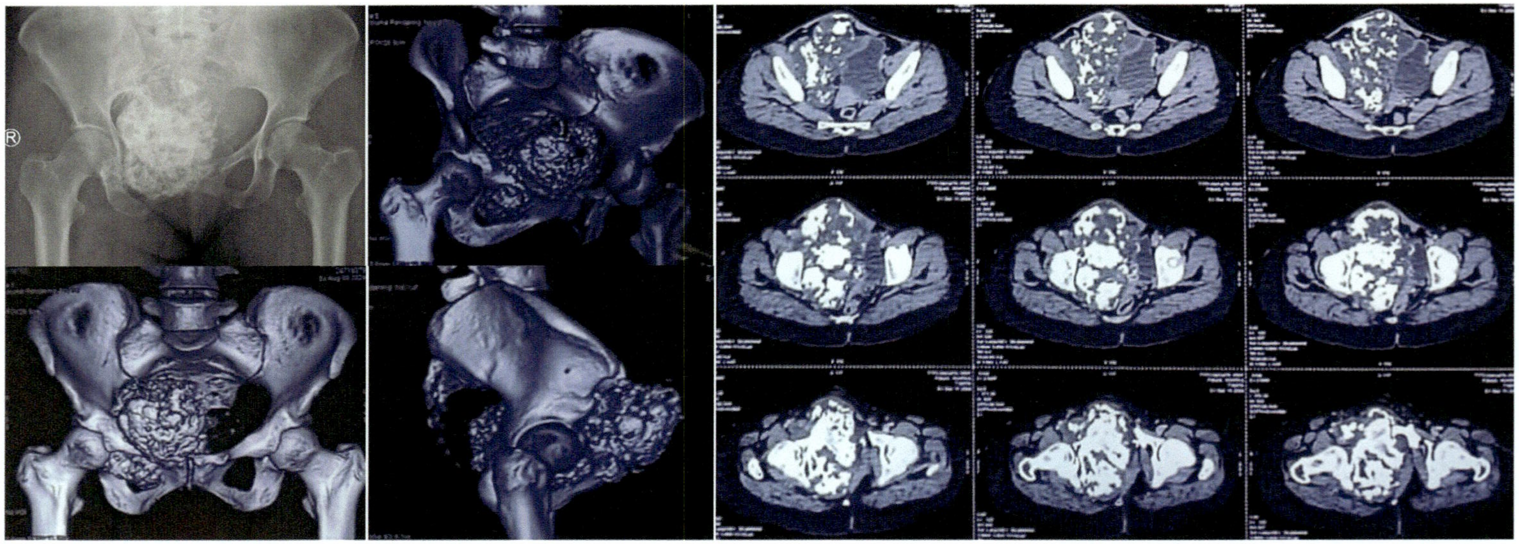

FIGURE 2.15 CT scan of a chondrosarcoma involving the pubis. (Left) Plain radiograph demonstrates a large expansile lesion with characteristic calcifications. (Middle) 3D CT reconstruction delineates the extent of bone destruction and the relationship of the tumor to the pelvic ring. (Right) Axial CT sections reveal an expansile chondroid tumor with cortical breach and areas of "rings-and-arcs" calcification, typical of cartilaginous neoplasms. CT plays a crucial role in evaluating lesions at anatomically complex sites such as the pelvis, where MRI assessment may be technically challenging. It provides superior delineation of cortical destruction, the pattern of mineralization, and the precise anatomical extent of the tumor, thereby serving as an essential tool for surgical planning.

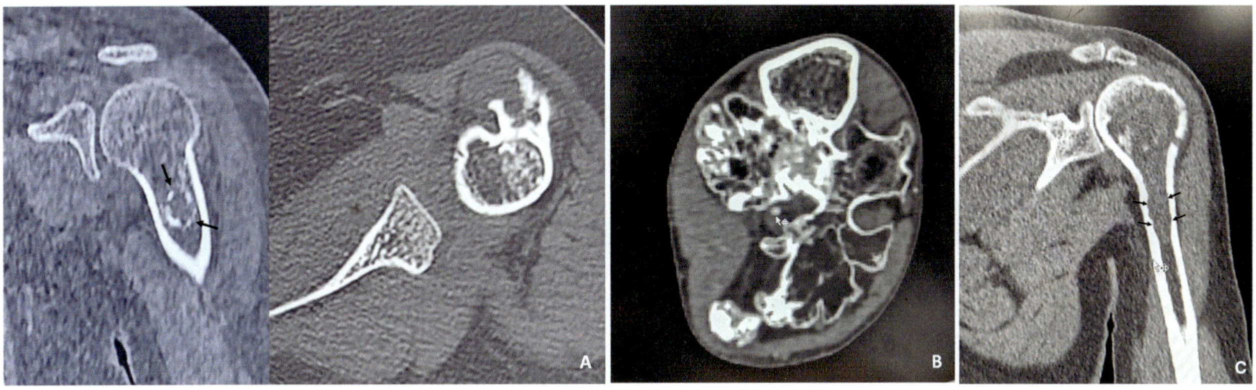

FIGURE 2.16 (A) CT scan demonstrating the characteristic "rings-and-arcs" pattern of calcification, a hallmark feature of chondroid tumors, representing mineralization within the cartilaginous matrix. (B) CT scan of an osteochondroma of the tibia, showing continuity of the cortex and medullary cavity between the lesion and the parent bone, which is diagnostic of osteochondroma. CT provides superior visualization of mineralization patterns in chondroid tumors and is essential in confirming the cortico-medullary continuity of osteochondromas, thereby aiding in accurate diagnosis and differentiation from other bone surface lesions. (C) CT scan of the proximal humerus in a case of chondrosarcoma, demonstrating characteristic endosteal scalloping with cortical erosion (black arrows). These findings are indicative of the locally aggressive nature of the tumor, highlighting its potential to compromise cortical integrity and extend into surrounding structures.

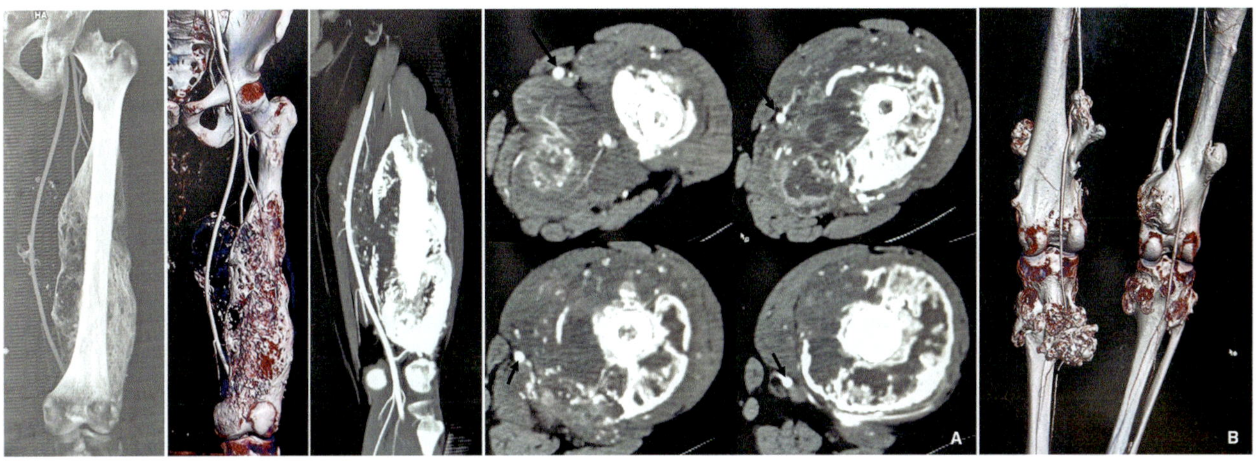

FIGURE 2.17 (A) CT angiography of a case of osteosarcoma of the femur demonstrating the relationship of the tumor mass with the femoral vessels. The black arrows mark the course of the superficial femoral artery in axial sections, showing close abutment to the tumor. 3D and coronal reconstructions further delineate the spatial orientation of the artery relative to the tumor, which is critical for surgical planning. (B) CT angiography in a patient with multiple osteochondromas of the lower limbs. The images clearly demonstrate the course of the femoral and popliteal vessels in relation to the tumor masses. Such vascular mapping is essential in planning surgical excision to avoid iatrogenic vascular injury. CT angiography not only aids in defining tumor–vessel relationships but also provides a detailed roadmap for limb-salvage procedures.

CTA offers several advantages, including shorter acquisition times, three-dimensional multiplanar reconstructions, and the ability to simultaneously assess adjacent bony and soft tissue structures. In cases where MRI angiography is contraindicated or unavailable, CTA serves as an effective alternative. In oncologic surgical planning, detailed vascular mapping aids in reducing intraoperative complications, optimizing incision planning, and determining respectability. CTA is especially useful in high-grade sarcomas and complex pelvic or shoulder girdle resections.

EVALUATION OF SYSTEMIC EXTENT

Assessment of the systemic spread of bone tumors is crucial for accurate staging and treatment planning. Most bone sarcomas metastasize hematogenously, with the lungs and skeleton being the most common sites. A multimodal imaging approach is therefore necessary.

CT Chest for Pulmonary Metastasis

The lungs are the most frequent site of metastasis in high-grade primary bone sarcomas, such as osteosarcoma and Ewing sarcoma. High-resolution CT of the chest is considered the gold standard for detecting pulmonary metastases, especially small nodules that may be missed on plain radiographs.

Key features include:

- Use of thin-slice, high-resolution images (≤1.25 mm) with multiplanar reconstructions
- Pre- and posttreatment comparison to assess response or progression
- Regular follow-up imaging during surveillance for early detection of recurrence

CT chest should be performed at diagnosis, post-chemotherapy, and periodically during follow-up as per clinical protocol. Contrast is generally not required unless evaluating associated lymphadenopathy or mediastinal involvement.

Whole-Body Imaging: Bone Scan and PET-CT

Two key imaging modalities are used for systemic skeletal staging:

- **Radionuclide Bone Scan (99mTc-MDP)**: Most patients with new bone lesions that elicit a high suspicion of primary malignancy undergo bone scintigraphy with technetium Tc-99 methylene diphosphonate (99mTc-MDP) to assess the primary lesion and screen for additional skeletal involvement or metastases.
  - Useful in identifying multiple skeletal lesions in polyostotic conditions such as fibrous dysplasia, enchondromatosis, or Langerhans cell histiocytosis.
  - Bone scans cannot detect soft tissue lesions or lesions confined to the marrow and have limited specificity.
  - Abnormal radiotracer uptake indicates increased osteoblastic activity but does not differentiate benign from malignant lesions.
  - Cold or negative scans may indicate latent or quiescent lesions, though exceptions like multiple myeloma or certain metastatic carcinomas (e.g., renal cell carcinoma) exist.
  - Benign lesions such as giant cell tumor or enchondroma may also show increased tracer uptake, limiting the scan's ability to characterize lesions.
  - Hence, routine use of bone scintigraphy is not recommended for suspected benign lesions.
- **18F-FDG PET or PET-CT**:
  - PET is a functional imaging technique that evaluates glucose metabolism using F-18 fluorodeoxyglucose (FDG), which accumulates in metabolically active cells.
  - It is now standard in staging, response assessment, and surveillance in many cancers and is increasingly used in bone tumors.
  - Particularly useful in Ewing sarcoma, which has a ~25% incidence of metastasis at diagnosis.
  - Provides both metabolic and anatomical information when combined with CT, allowing detection of subcentimeter lesions and better localization.
  - The standardized uptake value (SUV) offers a quantitative measure of metabolic activity; however, overlap between benign and malignant lesions, as well as technical variables, limit its diagnostic cutoff utility.
  - PET-CT has increasingly replaced bone scans in several institutions for initial metastatic workup due to its superior sensitivity for marrow and soft tissue involvement.

Whole-body MRI is an emerging technique, particularly in pediatric and radiation-sensitive populations, offering high sensitivity without ionizing radiation.

IMAGING ASSESSMENT OF THERAPEUTIC RESPONSE

Recent studies have investigated the potential of imaging—particularly MRI and PET-CT—as noninvasive markers of histological response to neoadjuvant chemotherapy in primary bone sarcomas. Dynamic contrast–enhanced MRI (DCE-MRI) has been evaluated for its utility in predicting tumor necrosis, with one study demonstrating that a reduction exceeding 60% in the slope of the enhancement curve was indicative of a favorable histologic response in osteosarcoma [3].

Additionally, DCE-MRI has been employed to assess tumor angiogenesis, revealing correlations between qualitative imaging parameters and the expression of vascular endothelial growth factor (VEGF). This suggests the potential of DCE-MRI as a surrogate marker for tumor grade and biologic activity [4, 5].

Similarly, 18F-FDG PET-CT has shown promise in early assessment of chemotherapeutic response. Parameters derived from PET imaging, such as SUV, have been correlated with the degree of histologic necrosis observed after tumor resection [6]. A retrospective study in Ewing sarcoma further supported these findings, revealing that higher pretreatment FDG uptake was associated with increased metastatic risk. Moreover, significant changes in metabolic activity post-chemotherapy were found to correlate with histological response, positioning FDG PET-CT as a valuable tool in predicting tumor behavior and treatment efficacy in Ewing sarcoma [7].

SURVEILLANCE IMAGING

Standard radiography remains the primary imaging modality for local surveillance following definitive tumor resection. However, the presence of metallic implants used in skeletal reconstruction often hampers the diagnostic utility of CT and MRI. Advances in MRI technology, particularly in metallic artifact reduction techniques, hold promise for improved postoperative surveillance in the near future [8].

In terms of systemic surveillance, the landscape has evolved considerably. Where previously detection of metastatic disease relied on technetium-based bone scintigraphy and chest radiography or CT, the introduction of hybrid imaging modalities such as FDG PET-CT and whole-body MRI has markedly improved both sensitivity and specificity.

Hybrid PET-CT has demonstrated superior accuracy compared to stand-alone PET in detecting occult metastases, largely by enabling precise anatomical localization of hypermetabolic lesions, thereby reducing the rate of false positives [9, 10]. In Ewing sarcoma, PET-CT has outperformed conventional bone scintigraphy in detecting both local and distant recurrence, prompting some experts to recommend discontinuation of bone scans in routine follow-up [11].

Whole-body MRI, which avoids ionizing radiation, has also gained traction, especially in pediatric populations. It has demonstrated comparable sensitivity and specificity to PET-CT in detecting skeletal metastases and is increasingly used in the surveillance of musculoskeletal tumors [12].

Collectively, these modalities enable early identification of disease recurrence and metastasis, thereby improving patient monitoring and informing timely therapeutic interventions.

SUMMARY

- Plain radiographs remain the first-line tool in bone tumor evaluation, offering essential insights into lesion characteristics, aggressiveness, and anatomical localization.
- MRI is the imaging modality of choice for local staging, biopsy planning, and assessment of tumor extent, with advanced techniques like DCE-MRI and DWI aiding in prognostication.
- CT is indispensable for assessing cortical integrity, mineralized matrix, and lung metastases, while CT angiography assists in preoperative vascular mapping for limb salvage.
- Systemic staging relies on PET-CT and radionuclide bone scans, with PET-CT providing superior sensitivity for marrow and soft tissue involvement and monitoring treatment response.
- Surveillance imaging is evolving, with PET-CT and whole-body MRI emerging as effective tools for detecting recurrence and metastases, especially in the setting of metallic implants and pediatric patients.

REFERENCES

1. Nichols RE, Dixon LB. Radiographic analysis of solitary bone lesions. *Radiol Clin North Am.* 2011;49(6):1095–1114.
2. Humphries PD, Sebire NJ, Siegel MJ, Olsen OE. Tumors in pediatric patients at diffusion-weighted MR imaging: apparent diffusion coefficient and tumor cellularity. *Radiology.* 2007;245(3):848–854.
3. Amit P, Patro DK, Basu D, Elangovan S, Parathasarathy V. Role of dynamic MRI and clinical assessment in predicting histologic response to neoadjuvant chemotherapy in bone sarcomas. *Am J Clin Oncol.* 2014;37:384–390.
4. Bajpai J, Sharma M, Sreenivas V, Kumar R, Gamnagatti S, Khan SA, et al. VEGF expression as a prognostic marker in osteosarcoma. *Pediatr Blood Cancer.* 2009;53:1035–1039.
5. Bajpai J, Gamanagatti S, Sharma MC, Kumar R, Vishnubhatla S, Khan SA, et al. Noninvasive imaging surrogate of angiogenesis in osteosarcoma. *Pediatr Blood Cancer.* 2010;54:526–531.
6. Bajpai J, Kumar R, Sreenivas V, Sharma MC, Khan SA, Rastogi S, et al. Prediction of chemotherapy response by PET-CT in osteosarcoma: correlation with histologic necrosis. *J Pediatr Hematol Oncol.* 2011;33:e271–e278.
7. Gupta K, Pawaskar A, Basu S, Rajan MG, Asopa RV, Arora B, et al. Potential role of FDG PET imaging in predicting metastatic potential and assessment of therapeutic response to neoadjuvant chemotherapy in Ewing sarcoma family of tumors. *Clin Nucl Med.* 2011;36:973–977.
8. Ai T, Padua A, Goerner F, et al. SEMAC-VAT and MSVAT-SPACE sequence strategies for metal artifact reduction in 1.5T magnetic resonance imaging. *Invest Radiol.* 2012;47(5):267–276.
9. Treglia G, Salsano M, Stefanelli A, Mattoli MV, Giordano A, Bonomo L. Diagnostic accuracy of 18F-FDG-PET and PET/CT in patients with Ewing sarcoma family tumours: a systematic review and a meta-analysis. *Skeletal Radiol.* 2012;41(3):249–256.
10. Gerth HU, Juergens KU, Dirksen U, Gerss J, Schober O, Franzius C. Significant benefit of multimodal imaging: PET/CT compared with PET alone in staging and follow-up of patients with Ewing tumors. *J Nucl Med.* 2007;48(12):1932–1939.
11. Walter F, Czernin T, Hall T, et al. Is there a need for dedicated bone imaging in addition to 18F-FDG PET/CT imaging in pediatric sarcoma patients? *J Pediatr Hematol Oncol.* 2012;34(2):131–136.
12. Aryal A, Kumar VS, Shamim SA, Gamanagatti S, Khan SA. What is the comparative ability of 18F-FDG PET/CT, 99mTc-MDP skeletal scintigraphy, and whole-body MRI as a staging investigation to detect skeletal metastases in patients with osteosarcoma and Ewing sarcoma? *Clin Orthop Relat Res.* 2021;479(8):1768–1779.

3 Biopsy of Bone Tumors

INTRODUCTION

Biopsy constitutes the definitive step in the diagnostic triad for bone tumors, complementing clinical evaluation and imaging. It is not a mere procedural formality but a critical determinant of treatment planning and prognosis. When meticulously planned and executed, biopsy enables accurate histopathological classification, guides the extent of surgical resection, and informs the use of adjunctive therapies such as chemotherapy or radiotherapy. In contrast, an inappropriately performed biopsy can jeopardize local control, increase morbidity, and potentially eliminate limb salvage options.

The diagnostic approach to musculoskeletal neoplasms relies on the concordance of clinical, radiological, and pathological findings; any discordance should prompt reevaluation. While certain lesions with characteristic imaging features (e.g., osteochondromas, nonossifying fibromas) may not require tissue sampling, histological confirmation is essential for differentiating benign, aggressive benign, and malignant tumors.

Biopsies should ideally be performed in specialized tertiary centers within a multidisciplinary framework, as procedures undertaken in nonspecialized settings are associated with higher rates of diagnostic error, complications, and adverse oncologic outcomes [1, 2]. The primary objective is to obtain adequate tissue with minimal contamination, preserving future surgical planes. This chapter outlines the principles, indications, preoperative considerations, techniques, and outcomes of biopsy in bone tumors, with emphasis on evidence-based practice and avoidance of common pitfalls.

PRINCIPLES OF BIOPSY

The success of a biopsy in bone tumor management depends on strict adherence to oncological principles designed to maximize diagnostic accuracy while minimizing local morbidity and the risk of tumor dissemination. These principles are grounded in tumor biology, compartmental anatomy, and the requirements of limb salvage surgery. A poorly planned or executed biopsy can compromise oncological outcomes and, in some cases, preclude the possibility of limb preservation.

- A biopsy should only be undertaken after thorough clinical assessment and detailed imaging, ensuring that the procedure is the final diagnostic step following integration of clinical, radiological, and pathological considerations. This triad is essential for diagnostic accuracy, and any discordance among its components should prompt reevaluation before proceeding [3].
- Decision-making regarding the need for biopsy, the optimal technique, and the surgical approach should be undertaken within a multidisciplinary team that includes orthopedic oncologists, musculoskeletal radiologists, and pathologists, ensuring coordinated care and preservation of definitive treatment options [3].
- Whenever possible, the biopsy should be performed at the same institution where definitive surgery will be carried out. Procedures done at non-specialist or referring centers have been linked to higher rates of diagnostic error, tumor contamination, and poor oncological outcomes, including unnecessary amputations [2].
- The biopsy tract must be planned in alignment with the definitive surgical approach so that it can be entirely excised during tumor resection. Incorrect placement across inappropriate anatomical planes or compartments can necessitate wider excisions or even amputation [3] (Figure 3.1 A–C).
- The least invasive yet diagnostically adequate method should be chosen. Image-guided core needle biopsy is preferred for many lesions due to its high diagnostic yield and low morbidity, while open incisional biopsy is reserved for anatomically complex or inconclusive cases [4, 5].
- Incisions must be longitudinal, confined to a single compartment, and avoid crossing multiple planes, as transverse or curvilinear approaches (Figure 3.2) can compromise limb-sparing surgery [3].
- Meticulous hemostasis is essential to prevent hematoma formation, which can serve as a conduit for tumor spread. If a tourniquet is used, it should be applied without prior exsanguination to avoid proximal tumor dissemination [3].
- Tissue sampling should target the viable, peripheral regions of the tumor rather than necrotic centers to reduce the risk of sampling error, especially in heterogeneous sarcomas [3].
- Close coordination with pathology services is critical. An experienced musculoskeletal pathologist should ideally be available for frozen section or rapid on-site evaluation to improve diagnostic yield [6].
- Specimens must also be handled appropriately for ancillary studies, with fresh, formalin-fixed, or frozen preservation as required by the suspected diagnosis [7].
- Finally, the biopsy site, including any associated drains or hematoma tracts, must be regarded as contaminated and excised en bloc during definitive surgery [3].

DOI: 10.1201/9780367822002-4

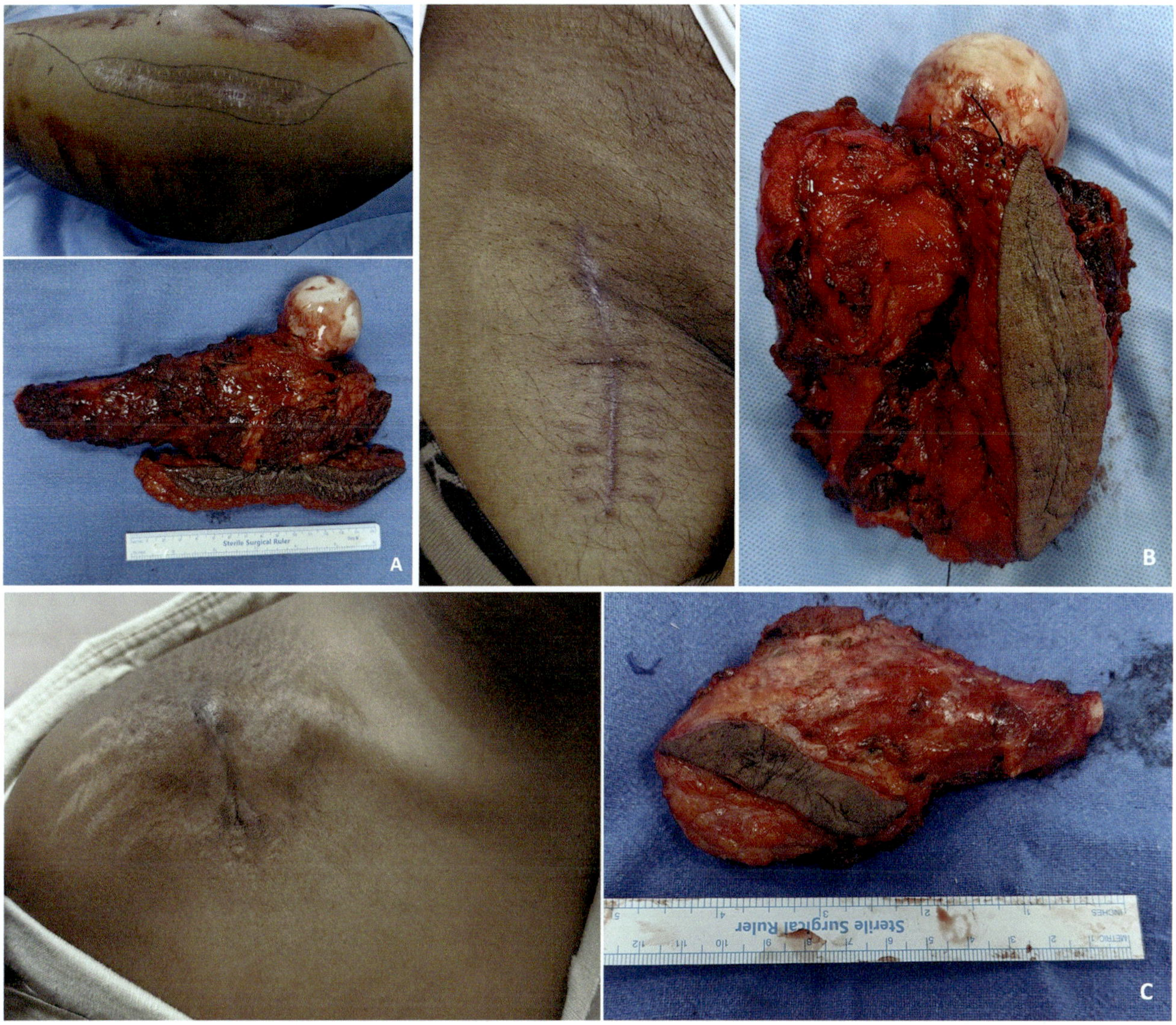

FIGURE 3.1 (A–C) Misplacement of biopsy incisions into incorrect anatomical planes or compartments should be strictly avoided, as it leads to contamination requiring more extensive excision and may jeopardize the possibility of limb salvage.

By adhering to these principles, biopsy serves not only as a diagnostic tool but as an integral part of the overall oncologic strategy, safeguarding both local control and functional outcomes.

TYPES OF BIOPSY TECHNIQUES

The choice of biopsy technique in bone tumors is influenced by the location and nature of the lesion, the need for ancillary studies, patient comorbidities, available imaging modalities, and institutional expertise. The goal is to obtain sufficient diagnostic tissue with minimal morbidity and maximal oncologic safety. Broadly, biopsy techniques are classified as **closed (percutaneous)** or **open (surgical)**, and each has specific indications and limitations (Table 3.1).

Fine-Needle Aspiration (FNA) Biopsy

Technique: A 20–25 gauge needle is used to aspirate cells from the lesion, often under ultrasound or CT guidance.

Indications:

- Suspected metastatic carcinoma involving bone
- Recurrence of previously diagnosed tumors
- Patients unfit for more invasive procedures

Diagnostic Accuracy:

- Variable; ranges from 60% to 90%, depending on tumor type and operator experience [8, 9].
- Lower diagnostic yield in sarcomas, especially round cell or myxoid tumors [5].

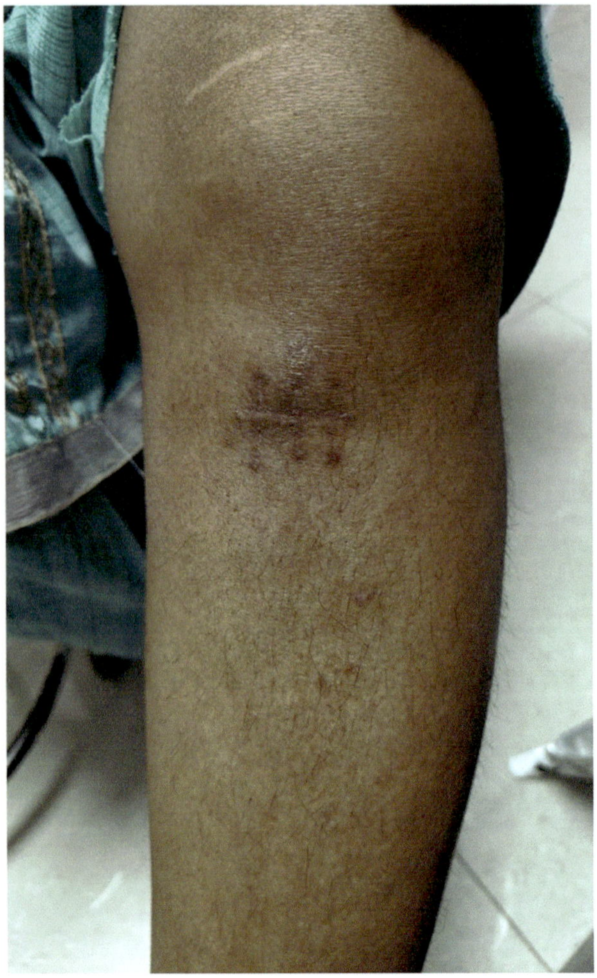

FIGURE 3.2 Transverse biopsy scars must be avoided as they necessitate wider excisions and can compromise limb-sparing surgery.

Pearls:
- Minimal morbidity, often performed under local anesthesia
- Rapid results possible, especially with on-site cytopathologic evaluation

Pitfalls:
- Limited tissue precludes evaluation of architectural features
- Insufficient for subclassifying sarcomas or performing immunohistochemistry in many cases
- High risk of nondiagnostic or equivocal results if not performed by experienced teams [10]

FNA has a more defined role in recurrent or metastatic disease but is generally **not preferred for primary diagnosis** of bone sarcomas.

Core Needle (Trocar) Biopsy

Technique: A larger bore needle (typically 14–18 gauge) is used to obtain tissue cores, usually with CT or MRI guidance.

Indications:
- Most primary bone tumors and soft tissue masses
- Lesions with extraosseous extension
- Deep-seated lesions where incisional biopsy is associated with greater morbidity

Diagnostic Accuracy:
- High: 85%–95% for bone lesions, >90% for soft tissue masses when performed with imaging guidance and immediate histologic evaluation [4, 11]

Pearls:
- Combines minimal invasiveness with sufficient tissue for histology, immunohistochemistry, and molecular studies
- Can often be done in an outpatient setting
- Allows precise targeting of viable tumor areas using cross-sectional imaging

Pitfalls:
- Sampling error in heterogeneous tumors or necrotic lesions
- Risk of inadequate hemostasis in vascular tumors
- Requires experienced radiologist or surgeon for accurate localization and trajectory planning

TABLE 3.1
Summary of Biopsy Types

Biopsy Type	Indications	Accuracy	Advantages	Limitations
FNA	Metastasis, recurrence	60%–90%	Minimally invasive, fast	Limited tissue, low utility for sarcomas
Core needle biopsy	Most bone and soft tissue tumors	85%–95%	High yield, image-guided, and outpatient feasible	Sampling error requires imaging and expertise
Incisional biopsy	Deep, inaccessible, or inconclusive needle biopsies	94%–98%	Direct visualization, large tissue sample	Morbidity, contamination risk, and the need for an OR setting
Excisional biopsy	Small superficial benign-appearing lesions	High	Entire lesion removed, one-step management	Oncologically unsafe if malignancy is misdiagnosed

Core needle biopsy has become the **preferred technique** in most musculoskeletal oncology centers for initial diagnostic workup [5].

Incisional (Open) Biopsy

Technique: A small surgical incision is made to directly visualize and sample tumor tissue. Usually performed in the operating room under regional or general anesthesia.

Indications:
- When needle biopsy is inconclusive or nondiagnostic
- Lesions with complex anatomy where imaging-guided biopsy is unsafe or unavailable
- Deep-seated tumors without extraosseous extension

Diagnostic Accuracy:
- Highest among all techniques: 94%–98% [3]

Pearls:
- Allows direct visual selection of viable tissue
- Enables collection of an ample sample size for histopathology and special studies
- Frozen section assessment can be done intraoperatively

Pitfalls:
- Greater soft tissue disruption and higher risk of contamination
- Requires careful planning: incision must lie within the definitive surgical field and be in line with the proposed resection
- Hematoma formation must be avoided through meticulous hemostasis
- Higher cost and resource requirement than percutaneous approaches

Open biopsy remains the **gold standard** in complex or equivocal cases and should be performed by the surgical team that will manage the definitive tumor resection.

Excisional Biopsy

Technique: Entire lesion is removed surgically, often with narrow margins, without prior histologic diagnosis.

Indications:
- Small (<3–5 cm), superficial lesions with classical benign imaging features (e.g., lipoma, osteochondroma)
- Masses located in surgically expendable regions with low suspicion of malignancy

Diagnostic Accuracy:
- High if properly selected; however, its role in primary malignant tumors is limited

Pearls:
- Provides a complete specimen for comprehensive analysis
- May eliminate the need for a second surgery in benign cases

Pitfalls:
- Oncologically unsafe if performed for malignant tumors under a benign assumption
- Risk of inadequate margins and contamination if malignancy is subsequently diagnosed
- Can convert a potentially resectable sarcoma into a case requiring more radical surgery or amputation [2]

Excisional biopsy should be undertaken **only in select benign-appearing cases** after complete imaging and clinical correlation.

PERCUTANEOUS CORE NEEDLE BIOPSY: TECHNIQUE AND STEPS (FIGURE 3.5)

Percutaneous core needle biopsy (CNB) has become the preferred technique for the diagnosis of most bone and soft tissue tumors, owing to its high diagnostic yield, minimal invasiveness, and ability to preserve oncologic planes. However, its success hinges on meticulous technique, anatomical understanding, and oncologic principles.

Preprocedural Preparation

- Not all lesions require biopsy; those with classic benign clinical and imaging features (e.g., osteochondroma, fibrous cortical defect) can be managed without histological confirmation.
- Biopsy is indicated for:
  - Lesions of uncertain etiology
  - Aggressive, destructive, or large masses
  - All suspected primary malignant bone tumors
- **Patient Assessment**: Includes evaluation of medical history, coagulation profile, and anesthetic fitness. Obtain informed consent discussing risks such as infection, bleeding, and possible nondiagnostic sampling.
- **Imaging Review**: Select the most viable and accessible area of the lesion—avoiding necrotic or cystic regions—and determine the safest trajectory. Prebiopsy imaging (MRI and CT) must be complete before tissue sampling (Figure 3.3).
- Because **bone and soft tissue sarcomas often show regional heterogeneity**, samples must be obtained from viable, representative areas—typically at the periphery of the lesion. Central regions may yield nondiagnostic samples due to necrosis and hemorrhage, a phenomenon leading to **sampling error**, where the tissue does not reflect the true nature of the tumor.

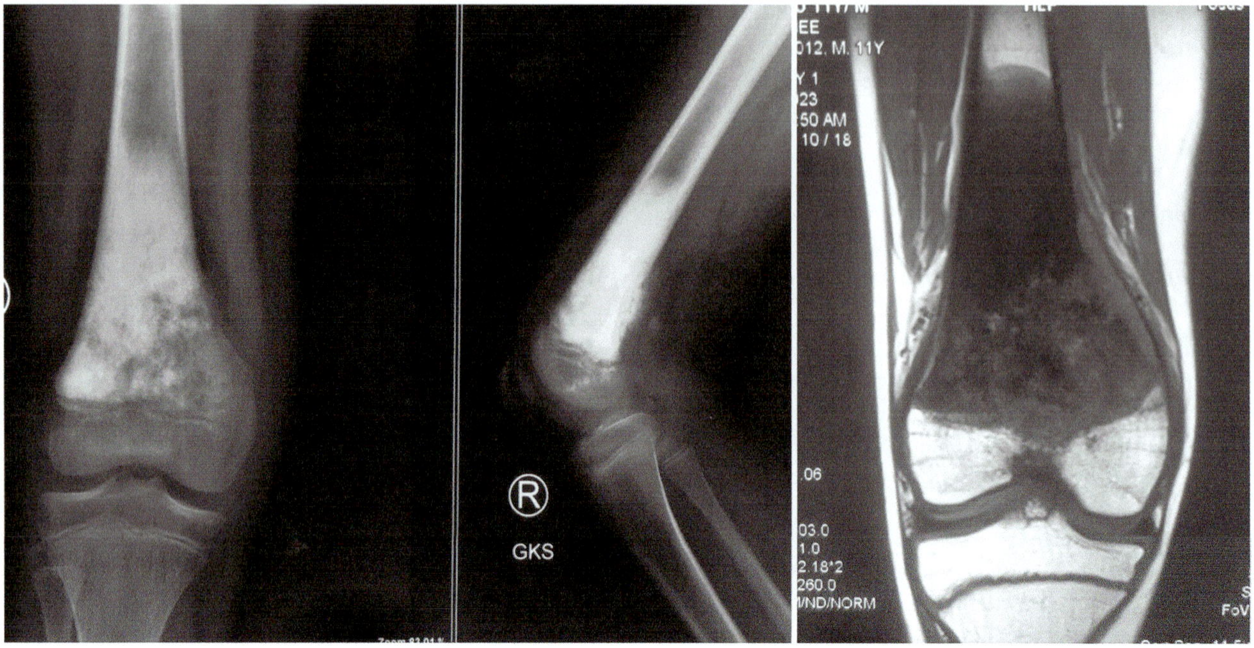

FIGURE 3.3 Pre-biopsy imaging must be complete and carefully reviewed before tissue sampling.

- If an extraosseous soft tissue component exists, it is often preferable for biopsy over violating the bone cortex, which could predispose the patient to a pathological fracture, especially in highly vascular or osteolytic tumors [3].

Patient Positioning

- Position the patient to provide the shortest and safest needle path to the lesion, simulating the orientation of the definitive surgical approach when feasible.
- The entry site should be planned such that the entire needle tract can be excised during the definitive tumor resection.

Biopsy System and Needle Selection

- **Gauge**: Typically, 14–16 gauge needles are used for bone and soft tissue lesions.
- **System**: Coaxial biopsy systems are preferred, as they allow multiple core samples via a single cortical entry point, minimizing tissue trauma.
- **Guidance**: Real-time image guidance with CT, MRI, fluoroscopy, or ultrasound is essential for accurate localization and to avoid critical structures [4].

Sterile Preparation and Anesthesia

- Check and ensure the availability of necessary instruments (Figure 3.4).
- Maintain strict aseptic technique (Figure 3.5A).

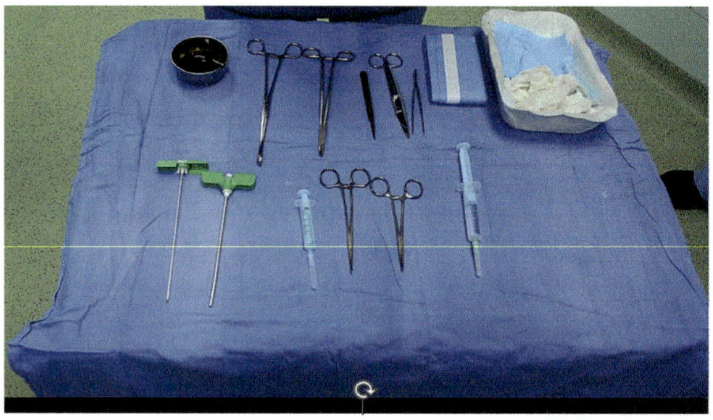

FIGURE 3.4 Check and ensure the availability of necessary instruments.

Execution of Biopsy

Incision and Trajectory

- The planned future incision for resection should be marked (Figure 3.5B).
- The possible site of biopsy is marked under C-arm guidance, aiming for the junction of tumor and normal bone to increase the possibility of sampling viable tumor cells (Figure 3.5C).
- Local anesthesia is infiltrated along the intended biopsy tract up to the periosteum or soft tissue surface (Figure 3.5D). Conscious sedation or general anesthesia may be administered in select patients (e.g., pediatric age group), though most CNBs are done with local anesthesia alone.

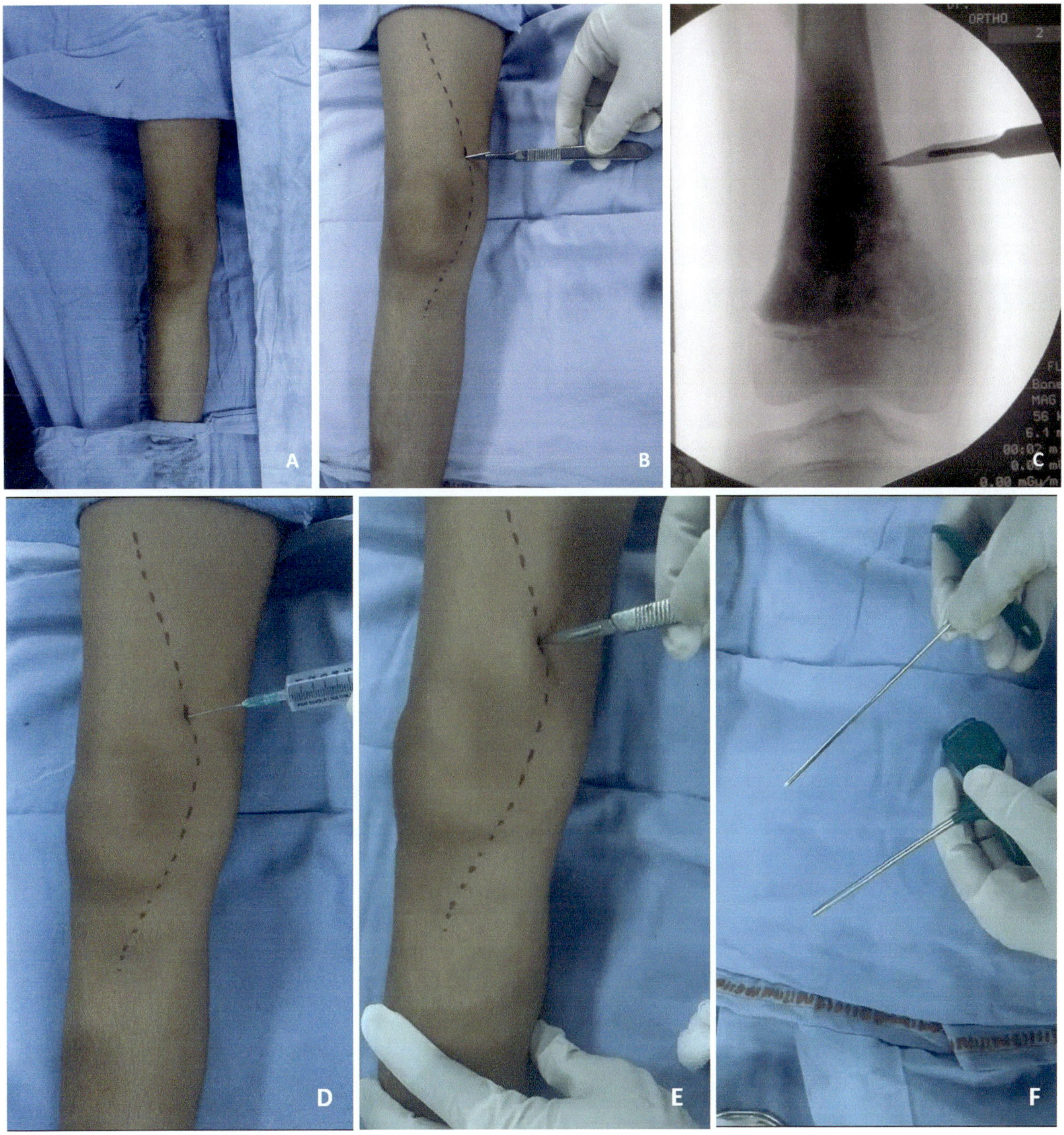

FIGURE 3.5 Percutaneous Core Needle Biopsy: Technique and Steps: (A) Clean and drape the biopsy site. (B) Mark the planned future incision for resection. (C) Mark the possible site of biopsy under C-arm guidance. Aim for the junction of tumor and normal bone to increase the possibility of sampling viable tumor cells. (D) Administer local anaesthetic and wait for the anaesthetic to take effect. (E) Make a 1 cm longitudinal incision in line with the future incision, extending deep to reach the bone. Introduce the core biopsy needle with the trocar (F), and reach the bone to be sampled

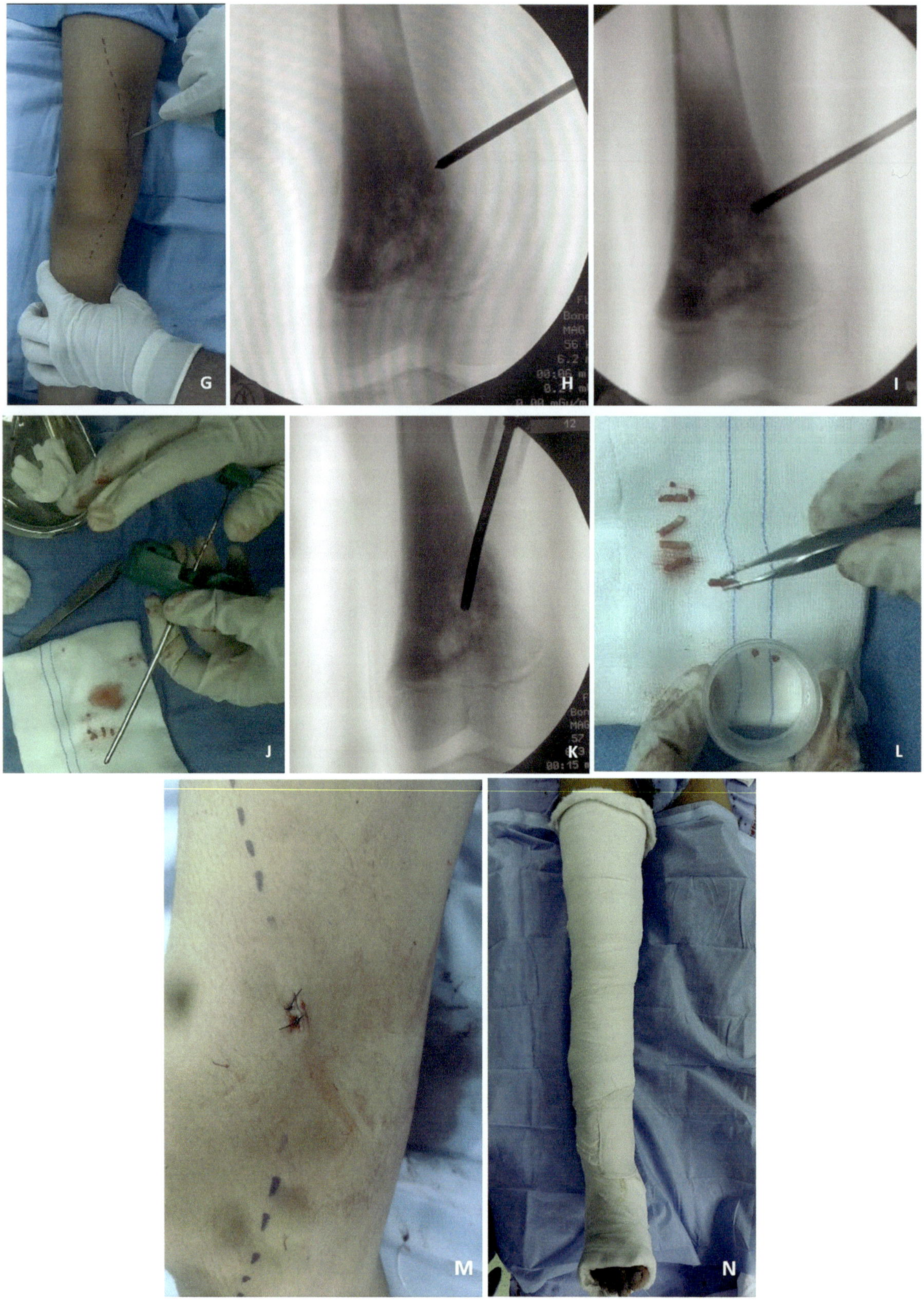

FIGURE 3.5 (Continued) (G). Confirm the zone of sampling again under the image (H). Use the core biopsy needle with the trocar to create a hole in the bone. Remove the trocar, and advance the needle under image guidance with a gentle semicircular motion (I). Use rotatory motion to break the captured core from its bed. Get the cores of bone out of the needle using a stilet (J). Repeat the same using the same tract while changing the angle to capture a sample from a different area (K). Obtain 4–6 good-quality cores (L), send for HPE in formalin/saline in a sterile container. Maintain haemostasis if there is any bleeding, and close the wound (M). Apply an appropriate plaster slab for immobilization to prevent a pathological fracture (N).

- A **small longitudinal skin incision** is made in line with the proposed surgical incision to accommodate the biopsy needle (Figure 3.5E). **Transverse incisions are contraindicated**, as they may complicate oncologic resection by requiring wider excisions and jeopardizing soft tissue reconstruction options [12].
- Traverse only one anatomical compartment.
- Avoid neurovascular bundles, tendons, ligaments, joints, and uninvolved tissue planes.

For Intraosseous Bone Lesions

- The outer cortex is penetrated with a bone trocar or drill to create a cortical entry window, followed by insertion of the biopsy needle. Avoid drilling through both cortices. Minimize hole size while ensuring adequate access.
- **Shape of the cortical window matters**:
  - **Clark et al**. demonstrated that **oblong holes with rounded ends** provide the **greatest residual strength** and least stress concentration, compared to square or rectangular holes with sharp corners [12].
  - If a small hole suffices, a **circular window** should be used. If a larger access is needed, the oblong design is preferred to preserve bone integrity [12].

Sampling Technique

- Insert the biopsy needle through the coaxial sheath into the viable peripheral portion of the tumor (Figure 3.5F–I).
- Obtain **multiple cores (typically 3–5)** from different angles through the same tract to reduce the risk of sampling error. Avoid multiple entries or back-and-forth passes (Figure 3.5J–L).
- For soft tissue components, biopsy is directed away from major neurovascular bundles and toward the most cellular, enhancing areas.
- **Avoid crushing or shearing** the specimen: Use a clean-cutting needle or curette to preserve histological architecture, which is critical for subtype classification.

On-Site Evaluation

- If feasible, a pathologist or cytopathologist should be present to perform **rapid on-site evaluation (ROSE)**, ensuring that adequate and viable tissue has been collected. This improves diagnostic yield and reduces the need for repeat procedures [6].

Postprocedural Measures

- **Hemostasis**: Apply manual pressure and avoid creating a hematoma (Figure 3.5M). Meticulous control of bleeding is essential because a **large hematoma can dissect tissue planes**, contaminate compartments, and **jeopardize limb-sparing surgery**.
- Apply a sterile occlusive dressing and a splint to immobilize the limb to prevent pathological fracture (Figure 3.5N).
- **Observation**: Monitor for signs of bleeding, pain, or neurologic changes in the immediate postprocedure period.

Specimen Handling and Documentation

- Properly label and preserve samples for histopathology, immunohistochemistry, microbiology, or molecular studies as needed.
- **"Biopsy what you culture and culture what you biopsy"**—in cases of infection suspicion, always send tissue for both pathological and microbiological analysis.
- Document the technique, number of passes, adequacy of tissue, and any complications. Clear communication with the pathology team is essential for tissue triaging—formalin fixation, fresh samples for microbiology, flow cytometry, or molecular studies as needed [7].

COMPLICATIONS AND PITFALLS OF BIOPSY

Biopsy, while an indispensable diagnostic step in the evaluation of bone tumors, is not without risk. Complications may arise from technical errors, improper planning, or failure to adhere to oncologic principles (Table 3.2). Importantly, many of these adverse outcomes are preventable. A thorough understanding of the potential complications and common pitfalls allows the treating team to minimize morbidity and preserve curative treatment options.

TABLE 3.2
Summary of Common Pitfalls in Biopsy

Pitfall	Impact	Prevention
Biopsy in the wrong plane/compartment	Tumor contamination, wider resection	Place the tract within the planned surgical incision
Inadequate sampling	Nondiagnostic result, repeat procedure needed	Target viable tumor; multiple cores; involve a pathologist
Hematoma formation	Tumor spread, infection, loss of limb salvage option	Meticulous hemostasis, compression, and avoiding large vessels
Transverse/curved incisions	Wider excision required	Use longitudinal incisions
Fracture following bone biopsy	Treatment delay, increased morbidity	Minimize window size; oblong holes with rounded edges
Neurovascular injury	Neurologic or vascular compromise	Use image guidance; avoid high-risk corridors

SUMMARY

- **Biopsy must be performed only after complete clinical and imaging evaluation** and should ideally be done at the treating center to avoid misdiagnosis and complications.
- **CNB is the preferred modality** for most lesions due to its high diagnostic accuracy, minimal invasiveness, and compatibility with image guidance.
- **Biopsy planning is critical**—the tract must be within the planned surgical field and confined to a single anatomical compartment to enable safe resection.
- **Target viable, peripheral areas of the tumor** to minimize sampling error; avoid necrotic, hemorrhagic, or cystic zones.
- **Meticulous hemostasis and tract control are essential** to prevent hematoma and tumor spread, which may compromise limb-sparing options.
- **All biopsy-related tissues, including tracts and drains, are considered contaminated** and must be excised en bloc during definitive surgery.
- **Common pitfalls and inadequate biopsies** can be avoided through multidisciplinary planning and adherence to oncologic principles.

REFERENCES

1. Mankin HJ, Lange TA, Spanier SS. The hazards of biopsy in patients with malignant primary bone and soft tissue tumors. *J Bone Joint Surg Am.* 1982;64(7):1121–1127.
2. Mankin HJ, Mankin CJ, Simon MA. The hazards of biopsy, revisited. *J Bone Joint Surg Am.* 1996;78(5):656–663.
3. Bickels J, Jelinek JS, Shmookler BM, Neff RS, Malawer MM. Biopsy of musculoskeletal tumors: current concepts. *Clin Orthop Relat Res.* 1999;(368):212–219.
4. Yang YJ, Damron TA. Comparison of needle core biopsy and fine-needle aspiration for diagnostic accuracy in musculoskeletal lesions. *Arch Pathol Lab Med.* 2004;128(7):759–764.
5. Rougraff BT, Aboulafia A, Biermann JS, Healey J. Biopsy of soft tissue masses: evidence-based medicine for the musculoskeletal tumor society. *Clin Orthop Relat Res.* 2009;467(11):2783–2791.
6. Virayavanich W, Ringler MD, Chin CT, et al. CT-guided biopsy of bone and soft-tissue lesions: role of on-site immediate cytologic evaluation. *J Vasc Interv Radiol.* 2011;22(7):1024–1030.
7. Rubin BP, Cooper K, Fletcher CD, et al; Members of the Cancer Committee, College of American Pathologists. Protocol for the examination of specimens from patients with tumors of soft tissue. *Arch Pathol Lab Med.* 2010;134(4):e31–e39.
8. Kilpatrick SE, Cappellari JO, Bos GD, Gold SH, Ward WG. Is fine-needle aspiration biopsy a practical alternative to open biopsy for the primary diagnosis of sarcoma? Experience with 140 patients. *Am J Clin Pathol.* 2001;115(1):59–68.
9. Fleshman R, Mayerson J, Wakely PE Jr. Fine-needle aspiration biopsy of high-grade sarcoma: a report of 107 cases. *Cancer.* 2007;111(6):491–498.
10. Liu K, Layfield LJ, Coogan AC, Ballo MS, Bentz JS, Dodge RK. Diagnostic accuracy in fine-needle aspiration of soft tissue and bone lesions: influence of clinical history and experience. *Am J Clin Pathol.* 1999;111(5):632–640.
11. Rimondi E, Staals EL, Errani C, et al. Percutaneous CT-guided biopsy of the spine: results of 430 biopsies. *Eur Spine J.* 2008;17(7):975–981.
12. Clark CR, Morgan C, Sontegard DA, et al. The effect of biopsy hole shape and size on bone strength. *J Bone Joint Surg Am.* 1977;59(2):213–217.

4 Fundamentals of Surgical Management of Bone Tumors

INTRODUCTION

Limb salvage surgery has emerged as a cornerstone in the multidisciplinary management of primary malignant bone tumors, offering a functional alternative to amputation without compromising oncological safety. The paradigm shift from ablative procedures to limb preservation has been driven by advancements in imaging, surgical techniques, and chemotherapy. Historically, the goal of surgery in bone tumors was to achieve complete oncologic excision, often through radical resections and amputations. However, with the increasing ability to achieve similar oncological outcomes through limb-sparing procedures, preserving the patient's function and quality of life has taken precedence.

Limb salvage procedures must achieve a delicate balance between adequate oncological clearance and optimal functional outcomes. This requires a thorough understanding of tumor biology, careful preoperative planning, meticulous surgical technique, and individualized reconstruction strategies. The principles of limb salvage surgery emphasize the need for achieving safe margins, utilizing barrier tissues effectively, and integrating appropriate reconstruction to restore form and function. This chapter aims to outline the fundamental principles governing limb salvage surgery in bone tumors, including oncological rationale, surgical planning, resection strategies, and reconstructive options.

GOALS OF LIMB SALVAGE SURGERY

Limb salvage surgery for osseous sarcoma was pioneered in North America in 1951 by Dallas Phemister at the University of Chicago [1]. Limb salvage is designed to serve two essential objectives:

1. **Oncological Control**: The foremost priority is complete tumor excision with negative margins. The adequacy of the surgical margin has a direct correlation with local recurrence rates and long-term survival. Achieving oncologically safe margins remains non-negotiable and forms the backbone of all limb salvage decisions [2].
2. **Functional Preservation**: Equally important is preserving meaningful limb function. The surgery should aim to maintain or restore skeletal integrity, joint mobility, and soft tissue coverage such that the salvaged limb is more useful than a prosthetic replacement would have been. This involves skeletal reconstruction, soft tissue restoration, and nerve preservation when feasible [3].

Additional goals include ensuring timely healing to facilitate early initiation of adjuvant therapy, providing durable soft tissue coverage, minimizing complications, and enabling early ambulation and return to normal activities.

INDICATIONS FOR LIMB SALVAGE SURGERY

LSS is considered appropriate when two critical prerequisites are met:

1. **Achievability of Adequate Surgical Margins**: Adequate margins are those that ensure a low likelihood of local recurrence.
2. **Functional Supremacy Over Amputation**: Limb salvage must provide a better functional outcome than an amputation would. A desensate, flail, or unstable limb—despite being oncologically cleared—may compromise quality of life more than a well-fitted prosthesis. Hence, if the reconstructed limb cannot offer adequate function or sensation, amputation may be the better option [3].

Every patient with sarcoma of the extremity should be considered for limb salvage if the tumor can be removed with an adequate margin and an adequate limb function can be maintained. Limb salvage is contraindicated if either of these conditions cannot be fulfilled. In some circumstances, the aggressiveness of the lesion or the extent of surgical excision precludes limb-sparing options and mandates amputation. Such indications for amputation include encasement of major neurovascular structures with inability to perform successful vascular bypass or extensive soft tissue involvement.

CONCEPT OF SURGICAL MARGINS

The concept of surgical margins is central to the oncological safety of limb salvage surgery in bone tumors. Surgical margins refer to the extent of healthy tissue excised around a tumor during surgery to achieve complete removal of microscopic disease. The adequacy of these margins is a key determinant of local control, recurrence risk, and long-term survival.

DOI: 10.1201/9780367822002-5

The traditional framework for surgical margins in musculoskeletal oncology was established by Enneking et al., who classified resections into **intralesional**, **marginal**, **wide**, and **radical**, based on the anatomical relationship of the tumor to the surrounding compartments and tissues (Table 4.1 and Figure 4.1) [4]. In general, benign bone tumors are adequately treated by either an intralesional procedure (e.g., curettage and burr drilling, cryosurgery) or by marginal excision. Primary bone sarcomas are treated with wide excision.

While widely adopted, the Enneking system lacked specificity in quantifying margin distances and did not describe the exact amount of "normal" tissue that defines a wide margin. In 1989, the Evaluation Method for Surgical Margins designated by the Japanese Orthopedic Association was accepted [5]. In this system, a surgical margin is evaluated according to the distance of the margin from the tumor's reactive zone, and consequently is classifiable into the four categories of curative, wide, marginal, or intralesional margin.

- **Intralesional Margin**: The plane of dissection passes through the tumor itself, and involves curettage or debulking. This type of resection is associated with a high risk of local recurrence and is typically avoided in malignant tumors.
- **Marginal Margin**: The excision passes through the reactive zone. It may be oncologically inadequate unless combined with adjuvant therapies such as radiotherapy.
- **Wide Margin**: The dissection plane lies outside the reactive zone and includes a cuff of normal tissue. It is further subdivided wide margins into:
    - *Inadequate wide*: 1 cm from the reactive zone.
    - *Adequate wide*: ≥2 cm from the reactive zone.
- **Curative Margin**: A margin of ≥5 cm from the reactive zone, or its equivalent when barrier tissues are present. This offers the highest assurance of local tumor control.

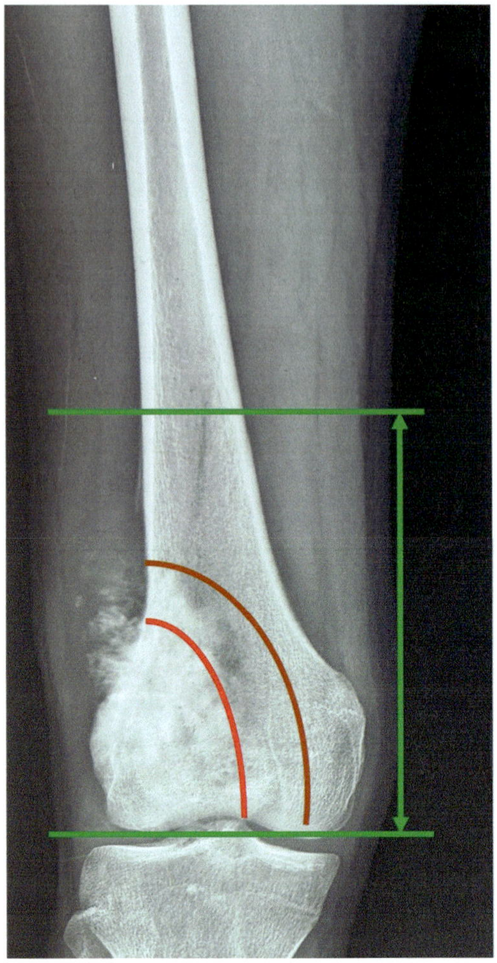

FIGURE 4.1 An illustration of Enneking's classification of surgical margins in musculoskeletal tumor surgery. The red line represents an intralesional excision, where the plane of dissection passes within the lesion and the pseudocapsule of the tumor is entered (e.g., curettage). The orange line denotes a marginal excision, in which the dissection passes through the reactive zone but does not enter the pseudocapsule, though microscopic disease may be left behind. The green arrows mark the extent of a wide excision, where the dissection passes through a cuff of normal tissue surrounding the lesion.

TABLE 4.1
Classification of Surgical Margins as Described by Enneking

Intralesional excision	Plane of dissection passes within the lesion. Pseudocapsule of the tumor is entered (e.g., curettage)
Marginal excision	Pseudocapsule of the tumor is not entered. Plane of dissection passes through the reactive zone. Microscopic disease may be left behind
Wide excision	Plane of dissection passes through a cuff of normal tissue
Radical excision	Removal of entire compartment of origin; complete extirpation of an entire bone

THE BARRIER EFFECT

Kawaguchi et al. described the concept of barrier in surgery for bone and soft tissue sarcoma [1]. Barrier refers to any tissue that has any resistance against tumor invasion and can include muscle fascia, joint capsule, tendon, tendon sheath, epineurium, vascular sheath, cartilage, pleura, and peritoneum. Except for joint cartilage, each of these tissues can be classified as either a thick barrier or a thin barrier (Table 4.2). Barriers are converted into the equivalent thickness of normal tissue. By considering barrier effects translated into concrete distance equivalents, surgery can be done at sites where barriers exist by using less margin than true physical distance. This approach allows for reduced resection distances when such barriers are intact, thereby minimizing unnecessary loss of function without compromising oncological safety.

TABLE 4.2
Types of Barriers

Barrier	Tissues	Equivalent Margin
Thin	Weaker membranous structure- Muscle fascia, adult periosteum, vessel sheath, epineurium, thin growth plates in older children	2 cm
Thick	Strong membranous tissue with a white tendinous luster- iliotibial band, presacral fascia, joint capsule, infant periosteum, thin growth plate in older children	3 cm
Joint cartilage	-	5 cm

MARGIN SELECTION IN PRACTICE

- For **high-grade tumors** with no or poor response to neoadjuvant therapy, margins >3 cm are recommended.
- If **preoperative chemotherapy is effective**, a 2 cm margin may suffice.
- For **low-grade tumors**, adequate wide or marginal margins are often sufficient, especially when anatomical barriers are present.
- In **recurrent tumors**, only curative margins consistently yield high rates of local control, irrespective of tumor grade.

The concept of surgical margins has evolved from a simplistic anatomical model to a biologically and anatomically nuanced framework. It offers a rational, quantifiable, and reproducible method for evaluating and planning resection margins in bone tumor surgery. By integrating the effects of tumor biology, neoadjuvant therapy, and anatomical barriers, it enables the surgeon to optimize the delicate balance between oncological safety and functional preservation.

RECONSTRUCTION STRATEGIES IN LIMB SALVAGE SURGERY

Endoprosthesis Reconstruction

Endoprosthetic reconstruction has revolutionized limb salvage surgery in musculoskeletal oncology, providing a reliable method to restore skeletal integrity and enable early mobilization following wide tumor resections. These modular metallic implants replace large bone segments and adjacent joints when necessary and are particularly valuable when resection involves the metaphyseal or epiphyseal regions of long bones.

Endoprostheses are primarily indicated in:

- Metaphyseal and epiphyseal resections (e.g., distal femur, proximal tibia, proximal humerus, proximal femur) (Figure 4.2).

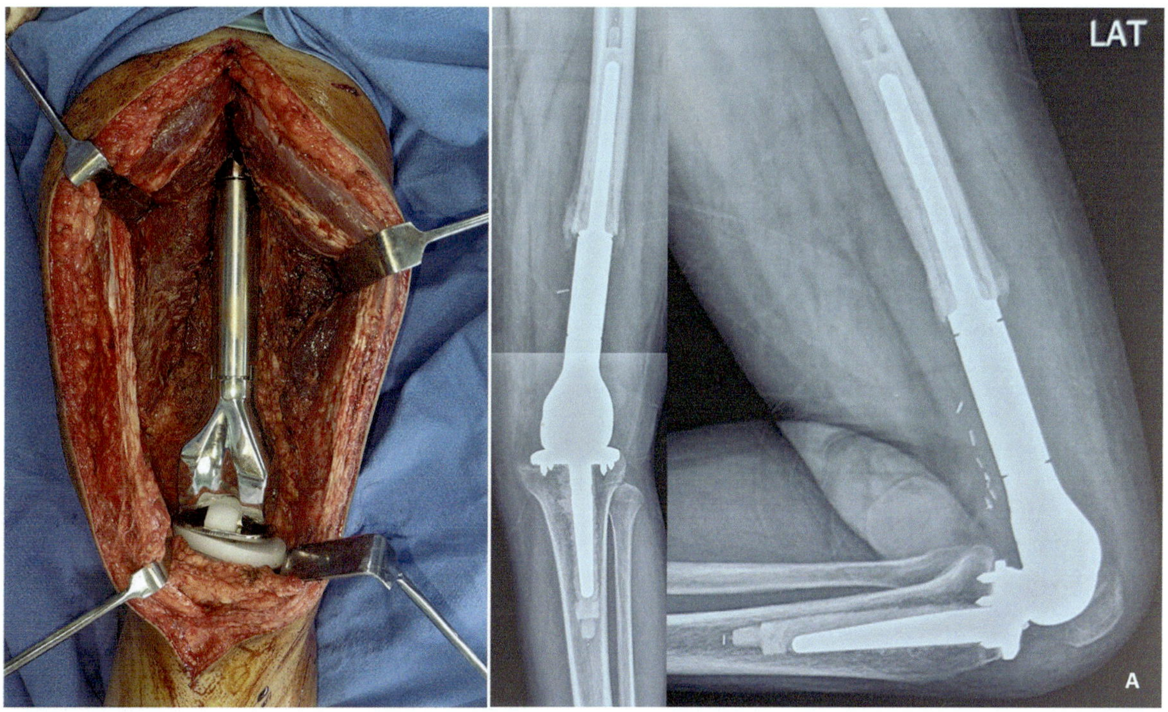

FIGURE 4.2 Endoprosthetic reconstructions following wide resection of peri-articular bone tumors at various anatomical sites. (A) Distal femur reconstruction with modular endoprosthesis – intraoperative image and postoperative radiograph. (B) Proximal tibia reconstruction with endoprosthesis – intraoperative image and postoperative radiographs. (C) Proximal humerus reconstruction with shoulder hemiarthroplasty-type endoprosthesis. (D) Proximal femur reconstruction with modular endoprosthesis. Endoprosthetic replacement is a mainstay of limb salvage surgery after wide resections of peri-articular bone tumors, offering immediate structural stability, restoration of joint function, and early mobilization, thereby significantly improving functional outcomes compared to ablative procedures.

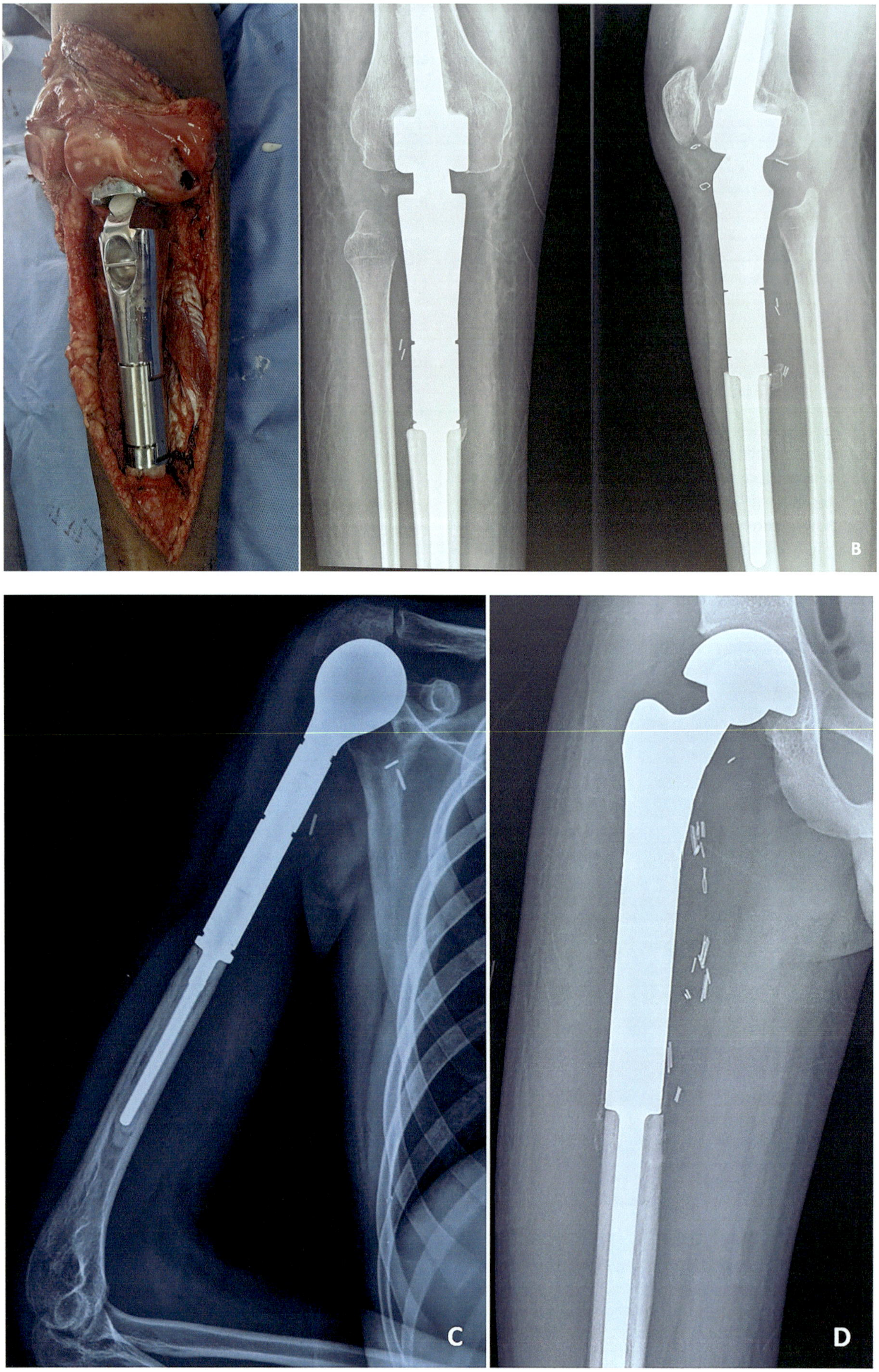

FIGURE 4.2 (Continued)

- Cases requiring immediate weight-bearing.
- Patients with poor biology for biological healing (e.g., post-chemotherapy or radiotherapy).
- Elderly patients or those with limited life expectancy, where long-term biological remodeling is not required.

Key advantages of endoprosthetic reconstruction include:

- Immediate mechanical stability
- Early weight-bearing and rehabilitation
- Customizability with modular designs
- Avoidance of donor site morbidity
- Good functional outcomes in well-selected patients

Modern tumor endoprostheses are modular, allowing intraoperative flexibility to accommodate different defect sizes and anatomical locations. Designs may include:

- **Fixed or rotating hinge knee mechanisms** for distal femur/proximal tibia resections
- **Expandable prostheses** for skeletally immature patients to accommodate future growth
- **Constrained or unconstrained hip components** for proximal femoral replacements

Materials used include titanium or cobalt-chrome alloys with porous-coated or hydroxyapatite-coated surfaces to promote osseointegration. The implants are anchored using cemented or uncemented stems.

Despite their benefits, endoprostheses are associated with a unique set of complications:

- **Infection**: One of the most feared complications, with rates ranging from 10–14% in large series [6].
- **Mechanical failure**: Including aseptic loosening, periprosthetic fracture, and component breakage, often necessitating revision surgery.
- **Instability**: Particularly in proximal femur and humerus reconstructions, influenced by poor soft tissue coverage or absence of muscular reattachment [7].
- **Dislocation and wear** in unipolar/bipolar hip replacements without acetabular resurfacing [8].

Long-term survivorship varies depending on anatomical site, fixation method, and patient-specific factors, but studies report implant survival ranging from 70% to 90% at five to ten years [7].

Endoprosthesis reconstruction is a mainstay in limb salvage surgery, offering predictable structural stability and allowing rapid return to function. Continuous innovations in modularity, materials, and soft tissue integration have significantly enhanced the safety and durability of these implants. Careful patient selection, surgical precision, and vigilant postoperative care are crucial to maximizing outcomes and minimizing complications.

Biological Reconstructions

Biological reconstruction techniques aim to restore skeletal continuity using living or processed bone, often allowing for long-term incorporation and remodeling. These methods are particularly favored in young patients, cases where longevity of reconstruction is prioritized, or in diaphyseal locations where endoprosthetic options may be limited. Biological reconstructions encompass **structural allografts**, **vascularized or nonvascularized fibular autografts**, and **recycled tumor-bearing autografts** (e.g., irradiated, pasteurized, or frozen). Each technique has distinct indications, advantages, and limitations.

Structural Allografts

Structural or osteoarticular allografts are cadaveric bone grafts used to replace resected bone segments, particularly in metaphyseal or diaphyseal locations.

Advantages:

- Restoration of bone stock
- Potential for biological incorporation
- Reattachment of ligaments, tendons, and joint capsules to native structures
- No donor site morbidity

Limitations:

- Risk of nonunion, fracture, or resorption
- Requires bone bank facilities
- Delayed rehabilitation and weight-bearing
- Immunologic rejection and risk of disease transmission [9]

Despite the potential for long-term durability, allografts have largely been supplanted by prosthetic reconstructions in joint-involving resections due to their fragility and high complication rates, particularly in the proximal tibia and humerus [10].

Vascularized or Nonvascularized Fibular Autografts

The fibula, due to its favorable length, cortical strength, and ease of harvest, is a commonly used autograft in the reconstruction of segmental bone defects, especially in intercalary resections. It can be used as a vascularized or nonvascularized graft depending on the defect characteristics and the host environment.

Vascularized Fibular Grafts:

- Ideal for large defects (>6 cm), irradiated surgical beds, or revision scenarios
- Possess intrinsic blood supply, enabling early union, graft hypertrophy, and long-term durability
- Facilitate biologic remodeling and resist resorption better than nonvascularized grafts
- Require microvascular expertise and longer operative time [11]

Nonvascularized Fibular Grafts:

- Technically simpler and suitable for smaller defects or well-vascularized host beds
- Often combined with internal fixation or structural allografts to enhance mechanical strength

These autografts are particularly favorable in young patients with high remodeling potential and non-weight-bearing upper limb reconstructions (Figure 4.3) [12].

Limitations:

- Inadequate mechanical strength, particularly in weight-bearing bones of the lower limb, making them prone to stress fractures, implant failure, or nonunion, especially in early phases post-surgery [13]
- Donor site morbidity, including ankle instability or peroneal nerve dysfunction

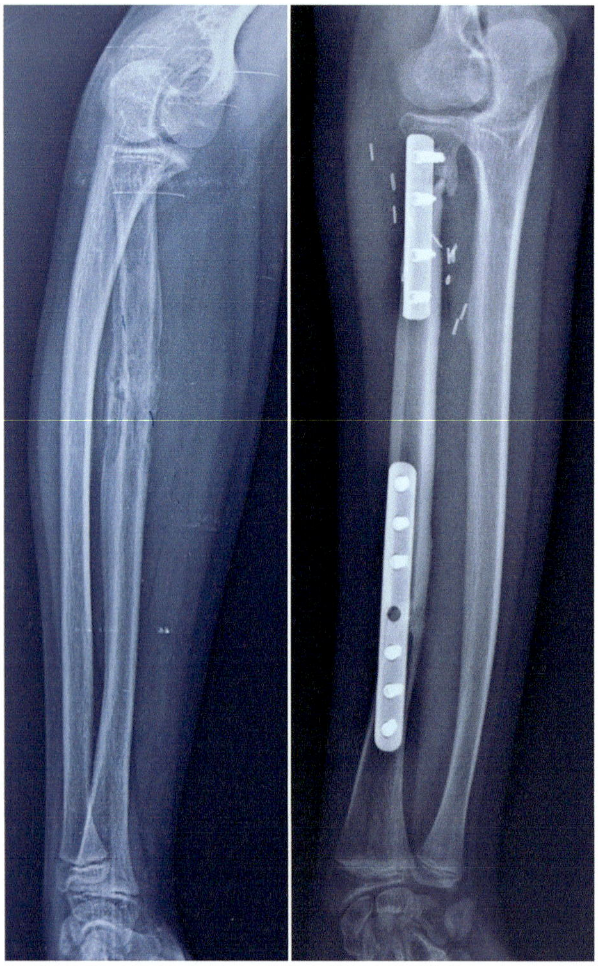

FIGURE 4.3 Reconstruction following wide resection of Ewing sarcoma of the radius using a fibular graft. (Left) Preoperative radiograph demonstrating Ewing sarcoma involving the radius. (Right) Postoperative radiograph showing reconstruction with fibular graft stabilized using a plate and screws. Biological reconstruction with a fibular graft provides structural stability and biological incorporation, making it a reliable method for reconstruction after oncological resection, especially in young patients where long-term durability is desirable.

- Prolonged time to full weight-bearing, often necessitating protected ambulation for several months
- Size mismatch in adult reconstructions, especially when used alone, limiting their ability to fill large bone gaps
- Technical demand in vascularized grafts, with the need for microsurgical expertise and risk of flap failure [12]

Composite Techniques (e.g., Capanna Technique):

- Combine vascularized fibula with massive allografts to overcome mechanical limitations and improve biological healing
- Show encouraging union rates and structural stability in long segment defects [14]

Recycled Tumor-Bearing Autografts

Reusing the patient's own resected bone, after devitalization to eradicate tumor cells, offers the advantage of a perfect anatomical match and preserved soft tissue attachments. Methods include:

- **Extracorporeal Irradiation (ECRT)**: Resected bone is sterilized with a high dose of irradiation (typically 50 Gy) and re-implanted (Figure 4.4) [15, 16]
- **Pasteurization**: Heating the specimen at 60°C–65°C for 30–40 minutes [17]
- **Liquid Nitrogen Freezing**: Tumor bone is frozen at −196°C and thawed before reimplantation [18, 19]

Advantages:

- Cost-effective and avoids allograft dependence
- Preservation of osteo-ligamentous architecture
- Potential for reattachment of tendons/ligaments [20]

Limitations:

- Risk of infection, fracture, and nonunion
- Long healing times and need for stable fixation
- Requires meticulous handling to prevent contamination

Biological reconstruction techniques offer unique benefits in preserving native bone stock, restoring ligamentous anatomy, and enabling potential long-term incorporation. While they demand longer rehabilitation periods and carry higher complication risks compared to endoprostheses, their role remains crucial in selected patients, particularly young, active individuals, and those with diaphyseal tumors. The choice of method must be individualized, balancing mechanical demands, biology of healing, and available expertise.

ALLOGRAFT-PROSTHESIS COMPOSITE RECONSTRUCTION

Allograft-prosthesis composite (APC) reconstruction is an innovative surgical technique designed to combine the advantages of structural allografts and modular endoprosthetic implants. This method is particularly useful

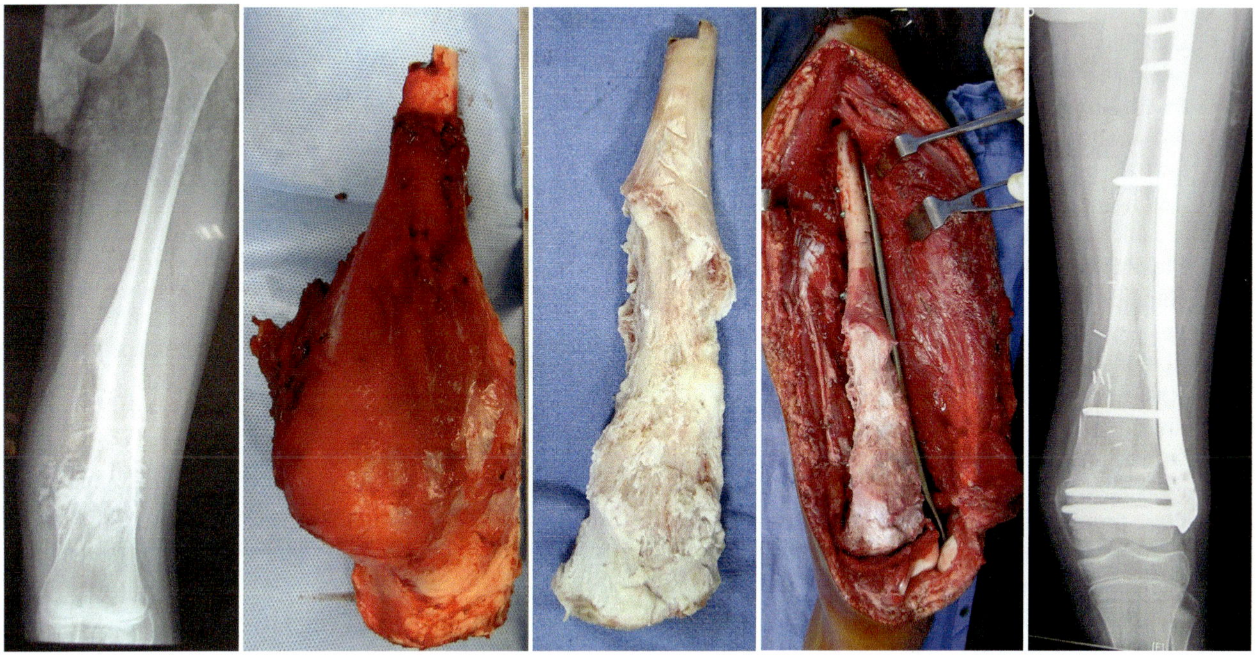

FIGURE 4.4 Extracorporeal irradiation and reimplantation (ECRT) for diaphyseal femoral tumor. (Left to right) Preoperative radiograph showing a diaphyseal tumor of the femur. Gross specimen following wide resection. The resected bone after extracorporeal irradiation (50 Gy) was used for sterilization. Reimplantation of the irradiated autograft with internal fixation. Postoperative radiograph demonstrating stable fixation of the re-implanted irradiated femoral segment. Extracorporeal irradiation (ECRT) provides a biological reconstruction option by sterilizing the patient's own bone with high-dose irradiation and reimplanting it, thereby preserving bone stock and joint surfaces while maintaining anatomical fit.

for reconstructing massive bone defects after oncological resections, especially in young patients or those requiring enhanced soft tissue reattachment and long-term durability [21–24].

CONCEPT AND RATIONALE

The APC technique involves integrating a segmental structural allograft with a prosthetic joint component. The allograft restores bone stock and provides a biological scaffold for soft tissue attachment, while the prosthetic element ensures joint stability and function without relying on the viability of allograft cartilage [22, 23].

Compared to osteoarticular allografts, APCs avoid problems related to graft cartilage degeneration and collapse. Additionally, unlike stand-alone prostheses, they offer better options for reattachment of ligaments and tendons and reduce the risk of aseptic loosening due to the load-sharing nature of the allograft [23, 24].

INDICATIONS

APC reconstruction is indicated in the following situations:

- Tumor resections involving the metaphysis or epiphysis of long bones (especially proximal femur, proximal tibia, and distal femur) [21–24].
- In young or active patients where long-term bone stock preservation is a priority [21].
- When soft tissue or ligamentous reattachment is necessary (e.g., knee joint reconstructions).
- In revisions of failed megaprostheses or allografts.

Types of APCs:

- **Cemented APC**: The prosthesis is fixed to the allograft using cement.
- **Uncemented APC**: The prosthesis is designed to integrate with the allograft without the use of cement.
- **Resurfaced APC**: A specialized technique where allograft is resurfaced to improve integration and function.

The procedure involves

- wide resection of the tumor with adequate oncological margins,
- shaping of a deep-frozen allograft to match the resected bone,
- fixation of a modular prosthesis within the allograft (cemented, uncemented or resurfaced),
- additional reinforcement using cortical strut allografts and plate fixation, and
- reattachment of the soft tissues.

This approach ensures mechanical stability and facilitates the re-establishment of soft tissue balance, particularly critical in joints such as the knee.

Advantages

- **Biological Integration**: Restores bone stock and facilitates soft tissue healing.
- **Load Sharing**: Reduces stress on the prosthesis, potentially prolonging implant longevity.
- **Soft tissue Reattachment**: Allows for bone-to-bone healing of ligamentous attachments, which is more reliable than soft tissue fixation to metal.
- **Flexibility in Reconstruction**: Can be tailored for complex resections and revision surgeries.

Limitations and Considerations

- **Risk of Nonunion and Fracture**: Particularly in the distal femur, where local blood supply is limited.
- **Infection Risk**: As with any massive reconstruction, especially with immunocompromised patients or those undergoing chemotherapy.
- **Technical Complexity**: Requires expertise in both oncologic and reconstructive surgery.
- **Graft Availability and Size Matching**: Dependence on bone bank resources and appropriate donor tissue.

APC reconstruction offers a viable limb salvage option for large skeletal defects after tumor resection. It balances the structural benefits of prostheses with the biological advantages of allografts. Despite some challenges, especially related to complications and surgical expertise, APC remains a key strategy in orthopedic oncologic reconstruction for select indications.

SOFT TISSUE CONSIDERATIONS IN LIMB SALVAGE SURGERY

Soft tissue reconstruction is critical for the overall success of limb salvage procedures, directly influencing implant survival, infection control, and functional outcomes. The goals are to ensure robust wound coverage, protect underlying prosthetic or biological reconstructions, restore muscle-tendon unit continuity, and create a stable platform for rehabilitation.

PRINCIPLES OF SOFT TISSUE RECONSTRUCTION

The fundamental goals include:

- Achieving **durable, tension-free wound closure**
- Ensuring **vascularized coverage** over implants or allografts
- Allowing **reconstruction of tendinous and muscular attachments**
- Facilitating **early mobilization and initiation of adjuvant therapy**
- Minimizing complications such as infection and wound necrosis

A multidisciplinary collaboration between orthopedic oncologists and reconstructive surgeons is vital, particularly in cases requiring complex reconstructions.

RECONSTRUCTION TECHNIQUES

Soft tissue reconstruction methods are selected based on the size of the defect, location, quality of the surrounding tissue, and presence of implants. These include:

- **Primary Closure**: Reserved for small resections with adequate surrounding soft tissue.
- **Local Muscle Flaps**: e.g., medial gastrocnemius flap for proximal tibial reconstructions.
- **Regional Rotational Flaps**: e.g., latissimus dorsi or rectus abdominis flaps for upper limb and pelvic defects.
- **Free Flaps**: e.g., anterolateral thigh (ALT), radial forearm, or gracilis flaps when local flaps are not feasible.

Muscle flaps provide bulk, promote vascularity, and reduce infection risks by filling dead space and separating the prosthesis from the external environment.

SITE-SPECIFIC APPROACHES

- **Proximal Tibia**: The medial gastrocnemius flap is the workhorse flap, commonly used for coverage and extensor mechanism reconstruction.
- **Proximal Humerus**: Requires restoration of shoulder stabilizers; muscle transfers like pectoralis major or latissimus dorsi are used.
- **Pelvis**: Large dead space often demands bulky flaps such as VRAM (vertical rectus abdominis myocutaneous).
- **Scapular/Shoulder Girdle**: Latissimus dorsi or trapezius-based flaps are preferred.

SOFT TISSUE INTEGRATION WITH PROSTHESIS

An essential component of soft tissue reconstruction in limb salvage surgery is **stable integration of the prosthesis with surrounding soft tissues**, which is particularly relevant for joint stability, prosthesis anchorage, and infection prevention.

1. **Use of Biomaterials (e.g., trevira tube, dacron sleeves, merselene tapes, synthetic mesh)**:
   a. Over time, **fibrous ingrowth** secures soft tissue to the implant, enhancing stability and reducing mechanical loosening.
   b. Particularly beneficial in shoulder and hip reconstructions where intrinsic muscular control is essential [25].
2. **Tendon-to-Bone or Tendon-to-Implant Fixation**:
   a. In reconstructions involving the knee (e.g., proximal tibia), patellar tendon can be **sutured to an anterior slot in the tibial prosthesis** or secured using a composite mesh for extensor mechanism continuity [25].
   b. For proximal femur, **abductor mechanism restoration** can be achieved by attaching gluteus medius and minimus to the prosthesis using nonabsorbable sutures or bone tunnels in the allograft.

3. **Anchorage Using Allograft-Host Junctions**:
   a. In APCs, muscle-tendon units can be sutured directly to the allograft, preserving the anatomical insertion site.
   b. This bone-to-bone or tendon-to-bone integration enhances mechanical strength compared to soft tissue-to-metal fixation.
4. **Biological Coating and Osseointegration Enhancements**:
   a. Use of **hydroxyapatite or porous coatings** on implant surfaces promotes soft tissue and capsular adherence, creating a sealed environment that prevents deep contamination and stabilizes the prosthesis.

These innovations have led to **improved functional outcomes** and **reduced dislocation or migration rates**, especially in anatomically mobile joints like the shoulder and hip.

Soft tissue reconstruction is a cornerstone of limb salvage surgery. It must be carefully planned and executed to ensure protection of underlying implants or grafts, restoration of function, and reduction of complications. Modern reconstructive principles emphasize not just coverage, but dynamic **integration of muscles and tendons with prosthetic components**, using techniques such as synthetic mesh sleeves and bone-tendon interfaces. The success of limb salvage lies not just in resecting the tumor or reconstructing the bone but also in **functionally reintegrating the limb into the patient's life** through meticulous and innovative soft tissue handling.

COMPLICATIONS OF LIMB SALVAGE SURGERY

Limb salvage surgery, though preferable to amputation in most musculoskeletal tumor cases, is associated with a distinct set of complications. These failures may be mechanical or biological and are broadly categorized using the updated **Henderson classification** [26] (Table 4.3).

SUMMARY

- Limb salvage surgery has become the standard of care for most resectable bone tumors, balancing oncological safety with functional preservation.
- A clear understanding of surgical margins and barrier tissues, as refined by Kawaguchi, is critical to achieving local control while minimizing morbidity.
- Reconstruction strategies must be individualized, with endoprosthetic and biological options each offering distinct benefits depending on patient factors, tumor location, and defect characteristics.

TABLE 4.3

Complications of Limb Salvage Surgery

Failure Type	Subtype	Description
A. Complications in Endoprosthetic Reconstructions		
Type 1: Soft Tissue Failure	1A: Functional	Dislocation, subluxation, tendon rupture, or poor attachment
	1B: Coverage	Aseptic wound dehiscence
Type 2: Aseptic Loosening	2A: Early (<2 years)	Poor initial bone-implant integration
	2B: Late (>2 years)	Bone resorption due to wear debris
Type 3: Structural Failure	3A: Implant	Breakage, wear, or expandable implant malfunction
	3B: Bone	Periprosthetic fracture
Type 4: Infection	4A: Early (<2 years)	Postoperative infection
	4B: Late (>2 years)	Hematogenous spread or post-revision infection
Type 5: Tumor Progression	5A: Soft Tissue	Local recurrence involving soft tissue
	5B: Bone	Bony recurrence, often requiring revision or amputation
Type 6: Pediatric Failure	6A: Physeal Arrest	Growth plate injury causing deformity
	6B: Joint Dysplasia	Malarticulation due to implant-host mismatch
B. Complications in Biological Reconstructions		
Type 1: Soft Tissue Failure	1A: Functional	Muscle detachment, instability
	1B: Coverage	Wound dehiscence
Type 2: Graft-Host Nonunion	2A: Hypertrophic	Abundant callus but mechanical instability
	2B: Atrophic	Poor biological healing response
Type 3: Structural Failure	3A: Fixation	Plate/screw breakage
	3B: Graft	Graft fracture, often periarticular
Type 4: Infection	4A: Early (<6 months)	Usually staphylococcal, post-op
	4B: Late (>6 months)	Often after reoperation or radiation
Type 5: Tumor Progression	5A: Soft Tissue	Local recurrence involving soft tissue
	5B: Bone	Intraosseous recurrence requiring graft removal
Type 6: Pediatric Failure	6A: Physeal Arrest	Growth disturbance
	6B: Joint Dysplasia	Altered joint morphology and function

- Techniques such as APCs and mesh-assisted soft tissue integration have significantly improved functional outcomes and prosthetic stability.
- Soft tissue reconstruction is integral to success, ensuring durable coverage, muscle reattachment, and early rehabilitation, especially in anatomically challenging sites.
- Multidisciplinary planning and patient-specific decision-making remain the cornerstones of achieving optimal oncological, functional, and quality-of-life outcomes.

REFERENCES

1. Phemister DB. Local resection of malignant tumors of bone. *AMA Arch Surg.* 1951;63:715–717.
2. Kawaguchi N, Ahmed AR, Matsumoto S, Manabe J, Matsushita Y. The concept of curative margin in surgery for bone and soft tissue sarcoma. *Clin Orthop Relat Res.* 2004;(419):165–172. doi:10.1097/00003086-200402000-00027
3. Puri A. Limb salvage in musculoskeletal oncology: recent advances. *Indian J Plast Surg.* 2014;47(2):175–184. doi:10.4103/0970-0358.138937
4. Enneking WF, Spanier SS, Goodman MA. A system for the surgical staging of musculoskeletal sarcoma. *Clin Orthop Relat Res.* 1980;153:106–120.
5. Japanese Orthopaedic Association Musculoskeletal Tumor Committee. Evaluation method of surgical margin for musculoskeletal sarcoma. In: JOA Musculoskeletal Committee, editor. *Evaluation method of surgical margin for musculoskeletal sarcoma.* 1st ed. Tokyo: Kanehara; 1989. pp. 3–22.
6. Meijer ST, Paulino Pereira NR, Nota SPFT, Ferrone ML, Schwab JH, Lozano Calderón SA. Factors associated with infection after reconstructive shoulder surgery for proximal humerus tumors. *J Shoulder Elbow Surg.* 2017;26(6):931–938. doi:10.1016/j.jse.2016.10.014
7. Smolle MA, Andreou D, Tunn PU, Leithner A. Advances in tumour endoprostheses: a systematic review. *EFORT Open Rev.* 2019;4(7):445–459. doi:10.1302/2058-5241.4.180081
8. Stevenson JD, Kumar VS, Cribb GL, Cool P. Hemiarthroplasty proximal femoral endoprostheses following tumour reconstruction: is acetabular replacement necessary? *Bone Joint J.* 2018;100-B(1):101–108. doi:10.1302/0301-620X.100B1.BJJ-2017-0005.R1
9. Errani C, Tsukamoto S, Almunhaisen N, Mavrogenis A, Donati D. Intercalary reconstruction following resection of diaphyseal bone tumors: a systematic review. *J Clin Orthop Trauma.* 2021;19:1–10. doi:10.1016/j.jcot.2021.04.033
10. Benevenia J, Kirchner R, Patterson F, et al. Outcomes of a modular intercalary endoprosthesis as treatment for segmental defects of the femur, tibia, and humerus. *Clin Orthop Relat Res.* 2016;474(2):539–548. doi:10.1007/s11999-015-4588-z
11. Campanacci DA, Totti F, Puccini S, et al. Intercalary reconstruction of femur after tumour resection: is a vascularized fibular autograft plus allograft a long lasting solution? *Bone Joint J.* 2018;100-B(3):378–386. doi:10.1302/0301-620X.100B3.BJJ-2017-0283.R2
12. Errani C, Ceruso M, Donati DM, Manfrini M. Microsurgical reconstruction with vascularized fibula and massive bone allograft for bone tumors. *Eur J Orthop Surg Traumatol.* 2019;29(2):307–311. doi:10.1007/s00590-018-2360-2
13. Houdek MT, Wagner ER, Stans AA, et al. What is the outcome of allograft and intramedullary free fibula (Capanna technique) in pediatric and adolescent patients with bone tumors? *Clin Orthop Relat Res.* 2016;474(3):660–668. doi:10.1007/s11999-015-4204-2
14. Capanna R, Campanacci DA, Belot N, et al. A new reconstructive technique for intercalary defects of long bones: the association of massive allograft with vascularized fibular autograft. *Orthop Clin North Am.* 2007;38(1):51–60. doi:10.1016/j.ocl.2006.10.008
15. Oike N, Kawashima H, Ogose A, Hatano H, Ariizumi T, Kaidu M, et al. Long-term outcomes of an extracorporeal irradiated autograft for limb salvage operations in musculoskeletal tumours: over ten years' observation. *Bone Joint J.* 2019;101-B(9):1151–1159. doi:10.1302/0301-620X.101B9.BJJ-2019-0090.R1
16. Outani H, Takenaka S, Hamada K, Imura Y, Kakunaga S, Tamiya H, et al. A long-term follow-up study of extracorporeal irradiated autografts in limb salvage surgery for malignant bone and soft tissue tumors: a minimum follow-up of 10 years after surgery. *J Surg Oncol.* 2020;121(8):1276–1282. doi:10.1002/jso.25918
17. Lee SY, Jeon DG, Cho WH, Song WS, Kim BS. Are pasteurized autografts durable for reconstructions after bone tumor resections? *Clin Orthop Relat Res.* 2018;476(9):1728–1737. doi:10.1007/s11999.0000000000000100
18. Igarashi K, Yamamoto N, Shirai T, Hayashi K, Nishida H, Kimura H, et al. The long-term outcome following the use of frozen autograft treated with liquid nitrogen in the management of bone and soft-tissue sarcomas. *Bone Joint J.* 2014; 96-B(4):555–561. doi: 10.1302/0301-620X.96B4.32629
19. Wu PK, Chen CF, Chen CM, Cheng YC, Tsai SW, Chen TH, et al. Intraoperative extracorporeal irradiation and frozen treatment on tumor-bearing autografts show equivalent outcomes for biologic reconstruction. *Clin Orthop Relat Res.* 2018;476(4): 877–889. doi:10.1007/s11999.0000000000000022
20. Krieg AH, Davidson AW, Stalley PD. Intercalary femoral reconstruction with extracorporeal irradiated autogenous bone graft in limb-salvage surgery. *J Bone Joint Surg Br.* 2007;89(3):366–371. doi: 10.1302/0301-620X.89B3.18508
21. Campanacci DA, Scanferla R, Muratori F, et al. Allograft-prosthesis composite after proximal femur bone tumor resection in pediatric age: is it effective in preserving bone stock? *J Child Orthop.* 2024;18(5):531–539. doi:10.1177/18632521241269338
22. Errani C, Tanzi P, Ferra L, Campanacci L, Donati DM, Manfrini M. Resurfaced allograft-prosthetic composite for distal femur reconstruction in children with bone tumor. *Eur J Orthop Surg Traumatol.* 2021;31(8):1577–1582. doi:10.1007/s00590-021-02995-1
23. Donati D, Colangeli M, Colangeli S, Di Bella C, Mercuri M. Allograft-prosthetic composite in the proximal tibia after bone tumor resection. *Clin Orthop Relat Res.* 2008;466(2):459–465. doi:10.1007/s11999-007-0055-9
24. Lozano-Calderón SA, Chen N. Proximal humerus allograft prosthetic composites: technique, outcomes, and pearls and pitfalls. *Curr Rev Musculoskelet Med.* 2015;8(4):324–333. doi:10.1007/s12178-015-9306-7
25. Kapoor L, Banjara R, Ragase A, Majeed A, Kumar VS, Khan SA. Outcomes of major musculoskeletal oncological reconstructions using prolene mesh: a retrospective analysis from a tertiary referral centre. *J Clin Orthop Trauma.* 2021;16:195–201.
26. Henderson ER, O'Connor MI, Ruggieri P, et al. Classification of failure of limb salvage after reconstructive surgery for bone tumours: a modified system including biological and expandable reconstructions. *Bone Joint J.* 2014; 96-B(11):1436–1440. 10.1302/0301-620X.96B11.34747

Section II

Upper Extremity

5 Proximal Humerus Resection and Reconstruction

INTRODUCTION

The proximal humerus is the most common site of primary bone tumors in the upper extremity and the fourth most frequent skeletal location overall, accounting for ~10%–15% of osteosarcomas, 10% of Ewing sarcomas, and ranking second only to the spine in metastatic bone involvement [1–3]. Surgical management aims to achieve oncologic clearance with adequate margins while preserving limb form and maximizing function.

The shoulder's functional complexity demands stability of the scapulohumeral articulation and preservation of motion for activities of daily living. The integrity of the rotator cuff, deltoid, and axillary nerve critically influences reconstructive choice and functional outcome [4]. Failure to restore these elements risks instability, subluxation, or functional pseudoparalysis.

Reconstruction options include:

- Biological (osteochondral allografts, autografts)
- Prosthetic (anatomical or reverse total shoulder prostheses)
- Allograft-prosthetic composites (APCs)

Each has distinct advantages and limitations regarding complication risk, durability, and postoperative function. No single method is universally optimal; selection should be individualized based on patient age, functional demands, resection extent, soft tissue availability, and neurovascular status.

This chapter reviews the management of proximal humeral tumors, emphasizing anatomy, resection classification, surgical techniques, reconstruction strategies, and an evidence-based analysis of outcomes and complications.

ANATOMIC CONSIDERATIONS

The proximal humerus and shoulder girdle form a complex anatomical region essential for upper limb function but challenging for tumor surgery. Its proximity to vital neurovascular structures, dependence on a coordinated muscular envelope, and role in glenohumeral motion demand precise surgical planning to achieve oncologic clearance and optimize postoperative function.

BONY AND ARTICULAR ANATOMY

The proximal humerus includes the humeral head, anatomical and surgical necks, and greater and lesser tuberosities, articulating with the glenoid fossa to form the glenohumeral joint. Stability is provided by the capsule, rotator cuff, and supporting ligaments. Tumors may remain intramedullary or extend beyond the cortex into soft tissue or the joint.

Glenohumeral involvement is a major determinant of resection type. Articular or capsular invasion, or glenoid involvement, requires extra-articular resection (Malawer V) to achieve margins and prevent recurrence. When the capsule and glenoid are preserved, intra-articular resection (Malawer I) permits joint-preserving reconstruction such as osteoarticular allograft or APCs. MRI is essential for assessing capsular disruption, intra-articular extension, or contamination from prior biopsy. Preserving the glenoid and capsule facilitates more functional reconstruction.

MUSCULAR ATTACHMENTS

The rotator cuff (supraspinatus, infraspinatus, teres minor, subscapularis) stabilizes the humeral head and inserts on the tuberosities, which are often resected. The deltoid, innervated by the axillary nerve, is the primary abductor and critical for postoperative shoulder elevation. Additional attachments—pectoralis major, latissimus dorsi, and teres major—are usually detached during exposure. The biceps brachii and coracobrachialis, with the musculocutaneous nerve, can often be preserved.

NEUROVASCULAR STRUCTURES

The axillary nerve and posterior humeral circumflex artery pass through the quadrangular space to supply the deltoid and teres minor; preservation is key for abduction and external rotation. The radial nerve, coursing posteriorly, requires protection during distal exposure. Medially, the brachial plexus, axillary vessels, and median, ulnar, and musculocutaneous nerves demand careful dissection. Neurovascular encasement or infiltration is a contraindication to limb salvage, often necessitating amputation or palliation.

SURGICAL IMPLICATIONS

- Preserve the axillary nerve and deltoid for functional reconstruction.
- Intra-articular resections are preferred when the capsule and glenoid are intact.
- Extra-articular resections are required for capsular or glenoid involvement, with more limited reconstructive potential.

DOI: 10.1201/9780367822002-7

- MRI is vital for defining tumor extent and resection planning.
- A robust soft tissue envelope is crucial for reconstruction stability and preventing instability or dislocation.

PREOPERATIVE CONSIDERATIONS

Clinical Assessment

Evaluation begins with a detailed history of pain, restricted motion, or a palpable mass (Figure 5.1). Neurological symptoms such as paresthesia or weakness may indicate brachial plexus or peripheral nerve involvement. Examination should assess:

- shoulder range of motion, swelling, or deformity;
- neurological status of axillary, radial, musculocutaneous, median, and ulnar nerves; and
- vascular status, including radial/ulnar pulses and collateral circulation (Allen's test).

Findings guide limb salvage feasibility and reconstruction planning.

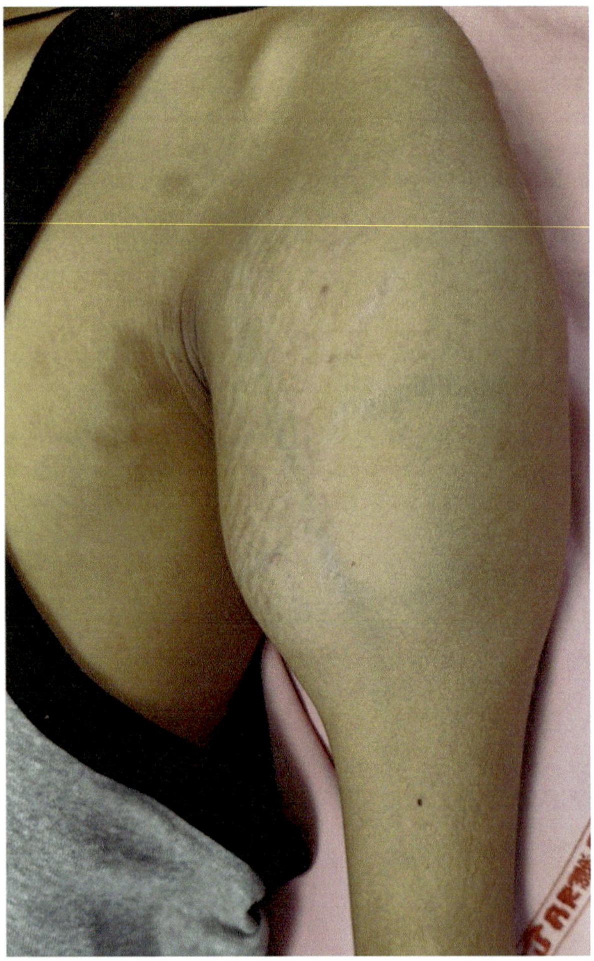

FIGURE 5.1 Clinical picture of a patient with Osteosarcoma involving the proximal humerus.

Imaging and Staging

Preoperative imaging defines tumor extent, involvement of adjacent structures, and resection margins:

- Plain Radiographs – AP, lateral, and axillary views to assess bone destruction, periosteal reaction, soft tissue extension, and guide biopsy trajectory (Figure 5.2).
- MRI – Gold standard for intramedullary extent, cortical breach, soft tissue and neurovascular involvement, and articular invasion; essential for resection planning (Figure 5.3).
- CT – Defines cortical bone loss, aids 3D reconstruction and prosthesis templating.
- Bone Scan (Tc-99m) – Detects skip lesions and multifocal disease.
- CT Chest – Mandatory for high-grade sarcomas to assess lung metastases.
- PET-CT – Useful for metabolic characterization, whole-body staging, and treatment response evaluation, especially in metastatic/Ewing tumors.

Biopsy

Performed only after definitive imaging, preferably by the treating surgical oncologist. Core needle biopsy is preferred. The tract should lie within future resection margins. Avoid the deltopectoral interval; traverse muscle planes to limit contamination of critical surgical approaches.

Multidisciplinary Planning

Neoadjuvant chemotherapy, indicated in osteosarcoma and Ewing sarcoma, is planned based on biopsy and imaging, potentially improving resectability, reducing soft tissue extension, and allowing joint-preserving resections with functional benefits.

SURGICAL MANAGEMENT

Principles

Proximal humerus tumor surgery prioritizes wide oncologic margins with maximal functional preservation. An extensile approach ensures safe neurovascular exposure, facilitates tumor removal, and permits reconstruction.

Patient Positioning

The patient is placed supine or beach-chair; for combined scapular or posterior involvement, a modified lateral decubitus tilt may be used. A scapular roll rotates the scapula laterally, enhancing exposure. The limb is prepped free for manipulation and intraoperative assessment. Extra-articular resections require 360° access to the glenohumeral joint.

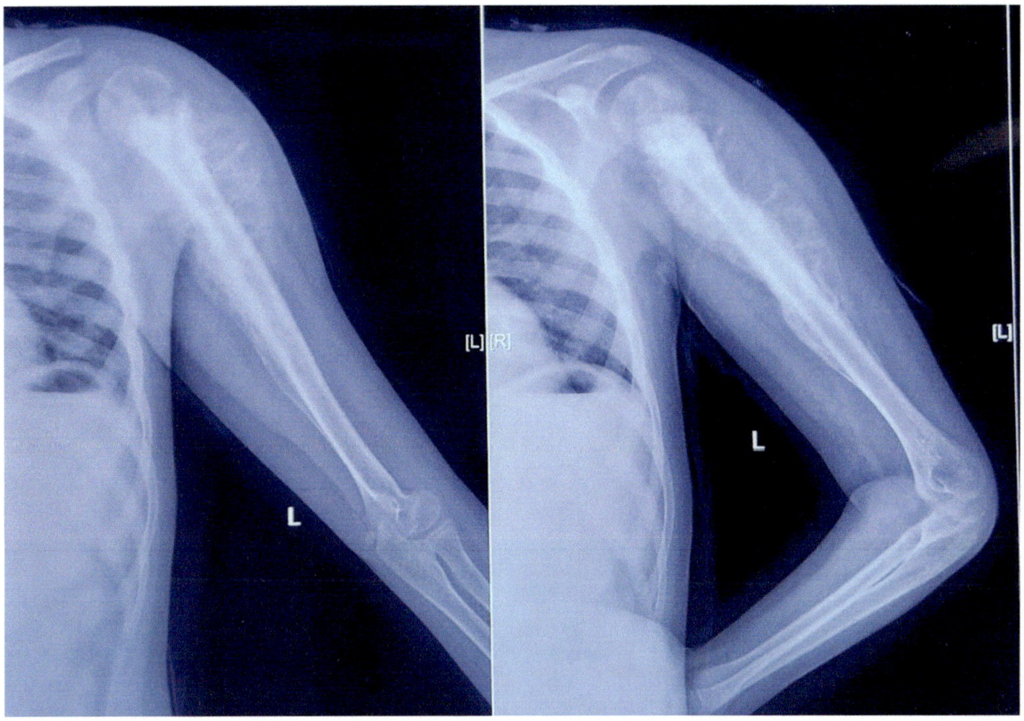

FIGURE 5.2 Plain radiographs of Osteosarcoma involving the humerus in a 9-year-old male.

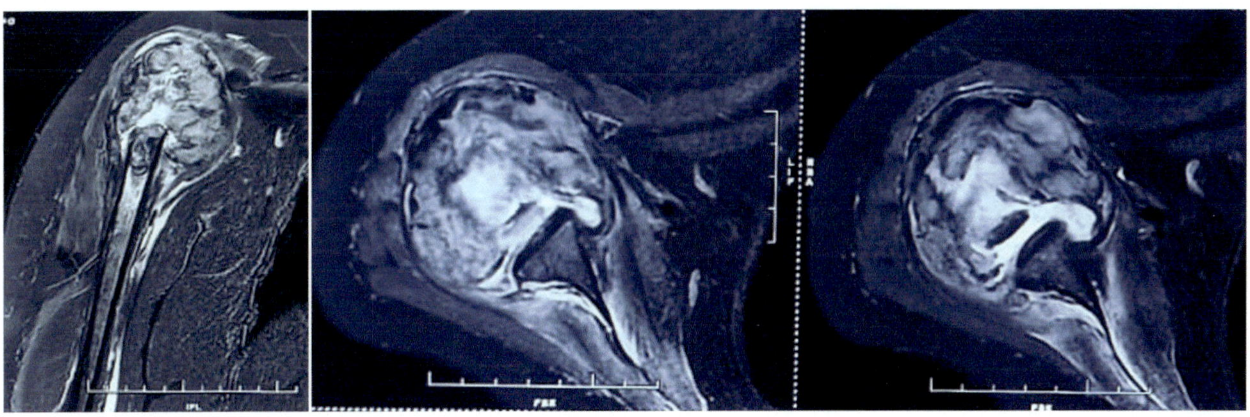

FIGURE 5.3 MRI images of Osteosarcoma proximal humerus. MRI facilitates the assessment of intramedullary tumor extent, soft tissue involvement, neurovascular proximity, and joint involvement.

Deltopectoral Approach

The deltopectoral interval is the standard:

- Make incision from coracoid to deltoid insertion (Figure 5.4A, 5.4B).
- Preserve the cephalic vein (retract laterally) or ligate.
- Develop the interval between the deltoid and pectoralis major to expose the proximal humerus, biceps tendon, and anterior capsule (Figure 5.4C, 5.4D).
- Extend distally for humeral shaft exposure or posteriorly for Type III–VI resections.
- Excise the biopsy tract en bloc with the tumor.

Soft tissue exposure:

- Raise skin flaps preserving fascia.
- Release pectoralis major from its insertion, reflect medially.
- Identify infraclavicular brachial plexus, axillary vessels, and coracoid process.
- Divide the pectoralis minor and retract the conjoint tendon (fusion of the short head of the biceps brachii muscle and the coracobrachialis muscle, attaching to the tip of the coracoid process).
- Identify the musculocutaneous nerve; preserve unless oncologically unsafe. Retract the divided muscles to expose the axillary sheath and neurovascular bundle.

- Tag and release rotator cuff tendons; detach pectoralis major, latissimus dorsi, and teres major and subscapularis (Figure 5.4E).
- Identify and mobilize the musculocutaneous nerve, brachial plexus, and axillary vessels early.
- Posteriorly, isolate the axillary nerve and posterior circumflex humoral vessels in the quadrangular space (Figure 5.4G).
- Protect the radial nerve during distal exposure.
- Preserve deltoid in Type A resections; detach in Type B.

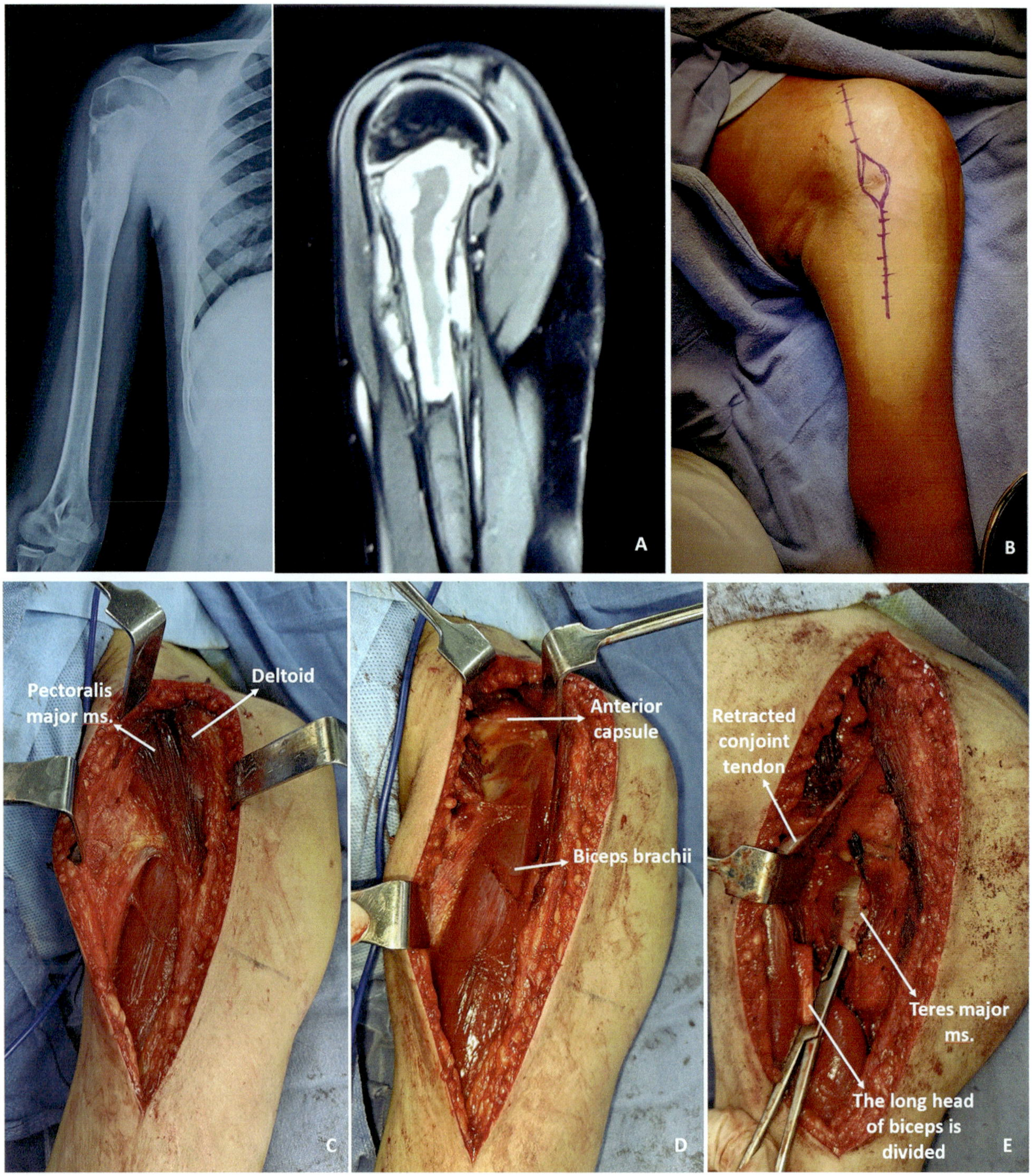

FIGURE 5.4 Radiographs and MRI (A) of Ewing sarcoma proximal humerus in a 14-year-old male. (B) The deltopectoral approach is the standard, with the incision starting from the coracoid to the deltoid insertion, depending on the length of resection. The interval between the deltoid and pectoralis major is developed to expose the proximal humerus, biceps tendon, and anterior capsule (C & D). The muscle attachments to the proximal humerus, including rotator cuff tendons, pectoralis major, latissimus dorsi, teres major, and subscapularis, are tagged and released (E).

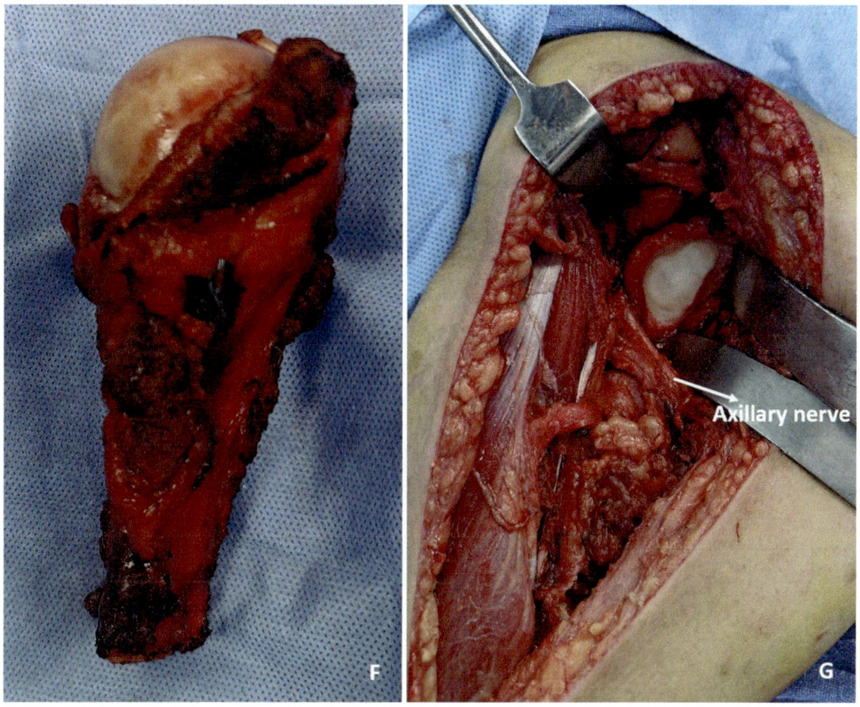

FIGURE 5.4 (*Continued*) The tumor is resected with wide margins (F). The axillary nerve is isolated and protected (G).

INTRA-ARTICULAR RESECTION (MALAWER TYPE I)

Indicated when the glenoid and capsule are tumor-free:

- Incise the anterior capsule; dislocate the humeral head anteriorly.
- Perform circumferential arthrotomy; release the inferior capsule with arm adducted/external rotation to protect the axillary nerve.
- Transect humerus 3–5 cm distal to tumor margin (per MRI) with oscillating saw; protect radial nerve.
- Deliver specimen anteriorly; send margins for frozen section.
- Preserves joint for reconstructive options such as osteoarticular allograft or APC.

EXTRA-ARTICULAR RESECTION (MALAWER TYPE V/VI)

Indicated for capsular, glenoid, or articular invasion or contamination from prior biopsy/fracture:

- Perform circumferential dissection around the joint, avoiding intra-articular entry.
- Detach anterior and posterior capsules in continuity from the scapula and glenoid.
- Divide the rotator cuff from scapular origins to ensure capsular clearance.
- Resect glenoid ± proximal scapula en bloc with humeral head and shaft.
- Dissect the quadrangular space; preserve or sacrifice the axillary nerve depending on tumor proximity.
- Type VI (total scapula) may require a separate posterior incision.
- Provides superior oncologic margin but precludes joint-preserving reconstruction; usually necessitates endoprosthetic or suspensory reconstruction.

BONE DIVISION AND MARGIN EVALUATION

- Protect the radial nerve during bone transection with retractors.
- Measure specimen; inspect gross margins (Figure 5.4C); obtain frozen sections as required.
- Excise biopsy site if outside main incision as a separate ellipse.

Key Technical Points:

- Maintain clear oncologic margins while preserving neurovascular structures when possible.
- Plan incision and muscle detachment to optimize later reconstruction.
- In extra-articular resections, accept functional compromise for oncologic safety.
- Use frozen section feedback to guide additional resection if margins are inadequate.

RECONSTRUCTION OF SKELETAL DEFECT

Prosthetic Reconstruction

Prosthetic reconstruction is the most commonly employed technique following proximal humerus resection for bone tumors. It offers immediate structural stability, restores limb length, and allows early mobilization without the need for biological integration. Its widespread adoption stems from its modularity, simplicity, and relatively predictable outcomes in comparison to biological reconstructions.

INDICATIONS

- Large defects not amenable to biological reconstruction
- Poor host biology or soft tissue cover
- Elderly patients with limited functional demands
- Situations with expected poor osteointegration or irradiated bone
- Metastatic tumors requiring quick recovery and pain relief

TYPES OF PROSTHESIS

Anatomical Endoprosthesis

Anatomical shoulder prostheses aim to replicate the natural shape and biomechanics of the glenohumeral joint. These are typically nonconstrained hemiarthroplasties or total shoulder prostheses that depend on an intact rotator cuff and deltoid for functional outcome. In oncologic settings, their use is often limited due to the sacrifice of soft tissues such as the rotator cuff, leading to reduced stability and function.

- Functional outcome is highly dependent on the preservation of soft tissues.
- Reported Musculoskeletal Tumor Society (MSTS) scores typically range from 18 to 23 out of 30, depending on deltoid and nerve status [5, 6].
- Shoulder abduction and elevation are often below 90°, particularly when the axillary nerve is compromised.

SOFT TISSUE RECONSTRUCTION

Reconstruction following proximal humerus tumor resection is frequently complicated by the loss of key dynamic stabilizers of the shoulder joint, particularly the rotator cuff, deltoid muscle, and often the axillary nerve. In such scenarios, ensuring mechanical stability of the shoulder becomes paramount to preserve distal limb function, especially elbow and hand movements. Traditional soft tissue reconstructions have focused on restoring a stable articulation between the prosthesis and glenoid; however, these methods are challenged by the lack of native muscular tension and attachment sites.

Several techniques have been proposed to address this issue. Marulanda et al. described the use of an aortic graft mesh (Gore-Tex) anchored with bioabsorbable screws for securing the prosthesis to the glenoid, reporting satisfactory outcomes with no instances of dislocation or subluxation and a low infection rate of 6.25% [7]. In contrast, Kitagawa et al. reported a 20% incidence of subluxation or dislocation with their method, which utilized synthetic sutures for attaching the prosthesis to remnants of the rotator cuff or acromion and Dacron tape for fixation to bony projections [8].

In a recent study by Kapoor et al. [9], 25 patients with proximal humerus tumors underwent wide resection followed by reconstruction using either an endoprosthesis or a nail-cement spacer construct, stabilized using Prolene mesh (Figure 5.5A–5.5D). Their technique provided robust anchorage to surrounding tissues and significantly reduced the risk of implant instability. Remarkably, no instances of dislocation or wound complications were reported. Moreover, the study recorded a mean MSTS score of 22.16, with excellent and good functional outcomes reported in 48% and 52% of patients, respectively. These results highlight the efficacy of Prolene mesh-based soft tissue reconstruction as a reliable and reproducible technique that compares favorably with other described methods. Similarly, Wang et al. demonstrated comparable results using polypropylene mesh, with no dislocations or infections observed in their cohort of 18 patients undergoing proximal humerus reconstruction [10].

OUTCOMES AND LIMITATIONS

While prosthetic reconstructions offer predictable pain relief and early function, they are limited in terms of active shoulder range due to loss of dynamic stabilizers. Dislocation rates vary from 10% to 25%, especially in deltoid-deficient cases. Long-term prosthetic survival is generally good in low-demand patients, but mechanical failure and loosening remain concerns in younger, active individuals. Reverse prostheses, when used with intact deltoid and axillary nerve, improve function significantly. MSTS scores in reverse total shoulder arthroplasty (RTSA) cases range from 21 to 25 [11, 12].

Prosthetic reconstruction, including anatomical and reverse designs, remains the mainstay of limb salvage for proximal humeral tumors. Its technical simplicity, modular design, and independence from biological integration make it a reliable and reproducible option. With advances in implant design and soft tissue reconstruction techniques, prosthetic solutions continue to evolve and offer functional outcomes that support both limb preservation and quality of life.

Reverse Total Shoulder Arthroplasty

RTSA reverses the normal anatomy of the shoulder: the glenosphere is placed on the scapular side and the concave component on the humerus. This design allows the deltoid muscle to act as the prime mover in shoulder elevation, bypassing the need for an intact rotator cuff.

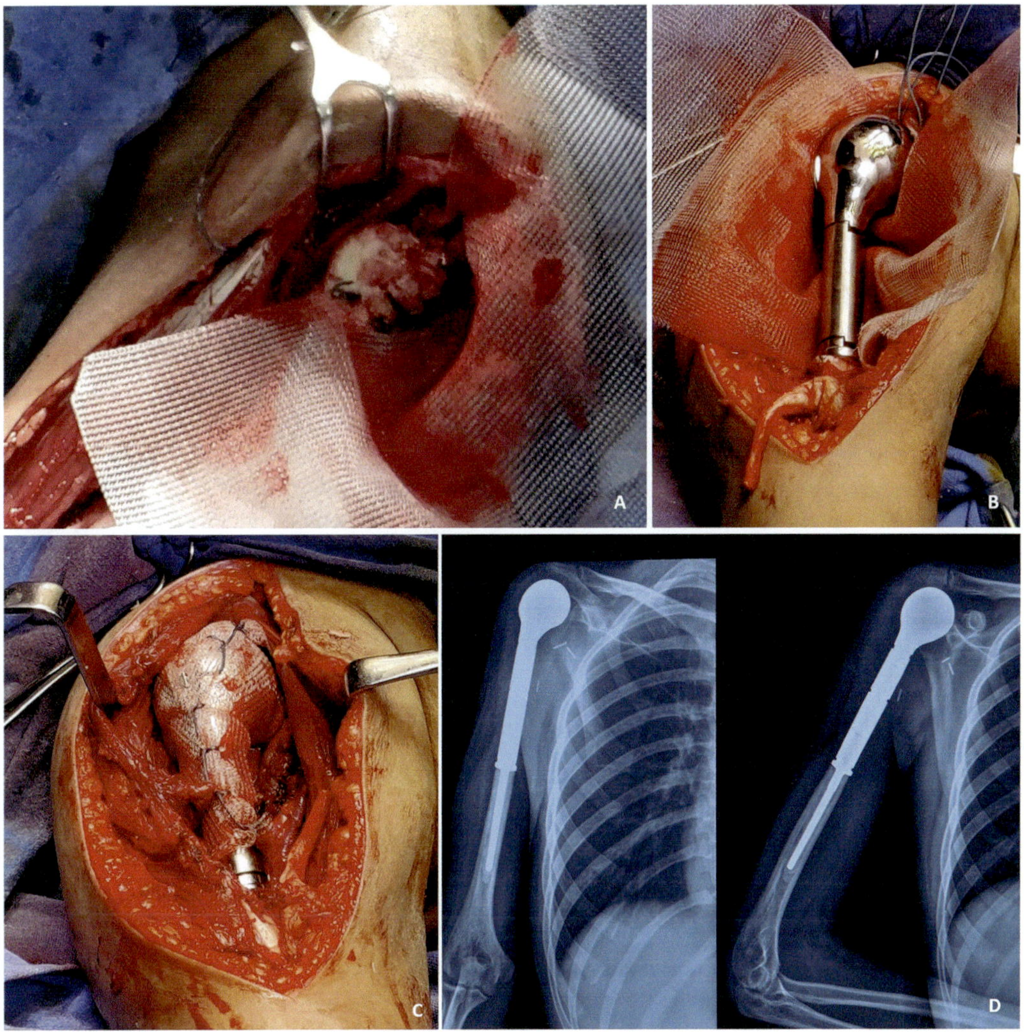

FIGURE 5.5 (A) Prolene mesh is anchored circumferentially to the remaining capsule and glenoid labrum with No. 5 Ethibond sutures. (B) Reconstruction of the defect with implantation of the proximal humerus endoprosthesis. (C) Mesh is then wrapped around the prosthesis to create a reinforced sleeve to which the residual muscles are reattached. (D) Post-operative radiographs following reconstruction with proximal humerus endoprosthesis.

- RTSA has gained popularity in limb salvage settings where the rotator cuff is sacrificed but the deltoid and axillary nerve are preserved.
- Studies report better active elevation and abduction, sometimes exceeding 90°, compared to anatomical prostheses [11, 12].
- Complications include scapular notching, instability, and loosening, though overall outcomes are favorable when patient selection is appropriate.

SURGICAL TECHNIQUE

Glenoid Component Placement: Accurate glenoid preparation and fixation form the cornerstone of reverse shoulder arthroplasty (RSA). The inferior glenoid rim is identified to guide optimal baseplate seating. The glenoid is reamed to a stable, flat subchondral bed, providing a secure foundation for implant fixation.

Baseplate positioning is critical, with superior tilt avoided due to its association with early loosening and scapular notching. Instead, an inferior inclination of approximately 10° has been shown to improve implant survival. Adequate native bone contact (at least 50%) is necessary for baseplate stability, and fixation is achieved with a central peg supported by multiple peripheral screws placed into dense cortical bone. This minimizes micromotion at the implant–bone interface and promotes long-term fixation.

Modern technologies, including CT-based or imageless navigation, augmented reality overlays, and patient-specific instrumentation (PSI), may further refine component positioning and screw trajectory, particularly in anatomically distorted or deficient glenoids.

Humeral Component Placement: Following tumor resection, humeral component placement is directed toward restoring joint mechanics, optimizing soft tissue balance, and ensuring stability. The humeral head is resected, typically at about 30° of retroversion, to create a suitable surface for component implantation. The humeral canal is sequentially reamed and broached to accommodate the selected stem, ensuring central alignment and stable fixation.

Offset and version are key determinants of joint kinematics. A humeral tray with an appropriate offset is chosen to optimize the center of rotation and achieve balanced soft tissue tension. The stem is usually positioned between 0° and 30° of retroversion, although the ideal orientation remains debated.

Intraoperative trialing with provisional components allows assessment of reduction, range of motion, and stability. Adjustments to offset, version, or glenosphere size may be undertaken to avoid impingement and restore functional mobility. Once satisfactory stability and motion are achieved, the definitive humeral stem and bearing are impacted into place.

Postoperative imaging is routinely employed to confirm component orientation and fixation, while also serving as a baseline for long-term surveillance of implant integrity and periprosthetic bone remodeling.

BIOLOGICAL RECONSTRUCTIONS

Biological reconstruction techniques offer the potential for skeletal integration, long-term durability, and preservation of host bone following proximal humerus resection. These techniques are particularly relevant in younger patients with longer life expectancy, where mechanical longevity and the potential for remodeling are prioritized over immediate stability. Biological methods include both allograft and autograft-based reconstructions, each with distinct indications, advantages, and limitations. However, these reconstructions are technically demanding and are associated with higher complication rates compared to prosthetic options.

Allograft Reconstruction

Osteoarticular allograft reconstruction involves replacing the resected proximal humerus with a cadaveric donor bone matched for size and morphology. This technique aims to anatomically restore joint contour and facilitate biological soft tissue reintegration by providing a scaffold for tendon and capsular attachment.

The allograft is typically secured to the host bone using compression plating or intramedullary fixation. Soft tissues such as the rotator cuff and deltoid are reattached using drill holes in the graft, enabling dynamic stabilization.

Despite its anatomical and biological appeal, allograft reconstruction is associated with a high incidence of complications, including graft fracture, subchondral collapse, nonunion, and infection. In a large series, DeGroot et al. reported a graft fracture rate of 37% and a mean MSTS score of 22.4 [13]. Potter et al. noted a graft failure rate exceeding 50% [14], while van de Sande et al. documented a 23% fracture risk at 228 months of follow-up [15]. These findings underscore the importance of careful patient selection and long-term surveillance.

Autografts

Autograft reconstructions utilize the patient's own tissues, either as vascularized or pedicled grafts, to bridge the skeletal defect following tumor resection. They offer the advantage of biological viability, reduced immunogenicity, and the potential for growth in pediatric patients.

Free Vascularized Fibula Graft (FVFG)

The free vascularized fibula graft is a microsurgically transferred bone flap, often harvested with the peroneal vessels, that provides living, osteogenic tissue capable of union and remodeling. This method is particularly advantageous in children and young adults with long diaphyseal defects and preserved recipient vasculature.

The fibula is secured to the humeral shaft using plate fixation, and vascular anastomoses are performed with thoracoacromial or axillary vessels. Wada et al. reported a mean MSTS score of 23.7 in 8 patients, although some developed graft resorption or fracture [16]. Bilgin similarly reported MSTS scores of 23 with preserved hand and elbow function following shoulder arthrodesis using FVFG [17]. Landau et al., in a recent systematic review, reaffirmed the durability and versatility of FVFG, despite the need for surgical expertise and donor site considerations [18].

Scapular Pillar Graft

The scapular pillar graft utilizes the lateral scapular border based on the circumflex scapular artery as a vascularized bone flap. This technique provides structural cortical bone and obviates the need for microsurgical harvest from a distant site.

Although less commonly employed, outcomes have been encouraging. Amin and Ebeid reported MSTS scores of 22.5 with a low complication profile [19]. Padiolleau et al. also reported acceptable results with a mean MSTS score of 21.3 [20]. This approach is especially useful in selected patients with small metaphyseal defects or in salvage situations.

Clavicula Pro Humero (CPH)

The clavicula pro humero reconstruction is a biological technique that repurposes the patient's clavicle to replace the proximal humerus. The clavicle is rotated inferiorly and fixed to the humeral shaft, functioning as a stable strut. It may be performed with or without vascular preservation.

This method is particularly suitable in pediatric and resource-limited settings. Barbier et al. reported good functional outcomes in 71% of patients with MSTS scores averaging 21.7 [21], while Calvert et al. documented MSTS scores exceeding 26 in pediatric cases [22]. Despite these advantages, concerns remain regarding shoulder contour deformity, restricted motion, and hardware-related complications.

Allograft-Prosthetic Composite Reconstruction

The allograft-prosthetic composite (APC) technique combines the advantages of both biological and prosthetic reconstruction by using a segmental allograft for biological integration and soft tissue reattachment, along with a modular prosthesis for immediate mechanical stability. APC reconstruction is especially useful in cases where the articular surface is sacrificed but soft tissue reintegration is desirable, such as in young patients or those undergoing extra-articular resection.

Indications

APC reconstruction is particularly indicated when

- rotator cuff or deltoid attachment is critical for restoring joint stability;
- the glenoid is preserved, and articular surface is sacrificed;
- the patient is young and functionally active, where long-term biological durability is desirable; and
- a compromised soft tissue envelope limits the efficacy of prosthesis alone.

SURGICAL TECHNIQUE

APC reconstruction involves the use of a diaphyseal or osteoarticular allograft combined with a prosthetic component, typically a modular humeral stem. The procedure generally proceeds as follows:

Host Bone and Allograft Preparation

After wide oncologic resection, the host humeral canal is reamed and irrigated in preparation for prosthetic insertion. A size-matched allograft is selected to replicate the length and contour of the resected proximal humerus. The intramedullary canal of the allograft is reamed and irrigated. A trial prosthesis is inserted to assess limb length, version, and alignment. Once confirmed, the final prosthetic stem is cemented into the allograft, ensuring rotational and axial stability.

Determination of Retroversion

Proper rotational alignment of the prosthesis is crucial to joint function and stability. Retroversion is typically set at 30 degrees from the epicondylar axis of the elbow to the prosthetic humeral head. Alternatively, intraoperative confirmation may involve orienting the prosthetic head directly into the glenoid with the forearm in neutral rotation. This chosen retroversion angle is marked at the junction between the host bone and the allograft, and fixation is performed accordingly.

Graft-Host Fixation

The allograft-prosthesis composite is inserted into the host humeral shaft and stabilized by

- cemented fixation, or
- mechanical compression plating with screws for biological union.

End-to-end cortical apposition is critical for union, and rotational alignment must match preoperative planning.

Soft Tissue Repair

The rotator cuff, deltoid, and capsule are reattached to the allograft via predrilled holes or with nonabsorbable sutures. When soft tissue quality is poor, a synthetic mesh sleeve may be wrapped around the allograft to provide a scaffold for tendon attachment. Tendons are tensioned with the arm positioned in 30–45° of abduction, simulating resting muscle length and preventing overtension.

Advantages

- Provides mechanical strength and structural continuity.
- Enables biological reattachment of soft tissues such as rotator cuff, deltoid, and capsule.
- Offers potential for biological remodeling and long-term durability, especially in younger patients.
- Better cosmetic and functional restoration compared to prosthesis alone.

Limitations

- Requires availability of a size-matched structural allograft from a bone bank.
- Increased surgical complexity and operative time.
- Risk of complications including nonunion at the host-graft junction, infection, and graft resorption or fracture.
- Monitoring for graft-host integration is essential over long-term follow-up.

CLINICAL OUTCOMES

Multiple studies have evaluated APC reconstruction of the proximal humerus, reporting variable complication rates and functional results. Dudkiewicz et al. demonstrated reliable tendon reattachment and functional gains, particularly with synthetic sleeves for soft tissue fixation [23]. Aseptic loosening was uncommon (0%–14%), while fracture rates ranged from 0% to 21%, with higher incidences reported by El Beaino et al. (5%) [24] and van de Sande et al. (20%) [15], likely reflecting longer follow-up. Instability remained a significant issue, especially in extra-articular resections, with rates of 57% in El Beaino et al. [24] and 36% in Moran and Stalley [25]. Infection rates were generally low (0%–13%), while pseudoarthrosis occurred in up to 30% of cases. Mean MSTS scores ranged from 66% to 79%, indicating satisfactory function when soft tissue reconstruction is optimized. Notably, APC combined with reverse shoulder prostheses (RSR) yielded superior function and avoided major complications [26, 27].

Overall, APC offers a durable, biologically integrated reconstruction balancing mechanical stability and tendon reattachment potential, with optimal results achieved in well-selected patients managed by experienced surgical teams with access to quality bone banking.

NAIL-CEMENT SPACERS IN PROXIMAL HUMERUS TUMOR RECONSTRUCTION

Nail-cement spacer reconstruction provides a simple, cost-effective alternative to modular endoprostheses after proximal humerus tumor resection, particularly in resource-limited settings. The technique involves inserting one or two Kuntscher nails into the reamed humeral canal, with a proximal polymethylmethacrylate (PMMA) cement head molded in situ (Figure 5.6). A Prolene mesh sleeve passed through the nail's eye is anchored to the glenoid using non-absorbable sutures, enhancing construct stability.

Although shoulder range of motion is generally inferior to that achieved with endoprostheses [28], functional outcomes are often comparable, with MSTS scores reported between 63% [29] and 75.33% [28]; Gulia et al. [30] achieved 71% using similar mesh augmentation. Comparative studies by Rafalla et al. [31] and Ebeid et al. [32] found no significant differences in function or complication rates between spacers and endoprostheses. Mesh augmentation plays a key role in preventing dislocation or subluxation, even without preserved rotator cuff or deltoid.

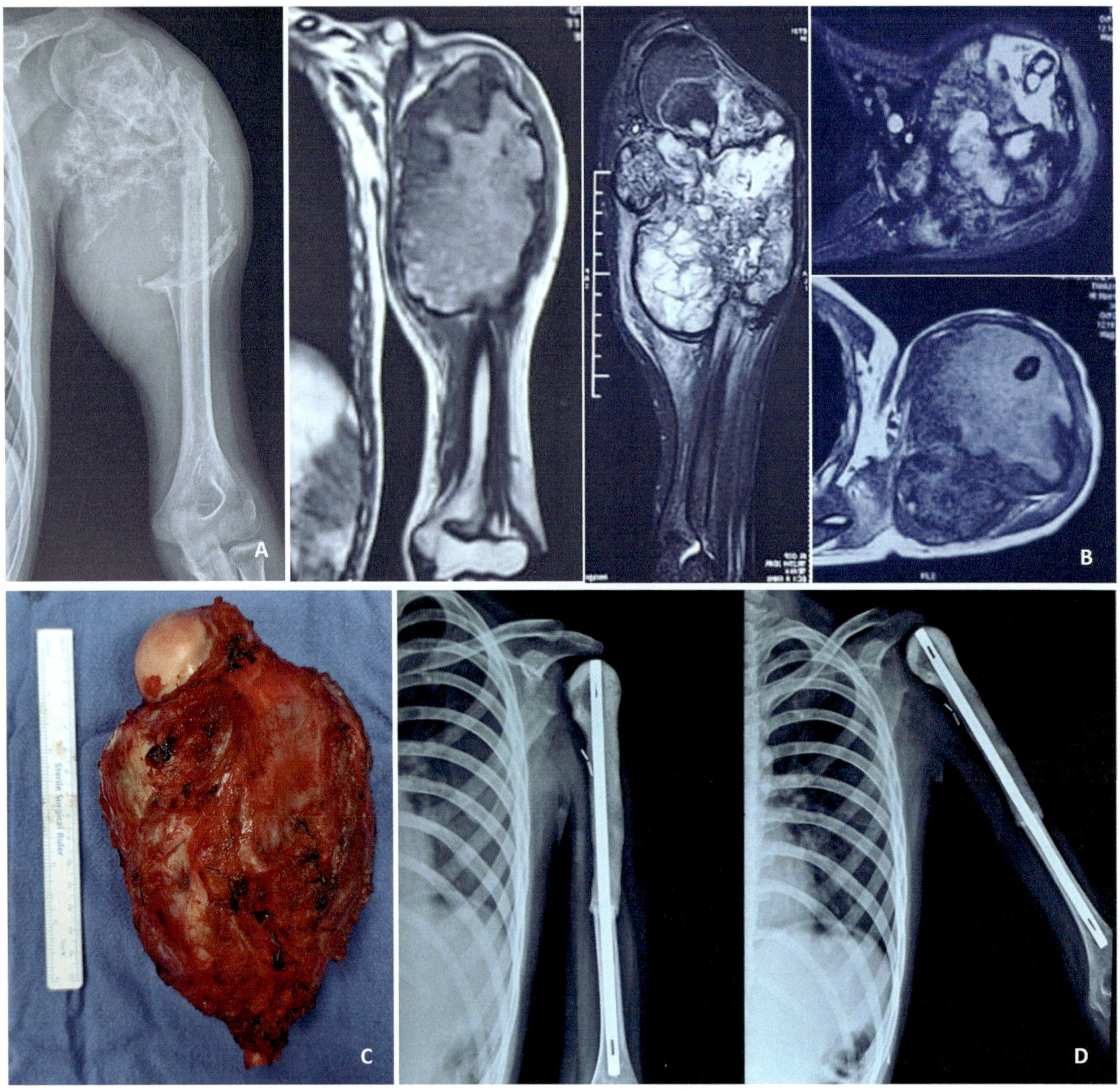

FIGURE 5.6 Radiographs (A) and MRI (B) images of Telengiectatic Osteosarcoma proximal humerus in a 19-year-old male, showing extensive soft tissue infiltration. (C) A wide resection was performed. (D) Post-operative radiographs with a nail–cement spacer used for reconstruction.

Despite limited active shoulder motion, this method reliably preserves elbow, wrist, and hand function, with complication rates—such as infection and nerve palsy—comparable to prostheses. Nail-cement spacers thus represent a pragmatic balance between oncological safety, functional utility, and affordability.

POSTOPERATIVE REHABILITATION

Rehabilitation after proximal humerus tumor resection and reconstruction is crucial for optimizing function and minimizing complications. Protocols are individualized based on resection extent, reconstruction type, and soft tissue status. Early mobilization of the elbow, wrist, and hand begins on the first postoperative day, while the shoulder is typically immobilized for four to six weeks, particularly after tendon or capsule reattachment. Passive shoulder range of motion is initiated at four to six weeks, progressing to active-assisted and active exercises as construct stability and soft tissue healing permit. Strengthening is generally introduced from 10–12 weeks, with further delays in biological reconstructions to protect graft union.

In prosthetic reconstructions, especially with preserved deltoid and axillary nerve, earlier range of motion is feasible, and reverse prostheses may expedite elevation recovery. Biological reconstructions, including allografts, autografts, and APCs, require a more conservative approach, delaying mobilization until radiographic signs of union, usually at six to eight weeks, and postponing strengthening for three to four months. Rehabilitation goals prioritize a stable, pain-free shoulder and functional independence of the limb, acknowledging that overhead activity is often limited. Long-term follow-up is essential for early detection of complications such as instability, nonunion, or graft failure.

SUMMARY

- The proximal humerus is a common tumor site requiring careful resection due to its complex anatomy and functional importance.
- Reconstruction strategy depends on tumor extent, patient profile, and soft tissue preservation.
- Prosthetic options, especially RSA, offer reliable outcomes when soft tissues are intact.
- Biological reconstructions (e.g., FVFG, CPH) are favored in young patients but are technically demanding with higher complication risks.
- APCs combine mechanical strength with biological integration for long-term durability.
- Soft tissue techniques using synthetic mesh improve stability and reduce dislocation risk.

REFERENCES

1. Wittig JC, Bickels J, Kellar-Graney KL, Kim FH, Malawer MM. Osteosarcoma of the proximal humerus: long-term results with limb-sparing surgery. *Clin Orthop Relat Res.* 2002;397:156–176.
2. Bielack SS, Kempf-Bielack B, Delling G, et al. Prognostic factors in high-grade osteosarcoma of the extremities or trunk: an analysis of 1,702 patients treated on neoadjuvant cooperative osteosarcoma study group protocols. *J Clin Oncol.* 2002;20(3):776–790.
3. Piccioli A, Maccauro G, Rossi B, Scaramuzzo L, Frenos F, Capanna R. Surgical treatment of pathologic fractures of humerus. *Injury.* 2010;41(11):1112–1116.
4. Sirveaux F. Reconstruction techniques after proximal humerus tumour resection. *Orthop Traumatol Surg Res.* 2019;105(1):S153–S164.
5. Raiss P, Kinkel S, Sauter U, Bruckner T, Lehner B. Replacement of the proximal humerus with MUTARS tumor endoprostheses. *Eur J Surg Oncol.* 2010;36(4): 371–377.
6. Angelini A, Mavrogenis AF, Trovarelli G, et al. Extra-articular shoulder resections: outcomes of 54 patients. *J Shoulder Elbow Surg.* 2017;26(11):e337–e345.
7. Marulanda GA, Henderson E, Cheong D, Letson GD. Proximal and total humerus reconstruction with the use of an aortograft mesh. *Clin Orthop Relat Res.* 2010;468(11):2896–2903. doi:10.1007/s11999-010-1418-1
8. Kitagawa Y, Thai DM, Choong PF. Reconstructions of the shoulder following tumour resection. *J Orthop Surg.* 2007;15(2):201–206. doi:10.1177/230949900701500216
9. Kapoor L, Banjara R, Ragase A, Majeed A, Kumar VS, Khan SA. Outcomes of major musculoskeletal oncological reconstructions using prolene mesh: a retrospective analysis from a tertiary referral centre. *J Clin Orthop Trauma.* 2021;16:195–201. doi:10.1016/j.jcot.2020.12.029
10. Wang B, Wu Q, Liu J, Yang S, Shao Z. Endoprosthetic reconstruction of the proximal humerus after tumour resection with polypropylene mesh. *Int Orthop.* 2015;39(3): 501–506. doi:10.1007/s00264-014-2597-2
11. De Wilde L, Boileau P, Van der Bracht H. Does reverse shoulder arthroplasty for tumors of the proximal humerus reduce impairment? *Clin Orthop Relat Res.* 2011;469(9): 2489–2495.
12. D'Arienzo A, Ipponi E, Ruinato AD, et al. Proximal humerus reconstruction after tumor resection: an overview of surgical management. *Adv Orthop.* 2021;2021:5559377. doi:10.1155/2021/5559377
13. DeGroot H, Donati D, Di Liddo M, Gozzi E, Mercuri M. The use of cement in osteoarticular allografts for proximal humeral bone tumors. *Clin Orthop Relat Res.* 2004;(427): 190–197.
14. Potter BK, Adams SC, Pitcher JD Jr, Malinin TI, Temple HT. Proximal humerus reconstructions for tumors. *Clin Orthop Relat Res.* 2009;467(4):1035–1041.
15. Bus MPA, van de Sande MAJ, Taminiau AHM, Dijkstra PDS. Is there still a role for osteoarticular allograft reconstruction in musculoskeletal tumour surgery? A long-term follow-up study of 38 patients and systematic review of the literature. *Bone Joint J.* 2017;99-B(4):522–530.
16. Wada T, Usui M, Isu K, Yamawaki S, Ishii S. Reconstruction and limb salvage after resection for malignant bone tumour of the proximal humerus: a sling procedure using a free vascularised fibular graft. *J Bone Joint Surg Br.* 1999;81-B(5):808–813.
17. Bilgin SS. Reconstruction of proximal humeral defects with shoulder arthrodesis using free vascularized fibular graft. *J Bone Joint Surg Am.* 2012;94(13):e94.
18. Landau MJ, Badash I, Yin C, Alluri RK, Patel KM. Free vascularized fibula grafting in the operative treatment of malignant bone tumors of the upper extremity: a systematic review of outcomes and complications. *J Surg Oncol.* 2018;117(7):1432–1439.

19. Amin SN, Ebeid WA. Shoulder reconstruction after tumor resection by pedicled scapular crest graft. *Clin Orthop Relat Res.* 2002;(397):133–142.
20. Padiolleau G, Marchand JB, Odri GA, Hamel A, Gouin F. Scapulo-humeral arthrodesis using a pedicled scapular pillar graft following resection of the proximal humerus. *Orthop Traumatol Surg Res.* 2014;100(2):177–181.
21. Barbier D, De Billy B, Gicquel P, Bourelle S, Journeau P. Is the clavicula pro humero technique of value for reconstruction after resection of the proximal humerus in children? *Clin Orthop Relat Res.* 2017;475(10):2550–2561.
22. Calvert GT, Wright J, Agarwal J, Jones KB, Randall RL. Is clavicula pro humeri of value for limb salvage of pediatric proximal humerus sarcomas? *Clin Orthop Relat Res.* 2015;473(3):877–882.
23. Dudlciewicz I, Velkes S, Oran A, et al. Composite grafts in the treatment of osteosarcoma of the proximal humerus. *Cell Tissue Bank.* 2003;4:37–41.
24. El Beaino M, Liu J, Lewis VO, Lin PP. Do early results of proximal humeral allograft-prosthetic composite reconstructions persist at 5-year follow-up? *Clin Orthop Relat Res.* 2019;477(4):758–765.
25. Moran M, Stalley PD. Reconstruction of the proximal humerus with a composite of extracorporeally irradiated bone and endoprosthesis following excision of high-grade primary bone sarcomas. *Arch Orthop Trauma Surg.* 2009;129(10):1339–1345.
26. King JJ, Nystrom LM, Reimer NB, Gibbs CP Jr, Scarborough MT, Wright TW. Allograft-prosthetic composite reverse total shoulder arthroplasty for reconstruction of proximal humerus tumor resections. *J Shoulder Elbow Surg.* 2016;25(1):45–54.
27. Lazerges C, Dagneaux L, Degeorge B, Tardy N, Coulet B, Chammas M. Composite reverse shoulder arthroplasty can provide good function and quality of life in cases of malignant tumour of the proximal humerus. *Int Orthop.* 2017;41(12):2619–2625.
28. Sehrawat S, Behera A, Kapoor L, et al. Endoprosthesis vs. nail-cement spacer application for reconstruction after oncologic proximal humeral resection: is there a difference in functional outcome? *JSES Int.* 2024;8(1):692–698. doi:10.1016/j.jseint.2024.01.018
29. Kundu ZS, Gogna P, Gupta V, Kamboj P, Singla R, Sangwan SS. Proximal humeral reconstruction using nail cement spacer in primary and metastatic tumours of proximal humerus. *Strategies Trauma Limb Reconstr.* 2013;8:149–154. doi:10.1007/s11751-013-0172-9
30. Gulia A, Amrath Raj BK, Gupta S, Patil A, Puri A. Implant cement spacer: a cost-effective solution for reconstruction of proximal humerus defects after tumor resection. *J Clin Orthop Trauma.* 2021;22:101574. doi:10.1016/j.jcot.2021.101574
31. Rafalla AA, Abdullah ES. Endoprosthetic replacement versus cement spacer in reconstruction of proximal humerus after tumor resection: cost and benefits. *J Orthop Surg (Hong Kong).* 2017;25(2):2309499017713937. doi:10.1177/2309499017713937
32. Ebeid WA, Eldaw S, Badr IT, Mesregah MK, Hasan BZ. Outcomes of modular endoprosthesis reconstruction versus cement spacer reconstruction following resection of proximal humeral tumors. *BMC Musculoskelet Disord.* 2022;23:484. doi:10.1186/s12891-022-05432-4

6 Scapular Resection and Reconstruction

INTRODUCTION

Tumors involving the scapula represent a distinct subset of shoulder girdle neoplasms, characterized by complex anatomical considerations and a historical trajectory that underscores the evolving philosophy of limb preservation. The scapula serves as a pivotal structure within the shoulder girdle, contributing to the origin or insertion of several muscles and facilitating a broad arc of motion including elevation, depression, protraction, retraction, and rotation of the upper extremity [1].

Historically, large malignant tumors of the scapula were managed by ablative procedures such as forequarter amputation, owing to concerns about local recurrence, neurovascular involvement, and the anticipated loss of function following extensive resection. However, this paradigm shifted significantly with advances in imaging, chemotherapy, surgical anatomy, and reconstructive options. Seminal work by Tikhoff and Linberg and later by Marcove and colleagues demonstrated that limb-sparing resections could offer equivalent oncological control with superior functional and cosmetic outcomes [2, 3].

The shoulder girdle is an anatomically dense region, containing the scapula, proximal humerus, and clavicle, enveloped by a complex network of muscles, nerves, and vessels. Scapular tumors, most commonly chondrosarcoma in adults and Ewing sarcoma in children, often remain asymptomatic until they reach considerable size due to the muscular coverage of the bone [4]. Contemporary management of scapular tumors prioritizes limb salvage, provided oncological principles are not compromised. Multiple surgical classifications have been proposed for scapular resections, with Malawer's system being the most widely adopted [5]. The goals of scapular resection and reconstruction are to achieve oncological clearance, preserve hand and elbow function, and, where possible, restore shoulder contour and mobility. This chapter aims to review the principles, techniques, and outcomes associated with scapular resections, emphasizing decision-making frameworks for limb salvage, nuances of surgical anatomy, and reconstruction modalities.

INDICATIONS FOR SCAPULAR RESECTION

Scapular resection is indicated for both low- and high-grade malignancies of the scapula, provided that adequate oncologic margins can be achieved while preserving essential neurovascular structures. It is most commonly performed for high-grade primary bone sarcomas not involving the brachial plexus or axillary vessels, low-grade chondrosarcomas with localized disease, and secondary bony invasion from soft tissue sarcomas in the periscapular region. Selected cases of metastatic disease or hematologic malignancies, such as myeloma or lymphoma refractory to systemic therapy or radiotherapy, may also benefit from resection for local control or symptomatic relief.

Preservation of elbow and hand function is a prerequisite for limb salvage, with a functional deltoid and intact musculature desirable though not mandatory, especially if alternative reconstruction strategies (e.g., static humeral suspension) are planned.

Absolute contraindications include encasement or invasion of the brachial plexus leading to a non-functional limb, tumor infiltration into the subclavian or axillary vessels when safe resection is not feasible, involvement of the thoracic outlet or posterior mediastinum, and unresectable chest wall invasion in patients with poor pulmonary reserve. Relative contraindications include the inability to obtain clear margins due to tumor proximity to vital structures, compromised soft tissue envelope from prior radiation or infection, extensive nodal disease, or advanced systemic metastases when resection is not palliative.

Importantly, the absence of axillary nerve or deltoid function—once considered a contraindication to prosthetic reconstruction—no longer precludes surgery. Alternative nonanatomic reconstructions such as mesh reinforcement, dynamic suspension, or soft tissue slings can provide stability and preserve upper limb function [6].

SURGICAL ANATOMY OF THE SCAPULAR REGION

A precise understanding of the complex anatomy of the scapular region is essential for safe and effective oncologic resection. The scapula is a flat, triangular bone articulating with the humerus at the glenohumeral joint and with the clavicle at the acromioclavicular joint. It provides an extensive surface for muscular attachment, contributing to upper limb mobility and stability, and is enveloped by a dense network of neurovascular structures that require meticulous preservation or controlled sacrifice during surgery [1].

Seventeen muscles originate or insert onto the scapula, including the trapezius, deltoid, rhomboids, latissimus dorsi, subscapularis, infraspinatus, and supraspinatus. The trapezius and deltoid are particularly important for maintaining postoperative contour and dynamic stability, especially when reconstruction is planned [2, 3].

DOI: 10.1201/9780367822002-8

The subclavian and axillary vessels, along with the brachial plexus, pass inferior to the clavicle and medial to the coracoid process. Branches such as the thoracoacromial, subscapular, and circumflex scapular arteries may tether tumors to adjacent structures, necessitating early ligation for safe mobilization. The suprascapular nerve, traversing the suprascapular notch to supply the supraspinatus and infraspinatus, is vulnerable in superior or posterior resections. The axillary nerve, accompanying the posterior humeral circumflex artery, should be preserved when possible to maintain deltoid function. The musculocutaneous nerve, located near the coracoid process, requires protection during anterior exposure [1–3].

Preoperative MRI, CT, and MR angiography facilitate mapping of tumor boundaries, vascular displacement, and soft tissue involvement. Identification of vascular anomalies or encasement of major neurovascular structures may alter surgical planning, influence the extent of resection, and determine reconstruction strategies.

CLASSIFICATION OF SCAPULAR RESECTIONS

Scapular resection classification has progressed from basic anatomical descriptors to integrated systems considering tumor location, joint involvement, soft tissue status, and surgical margins. The most widely adopted system is Malawer's 1991 classification, which defines six resection types (I–VI) based on the bones removed and whether the glenohumeral joint is resected intra- or extra-articularly (Table 6.1) [5]. Type III resections preserve the proximal humerus and joint, whereas Types IV and VI involve radical en bloc extra-articular removal of the scapula with part of the proximal humerus, typically for high-grade sarcomas or tumors breaching the joint or soft tissue.

The Enneking classification, endorsed by the Musculoskeletal Tumor Society [7], divides the scapula into Segment 1 (S1: scapular blade and spine) and Segment 2 (S2: glenoid, coracoid, acromion). S1 lesions often allow partial scapulectomy without reconstruction; S2 tumors require glenoid reconstruction, while combined S1+S2 involvement mandates total scapulectomy. Preservation of the glenohumeral joint generally supports good postoperative arm function.

Modifications to these systems account for soft tissue preservation, particularly of the deltoid and trapezius, as their retention is often essential for endoprosthetic reconstruction [8]. These classifications provide a common surgical language, guide resection extent, and help anticipate functional and oncological outcomes in modern limb salvage practice.

TABLE 6.1
Malawer Classification of Shoulder Girdle Resections

Type	Description	Abductor Status
Type I	Intra-articular proximal humeral resection	A: Abductors intact B: Abductors resected
Type II	Partial scapular resection	A: Abductors intact B: Abductors resected
Type III	Intra-articular total scapulectomy	A: Abductors intact B: Abductors resected
Type IV	Extra-articular total scapulectomy and humeral head resection (Classical Tikhoff–Linberg)	A: Abductors intact B: Abductors resected
Type V	Extra-articular humeral and glenoid resection	A: Abductors intact B: Abductors resected
Type VI	Extra-articular humeral and total scapular resection	A: Abductors intact B: Abductors resected

SURGICAL TECHNIQUE AND RESECTION APPROACHES

Scapular resection for bone tumors is among the most technically demanding procedures in orthopedic oncology, requiring meticulous preoperative planning, precise surgical execution, and a detailed understanding of the three-dimensional anatomy of the shoulder girdle. The primary objectives are complete oncologic clearance with negative margins while preserving maximal upper limb function.

PREOPERATIVE PLANNING

Preoperative workup includes plain radiographs, contrast-enhanced MRI, and CT scans to assess osseous and soft tissue tumor extent (Figure 6.1). CT or MR angiography is essential when the tumor lies near the subclavian or axillary vessels. MRI should include the neck, chest wall, and axilla to assess brachial plexus or thoracic involvement [1, 3]. For complex resections, 3D CT-based models aid in planning bone cuts and custom prosthetic designs [1]. Needle biopsy should be planned with the definitive incision to avoid contamination of uninvolved compartments.

PATIENT POSITIONING

The patient is placed in the lateral decubitus position with the operative side up. An axillary roll prevents brachial plexus compression on the dependent side. The arm is draped free to allow full manipulation and supported on a sterile stand or bolster.

SURGICAL APPROACHES

The combined anterior and posterior utilitarian approach is most commonly used for total and extended scapular resections. The incision begins at the junction of the medial and middle clavicle, extends laterally over the coracoid and deltopectoral groove, then curves posteriorly along the scapular spine toward the inferior angle. The biopsy tract is excised en bloc with the tumor. Skin flaps are elevated with care to preserve vascularity, especially in previously irradiated patients.

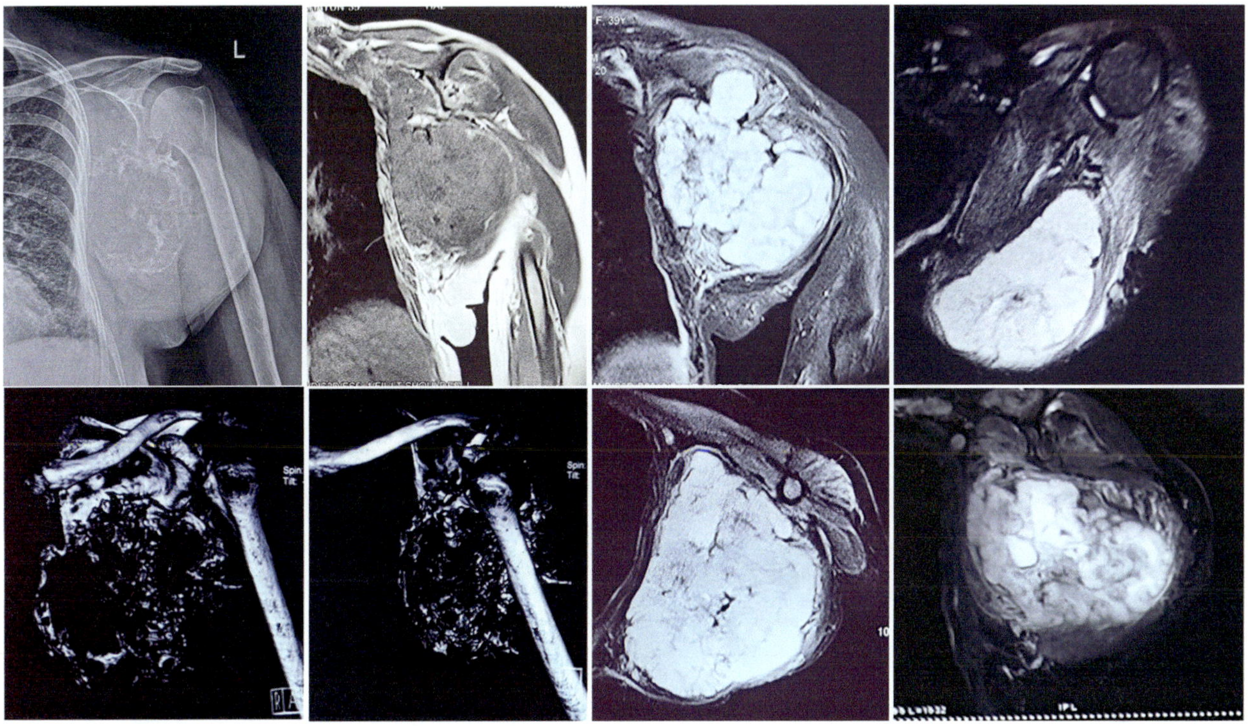

FIGURE 6.1 Radiological images of a 45-year-old female with chondrosarcoma of the scapula. The lesion appears as a large expansile, destructive mass involving the scapula, with areas of chondroid matrix calcification. There is cortical breach and thinning with extension toward the chest wall, though without gross intrathoracic invasion. The proximity of the tumor to the thoracic cage and surrounding soft tissues is well visualized, aiding in assessment of resectability and surgical planning.

DISSECTION AND EXPOSURE

- **Posterior Dissection**: The trapezius is detached from the scapular spine, followed by the deltoid, rhomboids, and latissimus dorsi. If uninvolved, these muscles are preserved for later reattachment to improve contour and stability.
- **Anterior Dissection**: The pectoralis major, pectoralis minor, coracobrachialis, and short head of the biceps are released from scapular attachments. The musculocutaneous and axillary nerves are identified and protected early.
- **Joint Resection**: In Type III resections, the glenohumeral joint is entered and divided. In Types IV and VI, the joint capsule and proximal humerus are removed en bloc with the scapula (Figure 6.2). The acromioclavicular joint is disarticulated, and if margin concerns exist, the distal clavicle may be excised.
- **Neurovascular Bundle**: Early ligation of the anterior/posterior circumflex humeral vessels, subscapular artery, and circumflex scapular artery facilitates mobilization of the axillary bundle. Thoracoacromial trunk branches are ligated for hemostasis.
- **Chest Wall Assessment**: The posterior approach permits palpation of the scapulothoracic interface to exclude chest wall invasion. Thoracic surgical assistance is sought if rib resection is required.

Once mobilized, the scapula is removed en bloc (Figure 6.3). Frozen section assessment of margins is performed, aiming for wide margins in high-grade sarcomas, with marginal or intralesional margins acceptable in selected metastatic or benign aggressive lesions when adjuvant therapy is planned.

RECONSTRUCTION OPTIONS AFTER SCAPULAR RESECTION

Reconstruction following scapular resection remains an area of ongoing debate in orthopedic oncology. The principal objectives are preservation of upper limb function—particularly elbow and hand dexterity—maintenance of shoulder stability, restoration of soft tissue contour, optimization of cosmesis, and provision of a stable, painless joint that allows the arm and hand to be positioned in space. The reconstructive strategy is determined by the extent of resection, quality of the remaining soft tissues, patient functional requirements, and institutional expertise.

Broadly, post-scapulectomy reconstruction options include:

- Humeral suspension (flail shoulder)
- Endoprosthetic (scapular or total shoulder) reconstruction
- Massive allografts
- Mesh-based static suspension techniques
- Nonreconstructive soft tissue closure

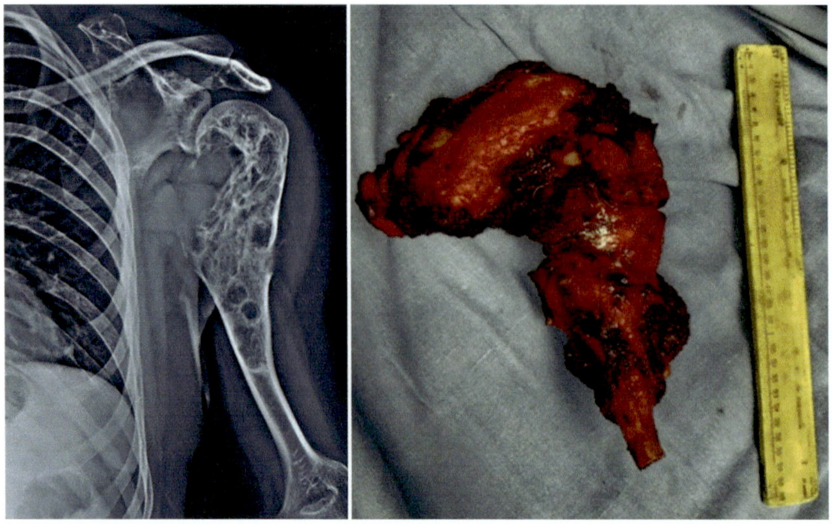

FIGURE 6.2 Extra-articular total scapulectomy and proximal humerus resection (Tikhoff–Linberg resection) in a case of chondrosarcoma of the scapula and the proximal humerus.

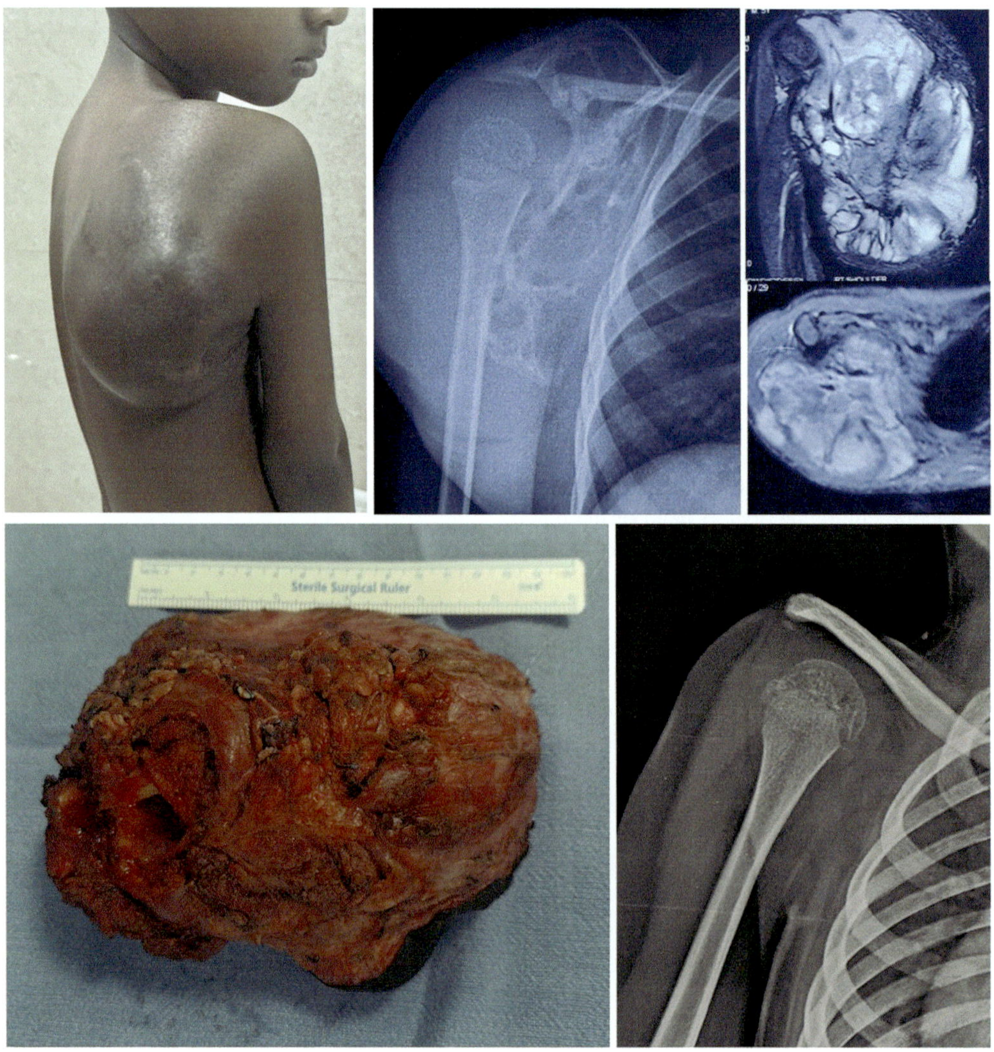

FIGURE 6.3 A 5-year-old male child with rhabdomyosarcoma of the scapula. Wide resection (total scapulectomy) was performed, followed by mesh-based static suspension of the humeral head to the clavicle.

Each technique offers distinct advantages and limitations in terms of function, complication profile, and feasibility.

HUMERAL SUSPENSION

Humeral suspension is a nonanatomic technique in which the proximal humerus is anchored to the clavicle or residual scapula using sutures, soft tissue, or mesh, often without prosthetic hardware. It is commonly employed in salvage situations where prosthetic reconstruction is not feasible due to inadequate soft tissue coverage, comorbidities, or resource limitations. The procedure is technically straightforward, cost-effective, and preserves hand and elbow function, although active shoulder motion is generally limited.

Bickels et al., in a series of 134 limb-sparing shoulder girdle resections, reported modest but acceptable functional outcomes with flail shoulder reconstruction, highlighting its reliability in achieving local control and patient acceptance [3]. Mayil Vahanan et al. [9] reviewed 23 patients undergoing scapulectomy without reconstruction, achieving excellent/good results in 13 and fair/poor in 10. Shoulder abduction was the major limitation, but wrist and hand function were preserved.

Mesh suspension techniques improve humeral stability. Salunke et al. [6] described using polypropylene mesh to create a static sling, wrapping the proximal humerus, and anchoring it to the clavicle and surrounding soft tissues. Their results showed comparable Musculoskeletal Tumor Society (MSTS) scores and mobility to patients undergoing traditional flail shoulder reconstruction.

DYNAMIC HUMERAL SUSPENSION

Dynamic suspension augments static fixation with tendon transfers—typically using the pectoralis major and latissimus dorsi—to restore partial active shoulder stability. This approach is most beneficial when the deltoid and trapezius are intact, facilitating better muscle integration. Hayashi et al. reported MSTS scores of 63%, similar to non-reconstructed shoulders, while Pritsch et al. observed improved manual dexterity and lifting ability compared to static suspension, albeit with modest shoulder abduction (generally <30°) [10, 11]. Complications include tendon rupture (5%–10%) and inferior humeral subluxation due to muscle atrophy.

In summary, humeral suspension—whether static or dynamic—remains a viable, low-cost solution, particularly in resource-constrained settings, with acceptable functional and cosmetic results.

MASSIVE BONE ALLOGRAFTS

Massive scapular allografts restore bony anatomy and provide a biological scaffold for host tissue integration. They are particularly advantageous in younger patients, glenoid-preserving resections, and cases requiring long-term durability. The graft is shaped to fit the defect and fixed to host bone with plates, screws, or synthetic ligaments such as the LARS (Ligament Augmentation and Reconstruction System) ligament for coracoclavicular fixation [12–14]. Secure soft tissue reattachment—especially of the rotator cuff, deltoid, trapezius, and periscapular muscles—is critical for functional recovery.

Reported MSTS scores range from 66.7% to 90% [12, 13, 15]. Zhang et al. [13] reported average scores of 80% in glenoid-sparing reconstructions, significantly outperforming glenoid-resected cases. Capanna et al. found superior abduction and forward elevation when the rotator cuff was preserved [12], while Biazzo et al. reported MSTS scores of 62%–82% with abduction between 30° and 45° [4]. Cosmesis is generally good, with restoration of shoulder contour and height.

However, complication rates are substantial. **Graft fracture** occurs in 10%–30%, **nonunion** in up to 33%, and **infection** in 5%–10%—rates higher than for prosthetic reconstructions [12, 13, 15]. Graft resorption, instability, and delayed incorporation can further compromise outcomes, particularly in irradiated tissues or with poor soft tissue coverage [16].

ENDOPROSTHETIC RECONSTRUCTION

Endoprosthetic reconstruction is the most anatomical method, replacing the resected scapula with a custom or modular prosthesis. Modern designs incorporate constrained or reverse shoulder mechanisms to improve stability, moving away from early designs that relied solely on soft tissue tenodesis. The aim is to restore lateral shoulder offset, prevent brachial plexus traction, and fill the defect after scapular resection [1, 8, 10].

Indications include resections involving the glenoid or extensive scapular loss (Malawer Type III/IV) where soft tissue preservation—particularly the deltoid, trapezius, rhomboids, and latissimus dorsi—is adequate. The prosthesis is fixed with multiple suture holes (typically 3 mm diameter, 10 mm spacing) for secure reattachment of preserved musculature using strong nonabsorbable sutures. The acromial surface articulates with the clavicle, and the humeral component may be a reverse-constrained prosthesis to optimize stability.

Muscle reattachment follows a layered approach:

- Teres major/minor laterally
- Rhomboids and levator scapulae medially
- Latissimus dorsi rotated over the prosthesis medially
- Trapezius and posterior deltoid tenodesis over the prosthesis for soft tissue coverage

In humeral replacement cases, Gore-Tex or polypropylene mesh may be used to reconstruct the joint capsule and minimize dislocation risk.

Reported MSTS scores range from 62% to 82% [1, 10, 17]. Tang et al. achieved a mean score of 76.7% in ten patients, with satisfactory daily function despite moderate

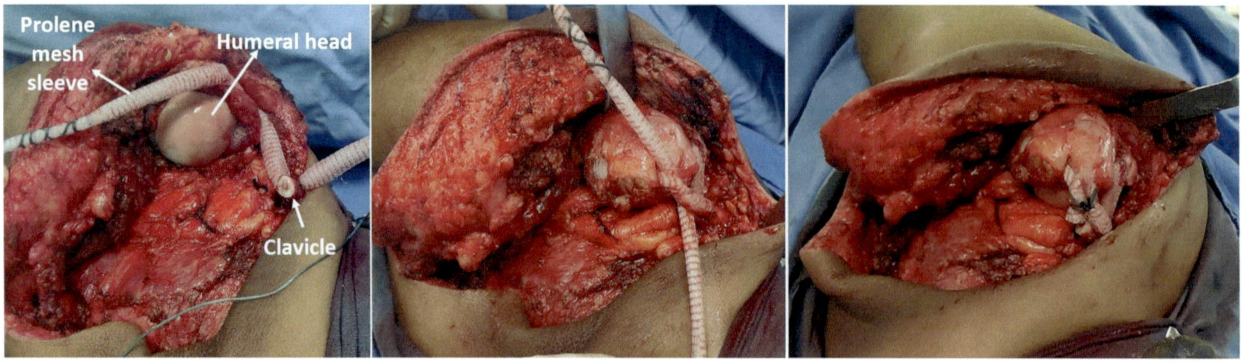

FIGURE 6.4 Mesh-based static suspension: A mesh is shaped into a sleeve around the proximal humerus and anchored to the clavicle with non-absorbable sutures.

shoulder restriction [17]. Shoulder abduction typically ranges from 30° to 45°, with limited external rotation.

Complications include **dislocation** (10%–20%), **infection** (~10%), and **mechanical failure** over time [18, 19]. Preservation of the deltoid correlates strongly with improved outcomes [18]. Compared to flail shoulder or allograft reconstruction, prosthetic reconstructions yield better cosmesis and MSTS scores—Pritsch et al. reported 79% for prostheses versus 62% for flail shoulders [10]. Advances in **3D-printed implants** have further enhanced customization and early functional outcomes [20].

MESH-BASED STATIC SUSPENSION

When prosthetic or allograft reconstruction is not feasible, static suspension with synthetic mesh offers a middle ground between flail shoulder and more complex reconstructions. Mesh is shaped into a sleeve around the proximal humerus and anchored to the clavicle, chest wall, or residual scapula with nonabsorbable sutures (Figure 6.4). This technique improves humeral head position, prevents inferior migration, and allows limited functional motion. Outcomes are generally similar to humeral suspension but with improved shoulder stability.

NONRECONSTRUCTIVE SOFT TISSUE CLOSURE

In certain palliative cases or when soft tissue is inadequate for anchoring, nonreconstructive closure is performed, leaving a flail shoulder. While shoulder motion is absent, hand positioning, elbow motion, and limb length are preserved, enabling patients to perform daily activities with compensatory movements.

POSTOPERATIVE REHABILITATION

Rehabilitation is critical to functional recovery and begins with **four to six weeks of immobilization** in a sling or abduction brace to protect reconstructions. During this period, patients maintain finger, wrist, and elbow mobility, with passive pendulum exercises introduced from weeks 2–3 in stable reconstructions.

From week 4, **passive and active-assisted shoulder motion** begins, progressing to active range and strengthening at 8–12 weeks. Therapy focuses on activating preserved or transferred muscles, restoring proprioception, and achieving independence in daily activities. Rehabilitation is individualized according to reconstruction type—dynamic reconstructions prioritize muscle re-education, while prosthetic reconstructions emphasize controlled mobility to prevent dislocation.

Long-term follow-up includes periodic imaging for reconstruction integrity, oncologic surveillance, and maintenance physiotherapy. While full shoulder motion is rare, meaningful improvements in limb positioning, stability, and hand use significantly enhance quality of life.

SUMMARY

- Limb salvage surgery of the scapula is technically demanding due to the region's complex anatomy and proximity to vital neurovascular structures.
- Scapular reconstruction aims to restore shoulder stability, ensure effective suspension of the humerus, and maintain good elbow, wrist, and hand function.
- Preservation of the deltoid and rotator cuff significantly enhances postoperative shoulder flexion and abduction.
- Reconstruction options—such as prosthetic replacement, massive allografts, and humerus suspension—should be tailored to the resection type and residual anatomy.
- Good functional, oncological, and cosmetic outcomes are achievable with meticulous soft tissue handling, appropriate reconstruction, and structured rehabilitation.

REFERENCES

1. Houdek MT, Wilke BK, Barlow JD. Management of scapular tumors. *Orthop Clin North Am.* 2023;54(1):101–108.
2. Malawer MM, Kellar-Graney K, Wittig JC. Total scapular resections with endoprosthetic reconstruction. In: Malawer MM, Sugarbaker PH, editors. *Musculoskeletal cancer surgery*. Dordrecht: Kluwer Academic Publishers; 2001. pp. 82–91.

3. Bickels J, Wittig JC, Kollender Y, et al. Limb-sparing resections of the shoulder girdle. *J Am Coll Surg.* 2002;194(4): 422–435.
4. Biazzo A, De Paolis M, Donati DM. Scapular reconstructions after resection for bone tumors: a single-institution experience and review of the literature. *Acta Biomed.* 2018;89(3): 415–422.
5. Malawer MM. Tumors of the shoulder girdle: technique of resection and description of a surgical classification. *Orthop Clin North Am.* 1991;22(1):7–35.
6. Salunke AA, Nandy K, Kamani M, et al. Is polypropylene mesh reconstruction functionally superior to non-reconstructive group following total scapular resection? A retrospective analysis of 16 patients and a systematic review of the literature. *J Orthop.* 2024;52:37–48.
7. Enneking WF, Dunham W, Gebhardt MC, Malawar M, Pritchard DJ. A system for the functional evaluation of reconstructive procedures after surgical treatment of tumors of the musculoskeletal system. *Clin Orthop Relat Res.* 1993;286:241–246.
8. Papagelopoulos PJ, Mavrogenis AF. Total scapulectomy and reconstruction using a scapular prosthesis. In: *Master techniques in orthopaedic oncology*. Lippincott Williams & Wilkins; 2021. pp. 313–323.
9. Mayil Vahanan N, Mohanlal P, Bose JC, Gangadharan R, Karthisundar V. The functional and oncological results after scapulectomy for scapular tumours: 2–16-year results. *Int Orthop.* 2007;31(6):831–836. doi:10.1007/s00264-006-0261-1
10. Pritsch T, Bickels J, Wu CC, Squires MH, Malawer MM. Is scapular endoprosthesis functionally superior to humeral suspension? *Clin Orthop Relat Res.* 2007;456:188–195. doi:10.1097/01.blo.0000238840.26423.b6
11. Hayashi K, Karita M, Yamamoto N, et al. Functional outcomes after total scapulectomy for malignant bone or soft tissue tumors in the shoulder girdle. *Int J Clin Oncol.* 2011;16(5):568–573. doi:10.1007/s10147-011-0229-z
12. Capanna R, Totti F, Van der Geest IC, Müller DA. Scapular allograft reconstruction after total scapulectomy: surgical technique and functional results. *J Shoulder Elbow Surg.* 2015;24(8):e203–e211. doi:10.1016/j.jse.2015.02.006
13. Zhang K, Duan H, Xiang Z, Tu C. Surgical technique and clinical results for scapular allograft reconstruction following resection of scapular tumors. *J Exp Clin Cancer Res.* 2009;28(1):45. doi:10.1186/1756-9966-28-45
14. Baran O, Havitçioğlu H. Extremity saving surgery and reconstruction for tumors of the scapula. *Acta Orthop Traumatol Turc.* 2007;41(3):195–201.
15. Mnaymneh WA, Temple HT, Malinin TI. Allograft reconstruction after resection of malignant tumors of the scapula. *Clin Orthop Relat Res.* 2002;405:223–229. doi:10.1097/00003086-200212000-00029
16. Chandrasekar CR, Mohammed R, Grimer RJ. Extracorporeally irradiated scapula as autograft in tumor surgery. *J Shoulder Elbow Surg.* 2009;18(3):e28–e32. doi:10.1016/j.jse.2008.07.014
17. Tang X, Guo W, Yang R, Ji T, Sun X. Reconstruction with constrained prosthesis after total scapulectomy. *J Shoulder Elbow Surg.* 2011;20(7):1163–1169. doi:10.1016/j.jse.2010.12.014
18. Schwab JH, Athanasian EA, Morris CD, Boland PJ, Healey JH. Function correlates with deltoid preservation in patients having scapular replacement. *Clin Orthop Relat Res.* 2006;452:225–230. doi:10.1097/01.blo.0000229323.37793.6d
19. Masamed R, Learch TJ, Menendez LR. En bloc shoulder resection with total shoulder prosthetic replacement: indications and imaging findings. *AJR Am J Roentgenol.* 2008;191(2):482–489. doi:10.2214/AJR.07.3286
20. Trikoupis IG, Mavrodontis II, Papadopoulos DV, et al. 3D-printed glenoid implant reconstruction after partial scapulectomy for malignant tumors: a case series. *Eur J Orthop Surg Traumatol.* 2024;34(3):1557–1562. doi:10.1007/s00590-024-03839-4

7 Distal Humerus Resection and Reconstruction

INTRODUCTION

Tumors involving the distal humerus represent a rare subset of musculoskeletal neoplasms, accounting for approximately 1% of all primary bone tumors and metastatic bone lesions [1]. While the incidence is low, the anatomical complexity of the elbow joint, compounded by the proximity of major neurovascular structures and limited soft tissue envelope, renders surgical management particularly challenging. Nonetheless, advancements in imaging, oncological therapies, and reconstruction techniques have rendered limb salvage a viable alternative to amputation in selected cases [2].

The goals of limb salvage surgery at the elbow include complete tumor excision with negative margins, preservation of critical neurovascular structures, and restoration of elbow stability and range of motion. This necessitates a multidisciplinary approach involving precise preoperative imaging, meticulous surgical planning, and the availability of a spectrum of reconstructive options, including endoprostheses, osteoarticular allografts, and allograft-prosthetic composites (APCs) [3, 4].

This chapter discusses the surgical indications, techniques, reconstructive options, complications, and outcomes associated with distal humeral resections. Drawing from current literature and institutional experience, it aims to provide a comprehensive overview for orthopedic oncologists involved in limb salvage surgery of the upper extremity.

SURGICAL ANATOMY

The distal humerus is a complex anatomical region, critical for elbow function and surrounded by essential neurovascular structures. Surgical resection in this area, particularly for oncologic purposes, requires an in-depth understanding of regional anatomy to facilitate safe dissection, achieve adequate oncologic margins, and ensure a viable reconstruction.

The distal humerus articulates with the ulna and radius to form the elbow joint and consists of two condylar columns—the medial and lateral columns—supporting the trochlea and capitellum, respectively. The osseous architecture provides limited canal diameter and cortical thickness, which presents technical challenges for secure fixation during prosthetic or allograft reconstruction.

From a neurovascular perspective, the region is densely populated. In the anterior compartment of the distal arm, the brachial artery travels alongside the median nerve, situated medial to the biceps tendon and anterior to the humerus. These structures course through the antecubital fossa and are particularly vulnerable during anterior surgical exposures. The ulnar nerve lies posterior to the medial epicondyle in the cubital tunnel and must be identified and protected intraoperatively, often requiring anterior transposition to prevent postoperative neuropathy. The radial nerve is especially at risk during the posterior and lateral dissection. It emerges from the spiral groove of the humerus in the mid-arm and traverses the lateral intermuscular septum to reach the anterior compartment, lying between the brachialis and brachioradialis muscles as it approaches the forearm.

The muscular coverage in this region is relatively limited compared to the proximal humerus or femur. The distal biceps and brachialis provide anterior bulk, while the triceps insert posteriorly. However, oncologic resections often necessitate resection of overlying soft tissue, particularly in cases of high-grade sarcomas or recurrent tumors, making postoperative wound healing and soft tissue coverage challenging.

During resection, neurovascular structures are ideally identified and mobilized proximally in uninvolved tissue planes and dissected distally along their natural course, with care to preserve the brachial artery and median and ulnar nerves, and minimize injury to the radial nerve. In selected cases, resection of a single nerve may be permissible if necessary for oncologic clearance; however, involvement of multiple major nerves or the main vascular bundle typically precludes limb salvage.

PREOPERATIVE PLANNING

Successful outcomes in distal humerus limb salvage surgery are highly dependent on meticulous preoperative planning. This includes tumor staging, surgical margin assessment, evaluation of limb salvage feasibility, and determination of the optimal reconstructive strategy.

A comprehensive clinical evaluation is the foundation, documenting pain characteristics, range of motion, preexisting deficits, and neurologic function. In cases of prior surgery or suspected recurrence, a detailed history of previous interventions is critical.

Plain radiographs help in the initial assessment of the lesion and bone destruction (Figure 7.1A). Magnetic resonance imaging (MRI) is the imaging modality of choice for local staging. T1-weighted sequences provide an accurate assessment of intramedullary tumor extent, while T2-weighted and contrast-enhanced sequences highlight soft tissue involvement and neurovascular proximity

DOI: 10.1201/9780367822002-9

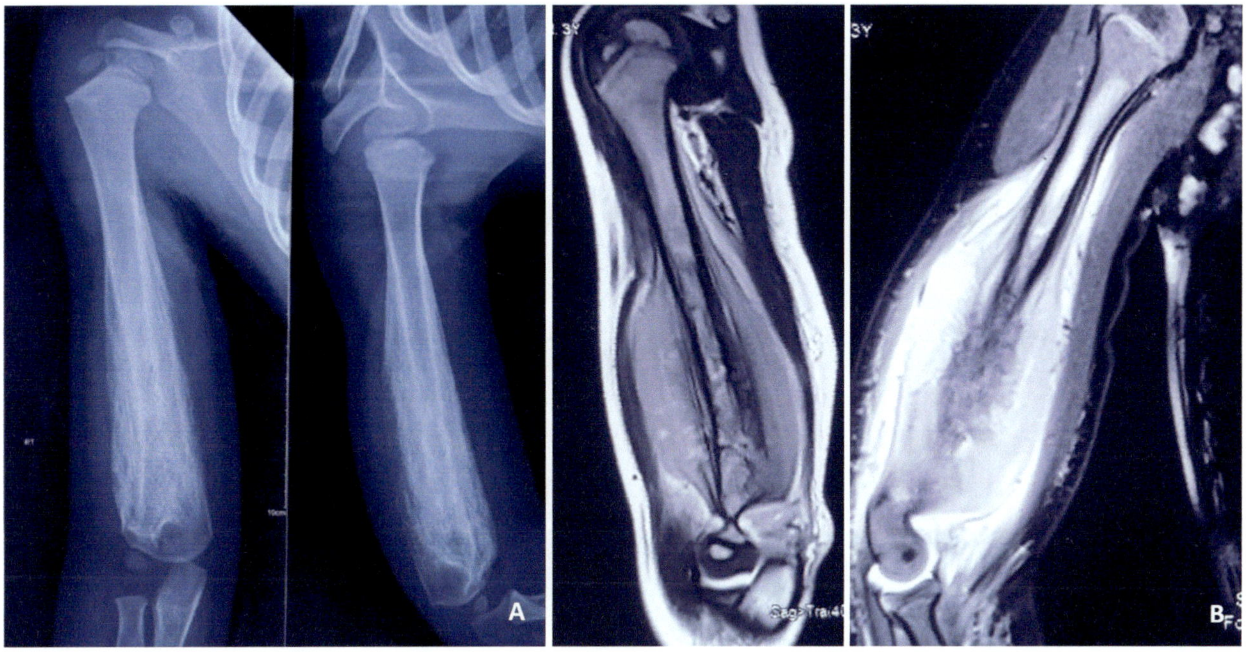

FIGURE 7.1 (A) Plain radiographs of a 5-year-old male with Ewing sarcoma of the humerus, showing a destructive diaphyseal lesion with permeative margins, cortical destruction, and periosteal reaction. (B) MRI images delineating intramedullary tumor extent, extraosseous soft tissue component, and proximity to the neurovascular bundle, providing essential information for surgical planning.

(Figure 7.1B). MRI is indispensable in determining the safety of resecting tumors near the brachial artery, median nerve, ulnar nerve, or radial nerve, and in evaluating the extent of any soft tissue extension across the elbow joint.

Computed tomography (CT) complements MRI by assessing cortical involvement and detecting subtle cortical erosions, periosteal reactions, or pathological fractures. In cases of metastatic disease, CT aids in determining the need for resection versus curettage and internal fixation. For preoperative planning of prosthetic or allograft reconstruction, CT imaging facilitates accurate templating of resection lengths and implant sizing.

Angiography or CT angiography may be necessary if neurovascular encasement is suspected. These modalities help distinguish between vascular displacement and encasement, particularly in high-grade sarcomas or soft tissue tumors that secondarily involve the bone. In cases with equivocal neurovascular involvement, angiographic findings may alter the surgical plan from limb salvage to amputation or influence decisions on vascular reconstruction.

Bone scintigraphy is useful in identifying skip metastases or multifocal lesions. It also assists in evaluating overall skeletal involvement, particularly in diseases such as Ewing sarcoma or multifocal osteosarcoma.

Preoperative biopsy must be performed judiciously, ideally using an image-guided core needle technique. The biopsy tract should be aligned with the planned surgical incision to ensure its complete excision at the time of definitive surgery. Anterior approaches through the brachialis are preferred; transgression of the biceps should be avoided to preserve elbow flexion capacity.

Furthermore, preoperative coordination with plastic surgery may be warranted in cases with inadequate soft tissue coverage, requiring rotational or free flap planning. Nutritional optimization, infection risk stratification, and anesthesia assessment are integral to the multidisciplinary planning process.

SURGICAL TECHNIQUE

Patient Positioning

The patient is positioned supine on a radiolucent operating table with the affected limb extended on an arm board. A small bolster under the ipsilateral scapula aids in shoulder external rotation, optimizing medial and anterior exposure. The limb is prepared from the shoulder to the fingertips. A pneumatic tourniquet may be used, although some surgeons prefer to avoid a tourniquet to maintain visualization of vascular landmarks, especially when tumor proximity to neurovascular structures is anticipated.

Incision and Approach

An S-shaped incision is commonly used for anterior or medial tumors involving the distal humerus. The incision starts at the mid-arm, aligned along the medial aspect of the biceps muscle, and is extended distally to the antecubital crease, incorporating the previous biopsy tract in an elliptical fashion to ensure oncological safety. From the antecubital crease, the incision curves laterally or medially across the volar surface of the elbow. Then it continues distally

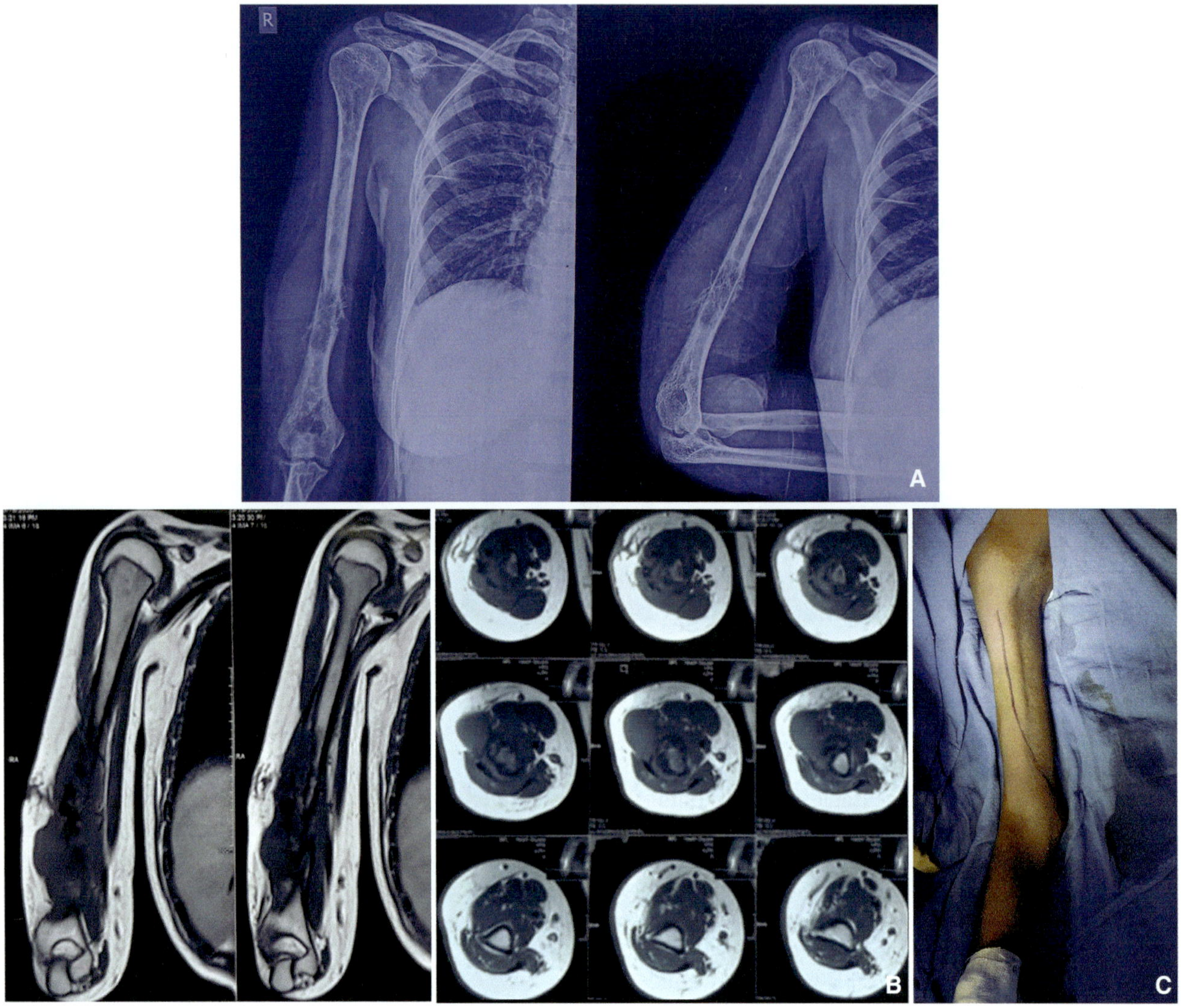

FIGURE 7.2 Radiological evaluation of Ewing sarcoma of the distal humerus in a 15-year-old male. (A) Plain radiograph shows a destructive diaphyseal–metaphyseal lesion with cortical destruction, permeative margins, and periosteal reaction. (B) MRI reveals intramedullary tumor extent with cortical breach and a large soft tissue component surrounding the distal humerus, while also demonstrating the relationship of the lesion to adjacent neurovascular structures. (C) The surgical management involves wide resection and endoprosthesis reconstruction. The incision starts at the mid-arm, aligned along the medial aspect of the biceps muscle, and is extended distally to the antecubital crease. The incision then curves laterally or medially across the volar surface of the elbow to continue distally for a short length of the proximal forearm.

for a short length along the dorsal aspect of the proximal forearm (Figure 7.2A–7.2C).

Medial and lateral fasciocutaneous flaps are developed, taking care to preserve the medial and lateral antebrachial cutaneous nerves. Adequate flap elevation facilitates exposure while maintaining vascularity and minimizing postoperative wound complications.

SOFT TISSUE DISSECTION

Neurovascular Dissection

The deep investing fascia overlying the neurovascular bundle is incised longitudinally. This facilitates the identification of key structures within their sheath:

- The brachial artery and its accompanying veins are palpated and dissected free along their course from the mid-arm to their bifurcation at the elbow. The biceps aponeurosis is incised to enhance visualization of the distal vasculature, including the ulnar and radial arteries, both of which are looped and protected. Minor branches, such as the inferior ulnar collateral artery and muscular twigs to the biceps and brachialis, are ligated as needed.
- The median nerve is traced from proximal to distal, mobilized across the antecubital fossa where it lies medial to the brachial artery, and followed distally to its branch point—the anterior interosseous nerve. Care is taken to avoid traction injury as it passes deep to the flexor digitorum superficialis.

- The ulnar nerve is identified proximally and followed distally through the medial intermuscular septum to the cubital tunnel, where the overlying fascial roof is released. Dissection continues to the level where the nerve passes between the humeral and ulnar heads of the pronator teres, allowing medial retraction with the brachial artery and median nerve.
- The radial nerve is approached in the interval between the brachialis and brachioradialis, traced distally across the elbow joint to its bifurcation into the superficial radial and posterior interosseous nerves. Proximally, the lateral intermuscular septum is opened, and the nerve is mobilized from the spiral groove up to the insertion of the latissimus dorsi.

Muscular Dissection

- Flexor-pronator muscles arising from the medial epicondyle are detached en bloc. If involved by tumor, resection is extended distally to achieve adequate margins. The branch of the median nerve to the flexor digitorum superficialis is identified and preserved when possible.
- Extensor musculature, including the brachioradialis and extensor carpi radialis longus, is similarly released from the lateral epicondyle. The posterior interosseous nerve is protected throughout, particularly if deeper dissection near the supinator or extensor origin is required.
- The biceps muscle is preserved if not involved (Figure 7.3). It is dissected free from the underlying brachialis and retracted for exposure. If the tumor invades the biceps, partial excision is considered, but care is taken not to compromise elbow flexion mechanics—particularly if the brachialis also requires resection.
- The brachialis muscle is often resected en bloc along with the tumor and serves as a tumor margin. In such cases, it may be released subperiosteally or transected distal to the elbow (Figure 7.4).
- The triceps muscle, particularly its medial head, may need partial resection depending on posterior tumor extension. The lateral and long heads are typically preserved. The triceps tendon remains attached to the olecranon, and routine olecranon osteotomy is avoided.

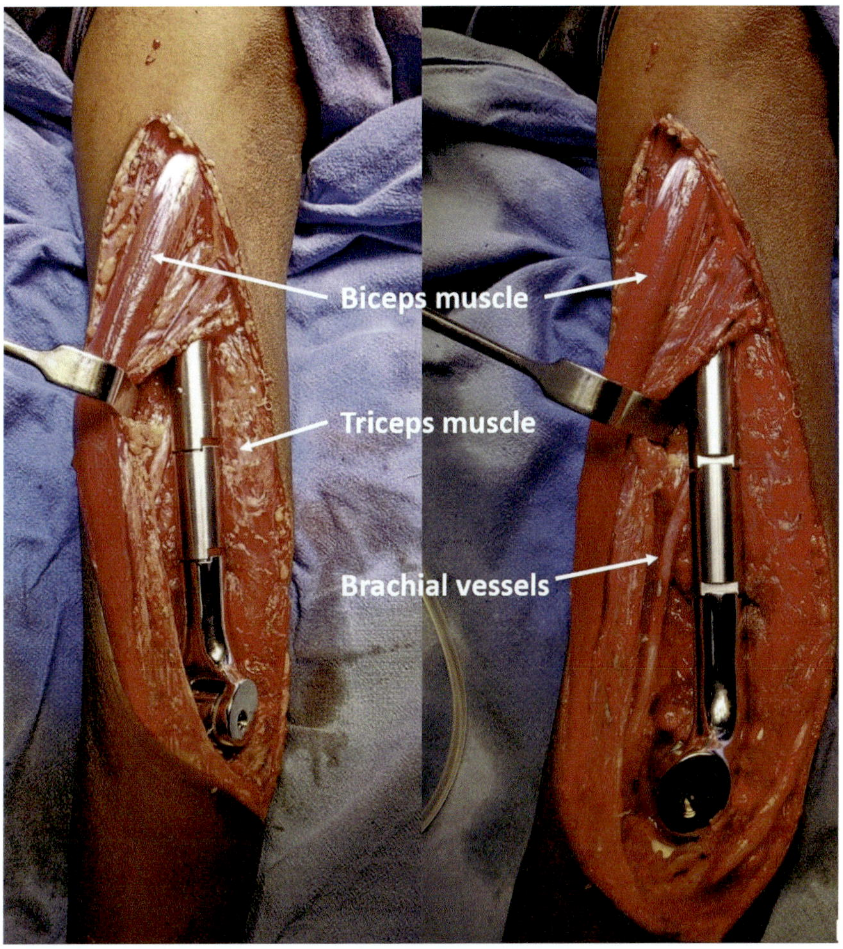

FIGURE 7.3 The biceps muscle is preserved if not involved. The lateral and long heads of the triceps are typically preserved. The brachial artery and its accompanying veins are palpated and dissected free along their course from the mid-arm to their bifurcation at the elbow. The defect is reconstructed using a distal humerus endoprosthesis.

Bone Resection

With soft tissues dissected and neurovascular structures looped and protected, the humerus is transected at least 2 to 3 cm proximal to the radiologically defined intramedullary tumor extent. The cut is made after the radial nerve is carefully visualized and protected. An oscillating or sagittal saw is used, and the bone is transected under continuous saline irrigation.

Posterior dissection is continued down to the olecranon fossa, and anteriorly to the coronoid fossa, ensuring circumferential release of soft tissues.

Elbow Joint Resection

For tumors extending into the articular region, an intra-articular resection is performed. The elbow joint capsule is circumferentially released from the olecranon and radial head. The humero-ulnar and radiohumeral joints are disarticulated. Preservation of the ulna and radial head is attempted unless directly invaded. Disarticulation is performed under direct vision, allowing en bloc removal of the distal humerus with attached soft tissue margins (Figure 7.4).

PREPARATION FOR RECONSTRUCTION

Following tumor removal, the reconstruction phase begins. The choice of technique—**endoprosthesis**, **osteochondral allograft**, or **APC**—is guided by preoperative planning and intraoperative findings.

- In prosthetic reconstruction, the **proximal humeral canal** is reamed for cemented or uncemented stem fixation. Trials are used to evaluate joint stability and alignment.
- For biological reconstructions, **contoured allografts** are secured with **locking plates**, and a **semi-constrained hinge prosthesis** may be cemented into the allograft if elbow articulation has been resected.
- **Soft tissue reconstruction** includes reattachment of preserved muscles using **nonabsorbable sutures** and sometimes the use of **local or free flaps** in case of deficient coverage.

Reconstruction following distal humerus resection is a critical component of limb salvage surgery and is guided by multiple factors, including patient age, tumor pathology, bone and soft tissue loss, neurovascular preservation, and surgeon expertise. The primary goals are to restore limb length, provide joint stability, enable functional elbow motion, and minimize complications. Several reconstructive strategies are available, broadly categorized into endoprosthetic reconstruction, biological options (e.g., osteoarticular allograft, APCs), and arthrodesis or resection arthroplasty in select scenarios. For extensive bone loss or elderly patients, megaprostheses offer shorter

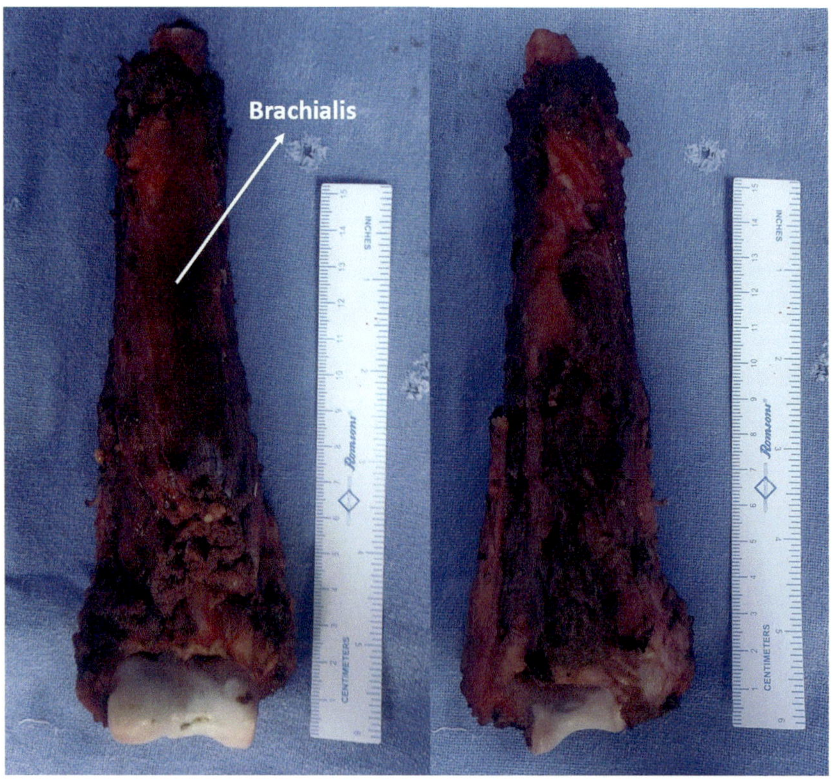

FIGURE 7.4 Resected tumor specimen. The brachialis muscle is often resected en bloc along with the tumor and serves as a tumor margin.

rehabilitation times and lower risk of nonunion. However, in younger patients or when the elbow joint can be preserved, osteoarticular allografts or APCs may provide better biological integration and allow reattachment of ligaments and tendons.

ENDOPROSTHETIC RECONSTRUCTION

Endoprosthetic reconstruction using modular or custom-linked elbow prostheses has become the most widely used technique for restoring elbow stability and motion following distal humeral tumor resection. It is particularly advantageous in patients with large bone loss, compromised bone quality, or where rapid functional restoration is desired. Modern systems typically incorporate linked, semi-constrained hinge mechanisms to replicate the articulation of the elbow while allowing some axial rotation and minimizing stress at the bone-implant interface.

Endoprosthetic reconstruction is particularly indicated in cases where wide excision is required for high-grade primary bone sarcomas involving the distal humerus. It is also well suited for patients with extensive bony destruction due to metastatic lesions, where immediate stability and early mobilization are essential. Furthermore, it serves as a reliable salvage option in cases of failed biological reconstructions, such as nonunion or structural allograft resorption. Elderly patients, especially those with diminished bone quality or limited functional demands, benefit from the predictable outcomes and rapid rehabilitation associated with endoprosthetic solutions.

However, this reconstructive approach has certain limitations. It is relatively contraindicated in young patients, owing to concerns regarding implant longevity. Additionally, endoprosthetic reconstruction may not be feasible in situations where adequate soft tissue coverage cannot be achieved, as insufficient coverage significantly increases the risk of wound complications and prosthetic exposure. Careful patient selection, therefore, remains paramount in optimizing outcomes.

TECHNIQUE OF ENDOPROSTHETIC RECONSTRUCTION

Endoprosthetic reconstruction of the distal humerus and elbow joint is most commonly performed using a modular, segmental tumor prosthesis. The prosthesis is designed to replicate the elbow's biomechanical function while allowing for intraoperative customization based on the extent of resection and the patient's anatomy.

The distal humeral prosthesis typically comprises a semi-constrained hinge mechanism that articulates with a corresponding ulnar component, recreating the elbow joint. Proximally, the humeral component is connected to a modular body segment through a Morse taper junction, which allows for selection of varying segment lengths to achieve the desired reconstruction span. This modular segment is then fitted onto a humeral stem, also via a Morse taper, and the entire assembly is cemented into the remaining proximal humeral canal.

The ulnar component, available in variable lengths, is similarly fixed with bone cement into the olecranon and proximal ulna. Prior to cementation, the ulnar canal is prepared by gently burring the olecranon fossa and reaming the medullary canal with hand instruments. The olecranon tip may be contoured slightly to facilitate direct and axial stem insertion. In prosthetic reconstruction, the proximal humeral canal is reamed for cemented or uncemented stem fixation. Trial components are used to confirm the optimal fit and alignment of both humeral and ulnar segments and to evaluate joint stability.

The prosthesis is assembled on the sterile field and inserted in a staged manner. The humeral stem is implanted first, ensuring that the hinge axis is aligned anteriorly and the component is seated in proper rotational orientation. The ulnar stem is then inserted and positioned to sit deeply within the canal while avoiding posterior cortical breach. After both stems have been cemented and allowed to cure, the hinge mechanism is securely linked, restoring joint continuity (Figure 7.5).

SOFT TISSUE RECONSTRUCTION

Following prosthetic implantation, meticulous soft tissue reconstruction is undertaken to ensure prosthesis coverage, preserve elbow function, and restore dynamic stability. The brachioradialis and extensor carpi radialis longus are mobilized and sutured to the remaining biceps and triceps musculature using heavy nonabsorbable sutures. This construct helps encase the flared humeral component and provide soft tissue bulk anteriorly and laterally.

A flexorplasty is performed to restore elbow flexion. With the elbow held in approximately 60° of flexion and the forearm fully supinated, the flexor-pronator muscle origin is transferred proximally and anchored to the biceps tendon. The biceps itself is pulled distally and placed under tension to reestablish its length-tension relationship, especially in cases where the prosthesis has been downsized to aid soft tissue closure. The origin of the flexor-pronator mass is secured to the medial edge of the biceps-triceps complex, recreating a stable medial soft tissue envelope. The remaining biceps-brachialis and triceps muscles are then sutured to one another, thereby enveloping the prosthesis and the protected neurovascular bundle. This layer provides essential coverage and structural integrity.

In instances of extensive soft tissue loss or inadequate coverage, the prosthesis may be shortened intraoperatively by 2–3 cm to facilitate wound closure without excessive tension. In such cases, retensioning of the biceps and proximal advancement of the flexor-pronator and brachioradialis origins becomes essential to restore elbow flexion mechanics and prevent lag.

Drains are placed, and the wound is closed in layers. The limb is supported in a hinged elbow brace, and a protocol of early but protected mobilization is initiated postoperatively.

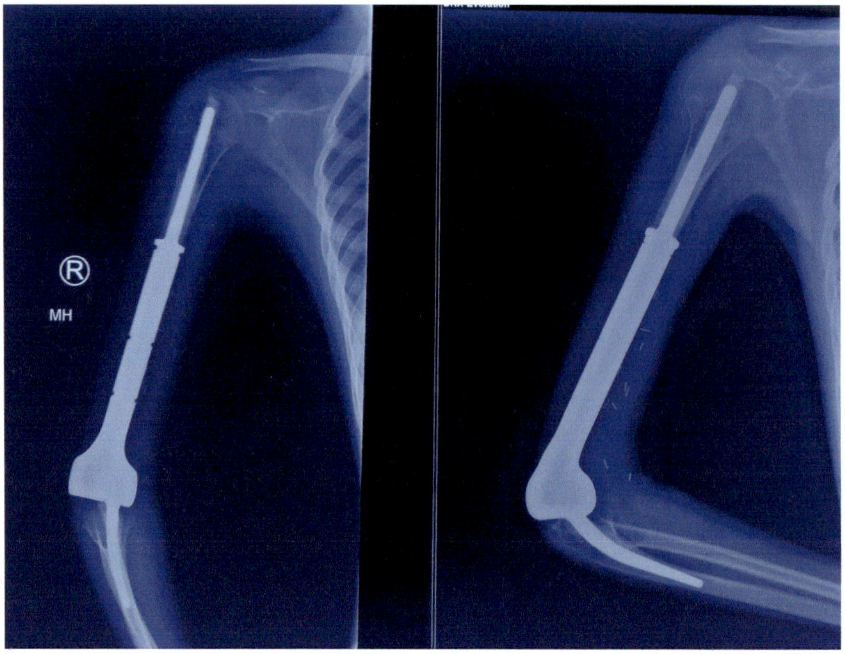

FIGURE 7.5 Post-operative radiographs following distal humerus tumor resection and endoprosthesis reconstruction.

Advantages

- **Immediate joint stability** due to the hinge mechanism
- **Early mobilization** and functional recovery
- **Predictable outcomes** in elderly or low-demand patients
- **Reduced risk of nonunion** and graft resorption compared to biological reconstructions

Outcomes

Several studies have reported favorable mid- to long-term outcomes with distal humeral endoprostheses. In a systematic review by Gonzalez et al., the mean Musculoskeletal Tumor Society (MSTS) score following distal humerus replacement for oncologic indications was 81.1%, with a five-year implant survival of 72% [2]. Henrichs et al. reported that limb salvage with endoprosthesis achieved good functional outcomes (mean MSTS 24/30), although prosthetic survival declined to 64% at five years, largely due to aseptic loosening and periprosthetic infections [1].

Complications

Despite its benefits, endoprosthetic reconstruction carries a notable risk of complications:

- **Aseptic loosening** is the most common cause of mechanical failure, particularly of the humeral stem. In a systematic review, aseptic loosening was the most common mode of failure, with a cumulative incidence of 12% (range 0%–33%) [2].
- **Periprosthetic infection**, although less frequent, remains a serious concern given limited soft tissue coverage around the elbow.
- **Radial or ulnar nerve palsy**, though usually transient, can occur due to extensive dissection or retraction.
- **Component failure or fracture** of modular junctions has been rarely reported in long-term follow-up [2].

OSTEOARTICULAR ALLOGRAFT RECONSTRUCTION

Osteoarticular allograft reconstruction involves replacing the resected segment of the distal humerus with a cadaveric allograft containing the native articular surface and adjacent diaphyseal bone. It offers the potential advantage of biological incorporation, preservation of bone stock, and reattachment of native soft tissue structures. This technique is especially relevant in younger patients, where long-term durability and avoidance of prosthetic complications are desirable.

Surgical Technique

The technique begins with the selection of a size-matched fresh-frozen or cryopreserved distal humerus allograft, typically based on radiographic templating and intraoperative comparison. The allograft is trimmed to match the osteotomy plane of the native humerus, and internal fixation is achieved using low-profile locking plates or compression plating constructs, often supplemented with cerclage wires when necessary. Care is taken to ensure precise alignment, rotation, and limb length restoration.

The ulna and radial components of the elbow are preserved, allowing the native elbow joint to articulate with the allograft's articular surface. If the native elbow is compromised or if instability persists, augmentation with soft tissue reconstruction or a constrained hinge implant may be considered.

Advantages

Osteoarticular allografts offer several theoretical and clinical benefits:

- Biological reconstruction with potential for host-graft bone union
- Soft tissue reattachment is facilitated, especially for the flexor-pronator and extensor origins
- Preservation of the native joint mechanics, provided articular congruity is maintained
- Avoidance of long-term mechanical complications such as prosthetic loosening

Outcomes

The long-term outcomes of osteoarticular allografts for distal humerus reconstruction remain variable, with reported complication rates higher than endoprosthetic alternatives. A systematic review by Kamalapathy et al. showed functional scores ranging from 65% to 80% of normal using MSTS criteria, but with high rates of complications such as nonunion, articular degeneration, and fracture [4]. The reported allograft survival rate was approximately 83%–86% at mid- to long-term follow-up (mean ~69 months). Structural failures including graft fracture, articular collapse, and resorption have been reported in up to 30% of cases, often necessitating secondary surgical intervention or conversion to endoprosthetic reconstruction [4].

Complications

Major complications associated with osteoarticular allografts include:

- **Nonunion at host-graft junction** (reported in 15%–30% of cases)
- **Graft fracture**, particularly in early postoperative rehabilitation
- **Articular cartilage degeneration**, resulting in stiffness and pain
- **Immune-mediated resorption** or graft collapse
- **Infection**, particularly in cases with large soft tissue dissection or prior surgery

Given these potential risks, the use of osteoarticular allografts has become less common and is now typically reserved for highly selected patients where joint preservation is prioritized and functional demands are high.

ALLOGRAFT-PROSTHETIC COMPOSITE RECONSTRUCTION

APC reconstruction is a hybrid technique that combines a modular tumor endoprosthesis with a structural osteoarticular or segmental allograft. This approach seeks to merge the mechanical reliability of prostheses with the biological advantages of allografts, particularly the potential for soft tissue reattachment, enhanced prosthesis stability, and biological integration at the host-graft junction. APCs are particularly useful when preserving joint articulation is not feasible and a complete elbow reconstruction is required.

APC reconstruction is particularly indicated in young or middle-aged patients where concerns regarding the long-term durability of standalone prostheses may influence reconstructive strategy. It is especially beneficial in cases requiring the simultaneous restoration of both bone and soft tissue units, such as when preservation or reattachment of key musculotendinous structures is critical for optimal upper limb function. APCs are also preferred in patients with adequate biological healing potential and where rigid internal fixation across the host-graft junction can be reliably achieved.

However, this technique is relatively contraindicated in certain clinical scenarios. Patients with compromised local vascularity, a history of prior radiation therapy, or previous infection at the surgical site are at higher risk for graft failure and nonunion. Additionally, the successful application of this method requires robust soft tissue coverage. Hence, in situations where soft tissue reconstruction is not feasible or reliable, alternative reconstructive strategies may be more appropriate.

Surgical Technique

The technique involves selecting a size-matched distal humerus allograft, which is then prepared to accept a modular prosthetic stem proximally. The prosthetic component is cemented or press-fit into the allograft, and the composite is then implanted into the host bone, typically secured with plate-and-screw fixation across the host-graft interface (Figure 7.6). The ulnar component may be either a prosthetic stem, cemented into the proximal ulna, or the patient's native articulation, depending on intraoperative findings.

A key technical step is achieving intimate contact at the host-allograft junction, which facilitates osteointegration. Where feasible, the APC is inserted as a single unit; alternatively, modular assembly may be performed in situ. The remaining muscle-tendon units, including triceps, brachialis, and forearm flexors/extensors, are sutured to the preserved periosteum and soft tissue of the allograft, aiding in functional recovery.

Advantages

- Biological fixation at the host-graft junction allows for long-term bone integration.
- Facilitates anatomic reattachment of soft tissues, contributing to better muscle tension and joint stability.

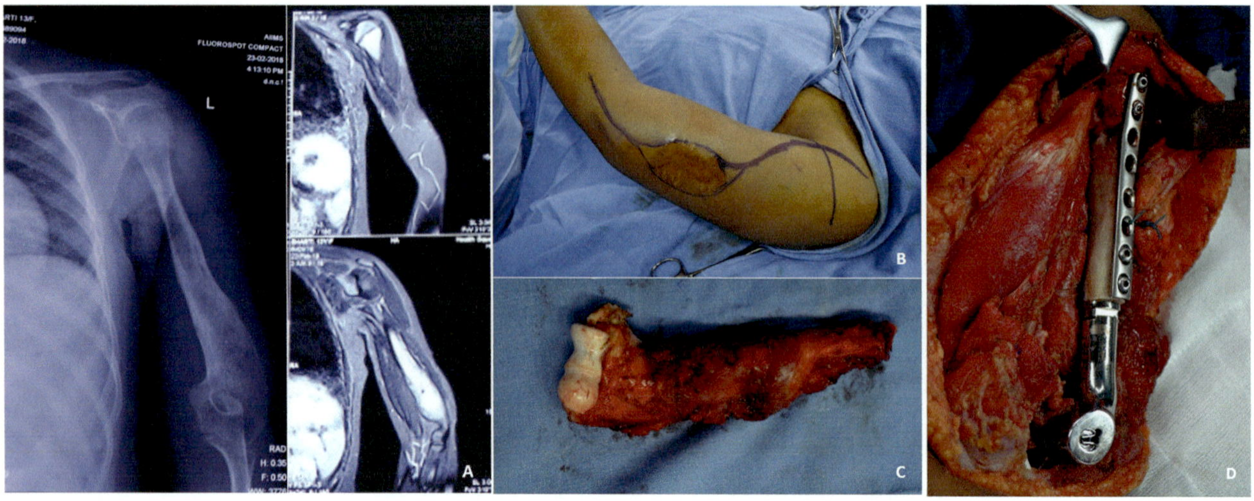

FIGURE 7.6 Radiographs and MRI (A) of Ewing sarcoma distal humerus in a 13-year-old female, showing long length of intramedullary involvement proximally. (B) The incision incorporates the previous biopsy scar. (C) A wide resection was performed. (D) An allograft-prosthesis composite was used for reconstruction.

- Reduces the risk of early prosthetic loosening seen with standalone endoprostheses.
- Suitable for younger patients requiring durable reconstructions with soft tissue integrity.

Complications

While APC reconstruction provides mechanical and biological benefits, it is not without challenges:

- **Host-allograft nonunion**, particularly if rigid fixation or compression is suboptimal.
- **Graft resorption** or fatigue fracture over time.
- **Infection**, especially in immunocompromised or previously irradiated patients.
- **Delayed functional recovery**, often necessitating prolonged rehabilitation.

Nevertheless, when successful, APCs can provide durable reconstruction with good joint mechanics and soft tissue integration.

SUMMARY

- Distal humerus resections are complex procedures requiring meticulous preoperative planning, precise soft tissue dissection, and protection of neurovascular structures to ensure oncological clearance and functional preservation.
- Endoprosthetic reconstruction offers immediate stability and predictable outcomes, making it ideal for elderly patients, metastatic lesions, or cases where rapid rehabilitation is desired.
- Osteoarticular allografts allow for joint preservation and biological integration but are associated with higher complication rates such as nonunion and graft fracture, making patient selection critical.
- APC reconstruction combines the mechanical strength of prostheses with the biological benefits of allografts, facilitating soft tissue reattachment and durable reconstruction in young or active patients.
- Each reconstruction method carries unique indications and limitations; endoprostheses suit elderly patients with poor bone stock, while allografts and APCs are preferable for biologically active and soft tissue favorable environments.
- Neurovascular preservation and soft tissue reconstruction are pivotal for achieving optimal functional outcomes post-resection.

REFERENCES

1. Henrichs MP, Liem D, Gosheger G, et al. Megaprosthetic replacement of the distal humerus: still a challenge in limb salvage. *J Shoulder Elbow Surg.* 2019;28(5):908–914. doi:10.1016/j.jse.2018.11.050
2. Gonzalez MR, Okay E, Sodhi AS, Lozano-Calderon SA. Reconstruction of the elbow with distal humerus endoprosthetic replacement after tumor resection: a systematic review of the literature and institutional case series. *J Shoulder Elbow Surg.* 2024;33(5):1104–1115. doi:10.1016/j.jse.2023.12.024
3. Hennessy DW, Raskin KA, Schwab JH, Lozano-Calderón SA. Endoprosthetic reconstruction of the upper extremity in oncologic surgery. *J Am Acad Orthop Surg.* 2020;28(8):e319–e327. doi:10.5435/JAAOS-D-19-00219
4. Kamalapathy P, Shah A, Raskin K, Schwab JH, Lozano-Calderón SA. Complications and survivorship of distal humeral allograft reconstruction after tumor resection: literature review and case series. *J Am Acad Orthop Surg Glob Res Rev.* 2021;5(2):e20.00256–e20.258. doi:10.5435/JAAOSGlobal-D-20-00256

8 Resections and Reconstructions around the Wrist

DISTAL RADIUS

Tumors of the distal radius, though relatively uncommon, present significant challenges for orthopedic oncologists due to the region's complex anatomy, proximity to vital neurovascular structures, and the high functional demands of the wrist. The distal radius ranks as the third most common site for giant cell tumors (GCT) of bone, accounting for approximately 10%–12% of all cases [1, 2] (Figure 8.1). While GCTs predominate, malignant primary tumors such as osteosarcoma, chondrosarcoma, and rare lesions like angiosarcoma, as well as metastatic deposits, may also occur at this site [3–6]. Distal radius GCTs, particularly Campanacci grade III lesions, are often managed with en bloc resection due to their aggressive nature, higher recurrence rates, and greater risk of pulmonary metastasis compared to other skeletal sites [7–9]. Malignant tumors similarly demand wide-margin resection to achieve local control.

Such resections create substantial osseous and soft tissue defects, necessitating carefully planned reconstruction to restore stability and function. Reconstructive strategies broadly include arthrodesis and arthroplasty, utilizing techniques such as total or partial wrist fusion, osteoarticular allografts, vascularized or nonvascularized fibular autografts, prosthetic replacement, and hybrid approaches [10, 11]. Selection depends on tumor biology, patient demands, and surgical expertise, with each method offering distinct advantages, limitations, and long-term implications.

TOTAL WRIST ARTHRODESIS

Total wrist arthrodesis remains one of the most time-tested and widely practiced reconstructive strategies following en bloc resection of the distal radius for bone tumors. Its primary objective is to achieve a stable, pain-free wrist capable of sustaining maximal grip strength and long-term durability, particularly in patients with high functional demands or when arthroplasty is contraindicated. This approach is especially suitable when tumor extent, location, or associated soft tissue compromise preclude the preservation of wrist motion, or in cases where previous arthroplasty has failed. It is often preferred in individuals engaged in heavy manual labor or those with limited life expectancy, where simplicity, predictable results, and implant survivorship outweigh the desire for motion restoration [11–13].

Several techniques have been developed to accomplish total wrist fusion, most of which involve bridging the defect between the proximal radius or its substitute and the carpus/metacarpals with a structural graft. Options include the use of massive allografts, nonvascularized fibular autografts, structural iliac crest bone grafts (ICBG), or use of ipsilateral ulna by ulnar translocation or centralization with ulnocarpal fusion.

Massive allografts offer the advantage of avoiding donor-site morbidity while providing immediate structural restoration. However, their limitations include the risk of delayed union, nonunion, graft fracture, and potential

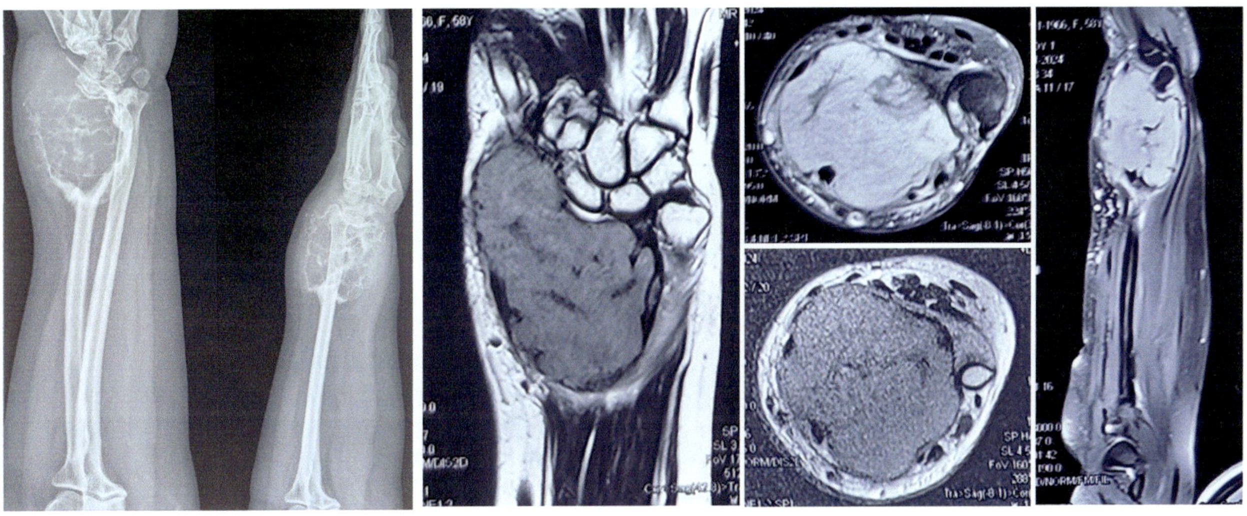

FIGURE 8.1 Radiological images of a giant cell tumor of the distal radius. Plain radiographs reveal an expansile, eccentric, lytic lesion extending to the subarticular region with cortical thinning and ballooning. MRI demonstrates intraosseous extent with cortical breach and associated soft tissue extension.

DOI: 10.1201/9780367822002-10

immunogenic response [14, 15]. **Nonvascularized fibular autografts** remain a widely adopted biological option due to their cortical strength and ease of shaping for arthrodesis. Qu et al. reported excellent results in eight patients treated with fibular autografts, noting a mean Musculoskeletal Tumor Society (MSTS) score of 93%, a Disabilities of the Arm, Shoulder, and Hand (DASH) score of 8, and recovery of grip strength to 71% of the contralateral side. Nevertheless, one graft fracture (12.5%) occurred [16]. Harvesting the proximal fibula introduces the risk of peroneal nerve injury, and avascular autografts, in general, carry complications such as delayed or nonunion, graft resorption, stress fracture, deformity, and fixation failure [17].

Structural iliac crest bone grafting is another reliable option, particularly for moderate-sized defects. Wang et al., in a series of 27 patients, reported a mean MSTS score of 96% and a DASH score of 9. Donor-site morbidity was minimal, but complications included fracture (3.7%), hardware failure (14.8%), and nonunion (7.4%) [18]. Its use, however, is generally restricted to defects less than 8 cm in length, making it less suitable for extensive resections [17].

Biological reconstruction using **ulnar translocation or centralization** techniques has gained attention, especially in resource-constrained settings or where donor-site morbidity is a major concern. These methods reposition the ipsilateral ulna to occupy the defect after distal radius resection, eliminating the need for free grafts or allografts and preserving native vascularity without the requirement for microsurgical anastomosis. The reconstruction is performed through the same surgical field, simplifying operative logistics.

Ulnar centralization, first described by Greenwood in 1932 [19], involves medial translation of the carpus to the distal ulna and performing ulnocarpal arthrodesis. The lunate is aligned with the third metacarpal, and fixation is achieved using a plate (Figure 8.2). This technique completely sacrifices forearm rotation but provides a robust, stable platform for hand function. Its simplicity and single union site contribute to faster rehabilitation. Bhagat et al. reported satisfactory function and 65% grip strength recovery in 25 patients [20], while Kapoor et al. achieved radiological union in 96% of 26 patients by six months, with a mean MSTS score of 26, grip strength reaching 74% of the contralateral side, and a low complication rate of 10.7% [21].

Ulnar translocation, on the other hand, preserves forearm rotation by mobilizing a segment of the distal ulna laterally to bridge the defect, while retaining its soft tissue and vascular attachments. The transferred segment is fixed from the radius across to the metacarpals (Figure 8.3). Puri et al. reported favorable results in 14 patients with Campanacci grade III GCTs, achieving a mean MSTS score of 87% and minimal complications [22].

Chalidis et al. described a modification using segmental plating for improved stability, though cosmetic results were less optimal and axial load-bearing capacity was reduced [23]. Zhang et al. further refined the technique with an ipsilateral double-barrel segmental ulnar graft combined with a modified Sauvé–Kapandji procedure, enabling one-bone forearm reconstruction while preserving limited pronation-supination. This yielded improved grip strength, higher functional scores, and reduced complication rates [24].

Overall, total wrist arthrodesis consistently provides reliable pain relief, restoration of grip strength, and long-term construct stability. However, the trade-off is the complete loss of wrist motion, which may limit fine motor skills and certain activities of daily living. While allografts and fibular autografts offer structural integrity, they are associated with risks of fracture and nonunion, and autografts also carry the additional risk of donor-site morbidity. Structural ICBG is effective for smaller defects, whereas ulnar-based reconstructions provide a cost-effective, biologically sound alternative, especially in situations where resources or graft availability are limited. Table 8.1 summarizes functional outcomes and complication rates across various wrist arthrodesis methods.

The choice of technique must be individualized, taking into account tumor biology, defect size, patient functional demands, and surgical expertise. Although complication rates such as nonunion, hardware failure, infection, and donor-site issues remain considerations, careful preoperative planning and meticulous technique can yield high rates of limb salvage with durable functional results.

PARTIAL WRIST ARTHRODESIS

Partial wrist arthrodesis offers a motion-preserving alternative to total fusion, suitable for patients whose functional needs require some wrist mobility. It involves selective fusion between carpal bones and the remaining host bone or reconstructive graft, with radio-scaphoid-lunate (RSL) arthrodesis most commonly favored for its ability to replicate normal wrist biomechanics [26].

Reconstruction typically employs nonvascularized or vascularized fibular autografts contoured to the carpal surfaces and fixed with plates or screws. Tibia cortical strut autografts (TCSA) are also used when fibular harvest is contraindicated. Zhu et al. reported on seven patients undergoing fibular-based arthrodesis, achieving a mean MSTS score of 85.3% and grip strength of 76.5% of the opposite side, though graft fracture occurred in 28.6% [6]. Van de Sande et al. achieved a mean MSTS score of 71.7%, DASH score of 9.2, and 75% grip strength recovery using TCSA, with only one fracture (5.9%) [6].

Partial arthrodesis preserves midcarpal and finger motion, benefiting activities of daily living. However, it is technically demanding, with a limited fusion surface, making fixation stability critical. Risks include delayed/nonunion, infection, and graft fracture [1]. When appropriately indicated, it can provide durable, motion-sparing reconstruction with acceptable strength and pain relief.

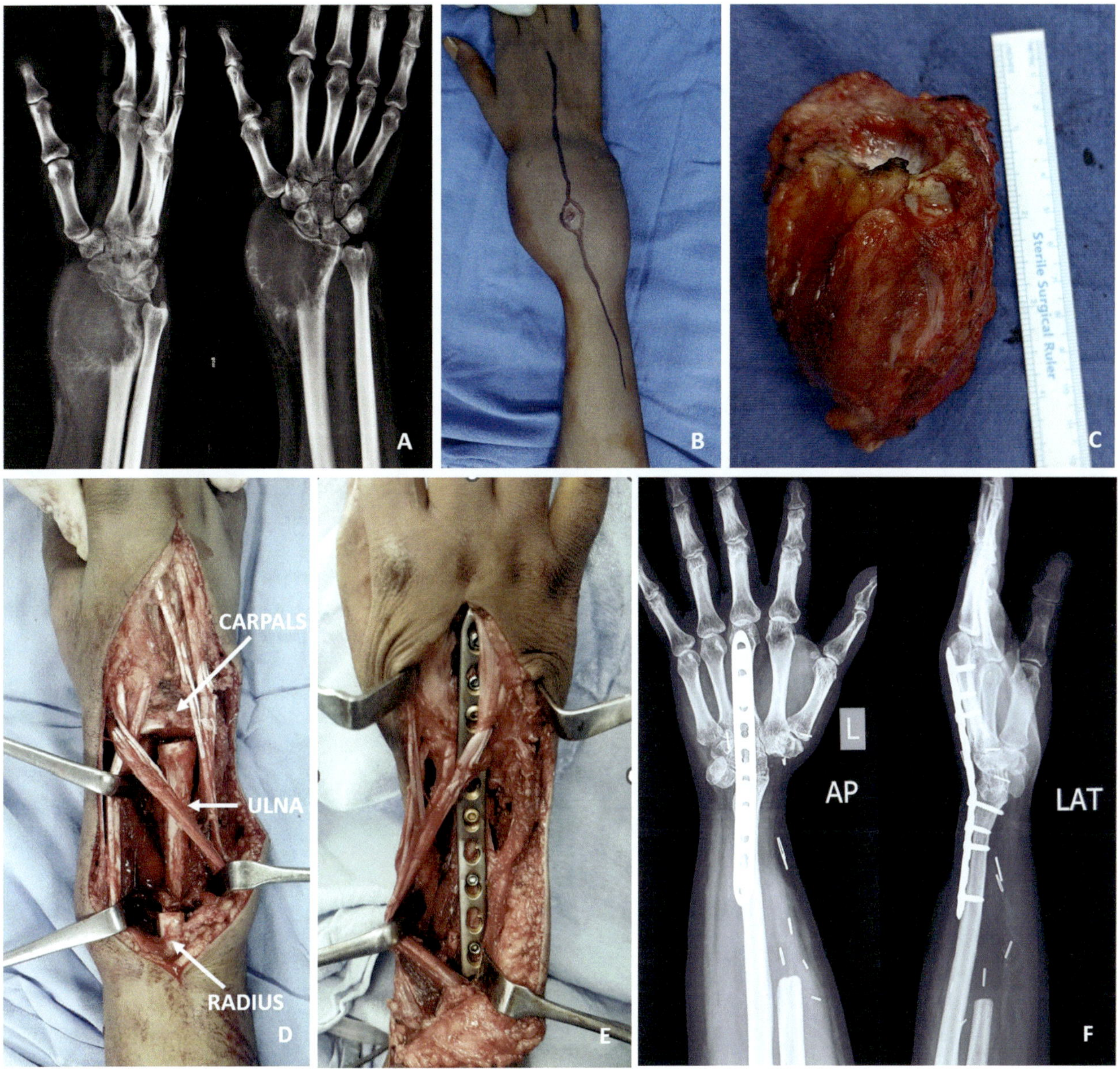

FIGURE 8.2 Preoperative radiographs of a patient with Campanacci grade 3 GCTB distal radius. The tumor was approached using a dorsal approach (B), and en bloc resection was performed (C). Reconstruction with centralization of the ipsilateral ulna and ulno-carpal fusion was performed. The articular cartilage of the distal ulna and lunate is removed to expose the cancellous bone underneath. Ulna is centralized and apposed to the prepared lunate in alignment with the third metacarpal (D), with the wrist in 20 degrees of dorsiflexion and forearm in mid-pronation. A 3.5 low-contact plate, prebent to 20 degrees at the ulnocarpal junction, is applied dorsally for fixation of the distal ulna to the third metacarpal (E). Post-operative radiographs after reconstruction (F).

WRIST ARTHROPLASTY

Wrist arthroplasty offers motion-preserving reconstruction after en bloc distal radius tumor resection, particularly in patients where mobility is prioritized over maximal strength. It is best suited for low-demand patients, children, or those requiring fine motor skills. Reconstruction options include:

1. Osteoarticular allograft arthroplasty
2. **Fibular head autograft arthroplasty** (vascularized or nonvascularized)
3. Prosthetic wrist replacement

OSTEOARTICULAR ALLOGRAFT ARTHROPLASTY

This method uses cadaveric distal radius segments with articular surfaces to restore joint anatomy while avoiding donor-site morbidity. Duan et al. reported in 15 patients a mean Mayo wrist score of 70 and grip strength of 27 kg, with no fractures when long locking plates were used [27]. Scoccianti et al. found a mean MSTS score of 86% at five-year follow-up [28]. However, nonunion rates up to 42.9% and progressive degenerative changes limit long-term success [25, 28, 29]. Allograft fractures remain a risk if fixation

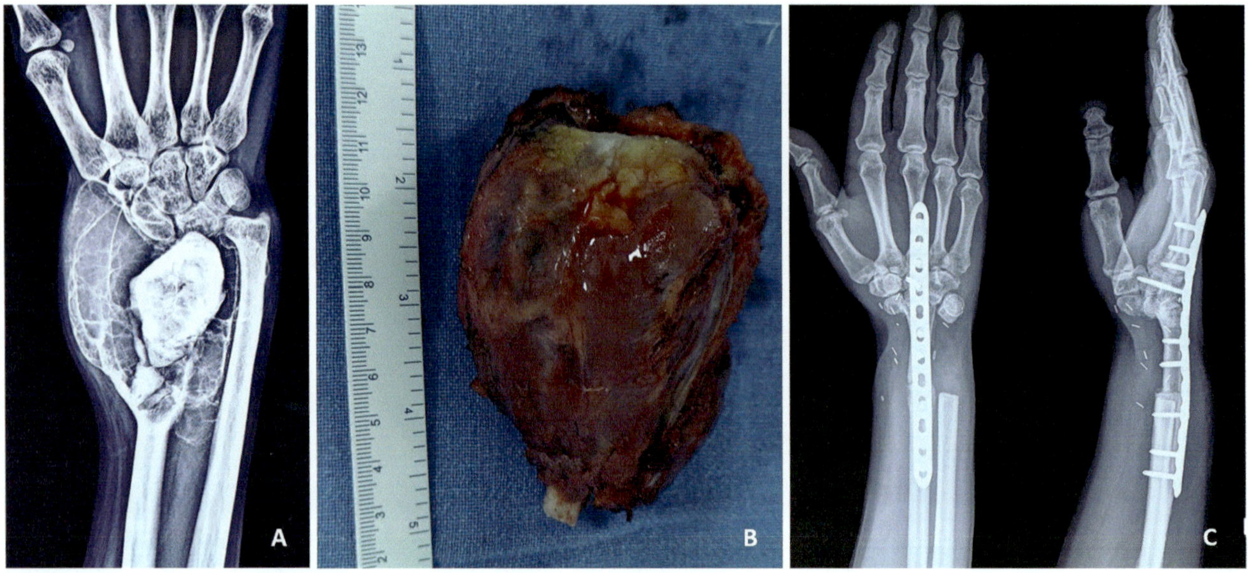

FIGURE 8.3 Preoperative radiographs of a patient with recurrent GCTB distal radius (A). En bloc resection was performed (B). Reconstruction with translocation of the ipsilateral ulna and ulno-carpal fusion was performed. The ipsilateral ulna is osteotomized. The transferred segment is fixed from the radius across to the metacarpals using a pre-bent 3.5 mm low-contact plate. Post-operative radiographs after reconstruction are shown in (C).

TABLE 8.1
Wrist Arthrodesis after En bloc Resection of Bone Tumors of the Distal Radius

Reconstruction	Author	Cases	Follow-Up (Months)	Functional Outcomes	Complications
Total Arthrodesis					
Nonvascularized fibula	Qu et al. [16]	8	80	MSTS 93%, DASH score 8, grip strength 71%	Fracture (12.5%)
Vascularized Bone Grafts	Clarkson et al. [17]	14	>12	MSTS 80%, DASH score 20	Peroneal nerve palsy (14.3%), flap necrosis (7.2%)
ICBG	Wang et al. [18]	27	56	MSTS 96%, DASH score 9, grip strength 51%	Fracture (3.7%), hardware failure (14.8%), nonunion (7.4%), hardware loosening (3.7%)
ICBG	Clarkson et al. [17]	13	>12	MSTS 90%, DASH score 17	Infections (15.4%)
Segmental ulna graft	Zhang et al. [24]	8	36	MSTS 83.3%, DASH score 48.9, grip strength 71%	Not mentioned
Ulna centralization	Bhagat et al. [20]	25	28.8	Grip strength 65%	Superficial wound infection (8%), additional bone grafting (8%)
	Kapoor et al. [21]	26	32.8	MSTS 86.6%, DASH score 10.1, grip strength 74%	Fracture of the ulna, hardware loosening, and reflex sympathetic dystrophy in one patient each, with an overall complication rate of 10.7%
Ulnar translocation	Puri et al. [22]	14	26	MSTS 87%	Radioulnar synostosis (7.1%), fracture (7.1%)
Partial Arthodesis					
Tibia cortical strut autograft	van de Sande et al. [6]	17	32	MSTS 71.7%, DASH score 9.2, grip strength 75%	Fracture (5.9%)
Nonvascularized/ vascularized fibula	Zhu et al. [25]	7	47.1	MSTS 85.3%, grip strength 76.5%	Fracture (28.6%)

Note: ICBG, iliac crest bone grafts; MSTS, Musculoskeletal Tumor Society scoring; DASH: disability of arm shoulder and hand scoring.

is inadequate [15]. This approach is more suitable for older, low-demand individuals or salvage cases.

FIBULAR HEAD AUTOGRAFT ARTHROPLASTY

Due to morphological similarity with the distal radius, the fibular head is a reliable autograft [30]. Nonvascularized grafts are technically simpler and avoid microsurgery; Saini et al. reported MSTS scores of 91.3% and grip strength of 71%, but subluxation (25%) and nonunion (16.7%) were notable [10]. Other studies reported grip strength recovery of 40%–70% with variable complications [8, 16].

Vascularized fibular head grafts, with intrinsic blood supply, improve incorporation in large defects or irradiated fields. Liu et al. achieved MSTS 92.3%, DASH 9, and grip strength of 71% with minimal subluxation or resorption [31]. Yang et al. [32] and Chung et al. [30] confirmed similar benefits. Drawbacks include technical demands, microvascular expertise, longer operative time, and risk of transient peroneal nerve palsy [29]. Long-term instability and degenerative changes can still occur.

PROSTHETIC WRIST REPLACEMENT

Indicated when graft reconstruction is unsuitable, especially in elderly or comorbid patients, prostheses may be unipolar (distal radius only) or total wrist replacements. Wang et al. reported Mayo wrist scores of 68 and grip strength of 68%, but 60% complication rates, including loosening, subluxation, and degeneration [33]. Advances in 3D-printed, custom uncemented designs have shown promise. Lu et al. reported a Mayo score of 72, DASH 18.7, and a few short-term complications at 14.5 months [34]. However, long-term survivorship remains uncertain, and high complication rates limit use in young, active patients.

Wrist arthroplasty offers functional mobility but with risks of nonunion, degeneration, instability, and implant failure (Table 8.2). Osteoarticular allografts restore anatomy but have high nonunion rates; fibular head autografts (especially vascularized) offer better incorporation but require technical expertise; prosthetic replacements are viable in select elderly or salvage cases but have high

TABLE 8.2
Wrist Arthroplasty after En bloc Resection of Bone Tumors of the Distal Radius

Reconstruction	Authors	Cases	Follow-Up (Months)	Functional Outcomes	Complications
Osteoarticular allograft	Asavamongkolkul et al. [35]	8	60	MSTS 93%, grip strength 72.2%	Nonunion (25%), fracture (12.5%), pain (12.5%)
	Bianchi et al. [15]	12	52	MSTS 91.7%	Nonunion (8.3%), joint instability (66.7%), subchondral bone alterations (100%)
	Duan et al. [27]	15	62.4	Mayo score 70, grip strength 27 kg	Pain (6.7%), degenerative changes (100%)
	Scoccianti et al. [28]	17	58.9	MSTS 86%	Fracture (5.9%), degenerative changes (100%)
	Kocher et al. [36]	24	130	Grip strength 64.8%	Fracture (16.7%), pain, need revision (8.3%), tolerable pain (54%), volar dislocation (4.2%)
	Li et al. [37]	10	84.7	MSTS 72%, grip strength 57.3%	Fracture (40%), subluxation (30%), nonunion (42.9%)
	van de Sande et al. [6]	7	32	MSTS 73.3%, DASH score 10.9, grip strength 80%	Plate loosening (14.3%), fracture (14.3%), nonunion (42.9%)
Vascularized fibula arthroplasty	Yang et al. [32]	17	51.6	Mayo Wrist scores 77.3, grip strength 77.2%	Pain (47%)
	Chung et al. [30]	12	75.1	MSTS 88%, grip strength 57.2%	Joint instability (41.7%)
	Liu et al. [31]	26	66.9	MSTS 92.3%, DASH score 9, grip strength 71%	Subluxation (11.8%), graft resorption (11.1%), degenerative changes (19%)
	Innocenti et al. [38]	6	52.8	Unavailable	Peroneal nerve palsy (33.3%)
Nonvascularized fibula arthroplasty	Chadha M et al. [8]	9	56	Unavailable	Fracture (22.2%), subluxation (11.1%), graft resorption (11.1%)
	Saini R et al. [10]	12	69.6	MSTS 91.3%, grip strength 71%	Subluxation (25%), nonunion (16.7%)
	Qu et al. [16]	13	80	MSTS 83%, DASH score 17, grip strength 40%	Subluxation (30.7%), nonunion (7.7%), flap necrosis (7.7%), CPN paralysis (7.7%)
	Asavamongkolkul et al. [35]	7	60	MSTS 93%, grip strength 69%	Pain (28.6%)

(Continued)

TABLE 8.2 ***(Continued)***
Wrist Arthroplasty after En bloc Resection of Bone Tumors of the Distal Radius

Reconstruction	Authors	Cases	Follow-Up (Months)	Functional Outcomes	Complications
	Humail et al. [29]	12	24	Grip strength 60%	Peroneal nerve palsy (16.7%), subluxation (16.7%), superficial wound infection (25%)
	Qi et al. [39]	12	39.6	MSTS 84.1%, DASH score 13, grip strength 55.2%	Carpal bone subluxation (25%), dislocation (8.3%), osteoarthritis (91.7%)
	Saikia et al. [40]	24	79.2	Grip strength 67%	Deep infection (4.1%), fracture (4.1%), subluxation (12.3%)
	Zhu et al. [25]	7	48	MSTS 86.3%, grip strength 59.2%	Subluxation (28.6%), degenerative changes (17.9%)
Prosthesis replacement	Wang et al. [33]	10	52	Mayo Wrist scores 68, grip strength 68%	Loosening (10%), subluxation (20%), degenerative changes (30%)
	Zhang et al. [41]	11	55.5	MSTS 80.3%, grip strength 72%	Superficial infection (9%), tolerable pain (9%)
	Natarajan et al. [42]	24	78	MSTS 74%	Flap necrosis (8.3%), deep infection (8.3%)
	Lu et al. [34]	11	14.5	Mayo Wrist scores 72, DASH score 18.7, grip strength 69.9%	NA

MSTS, Musculoskeletal Tumor Society scoring; DASH: Disability of Arm, Shoulder, and Hand scoring; CPN, common peroneal nerve.

complication risks. Careful patient selection and precise surgical technique are crucial for optimizing long-term outcomes.

STABILIZATION STRATEGIES IN WRIST RECONSTRUCTION

Joint instability is a major concern in wrist arthroplasty, particularly with biological reconstructions such as fibular head or osteoarticular allografts. Loss of key stabilizers—the capsule, radiocarpal ligaments, triangular fibrocartilage complex (TFCC), and distal interosseous membrane—necessitates targeted reconstruction.

The biceps femoris tendon, attached to the fibular head, can be woven into residual capsular and interosseous structures to restore stability [40]. Alternative methods utilize the fibular head capsule, lateral collateral ligament, or flexor carpi radialis tendon [43]. For distal radioulnar joint (DRUJ) instability, the Adams–Berger tendon graft technique through bone tunnels provides rotational stability [44].

Preserving or reconstructing the wrist's three-column support improves mechanical outcomes. The Sauvé–Kapandji (S-K) procedure, combined with distal radial allograft and DRUJ arthrodesis, offers a stable yet mobile construct. Szabo et al. reported enhanced grip strength, range of motion, and fewer degenerative changes [45], with Li et al. confirming superior outcomes over non-modified reconstructions [37].

DISTAL ULNA

Tumors of the distal ulna are rare but present unique challenges due to the anatomical and functional role of this region in forearm rotation, wrist stability, and load transmission through the DRUJ. Giant cell tumor of bone (GCTB) involving the distal ulna accounts for only 0.45%–3.2% of all GCTB cases. In Campanacci grade 3 lesions with cortical destruction, soft tissue extension, or recurrence after curettage, en bloc resection is frequently required [46].

While the distal ulna is often described as "expendable," its removal can lead to significant biomechanical consequences. The residual ulnar stump may impinge on the radius during rotation, displace dorsally, causing extensor tendon irritation or rupture, and contribute to ulnar translocation of the carpus with impaired load sharing. The DRUJ and the TFCC are critical components in maintaining the dynamic stability of the wrist and forearm. Together, they facilitate smooth pronation and supination, transmit axial loads across the wrist, and stabilize the distal ulna against the radius during movement. The TFCC acts as a suspensory and cushioning structure for the ulnar side of the carpus, contributing to both load-bearing and rotational control. Loss of the DRUJ and TFCC disrupts forearm stability, smooth pronation-supination, and axial load transfer, particularly during grip-intensive activities [47].

Dynamic radioulnar convergence is a common sequela after ulnar head resection, with the radius shifting ulnarward during rotation, causing painful impingement, instability, and reduced grip strength. Although some studies have reported acceptable results without reconstruction [48], growing recognition of the functional deficits associated with DRUJ loss has shifted attention toward reconstructive or stabilizing techniques in selected patients [47, 49].

ULNAR BUTTRESS ARTHROPLASTY

This technique involves placement of a tricortical iliac crest autograft adjacent to the carpal-ulnar junction to provide a static buttress, preventing carpal-ulnar translocation and stump impingement (Figure 8.4). Internal fixation secures the graft, which does not restore the DRUJ but preserves wrist alignment and load distribution. Kapoor et al. [46] reported 100% radiologic union, favorable MSTS and QuickDASH scores, and no instability or recurrence. The method is technically straightforward, avoids microsurgical complexity, and has minimal donor-site morbidity, making it a practical option in oncologic settings.

STABILIZATION OF THE ULNAR STUMP

An unstabilized stump may displace dorsally, irritating soft tissues and jeopardizing tendon function. Multiple soft tissue stabilization techniques have been described:

- **Extensor Carpi Ulnaris tenodesis** (ECU) using a distally based extensor carpi ulnaris strip (Goldner and Hayes [50]; Kayias et al. [51])
- **Lasso tendon grafts** (Gainor [52])
- **Dual tendon stabilization** using portions of FCU (flexor carpi ulnaris) and ECU threaded into the stump canal (Breen and Jupiter [53])
- **Pronator quadratus advancement** (Johnson [54])
- **Various autograft and fascial wraps**, including fascia lata or plate arthrodesis (Ferracini et al. [55])

These aim to reduce stump mobility, minimize dorsal displacement, and protect extensor tendons. However, their necessity is debated. Wolfe et al. [56] and others [57–59] reported comparable outcomes without stabilization, and cadaveric studies have shown no consistent biomechanical advantage. Therefore, stump stabilization should be individualized, based on patient activity demands, intraoperative stability, and soft tissue status.

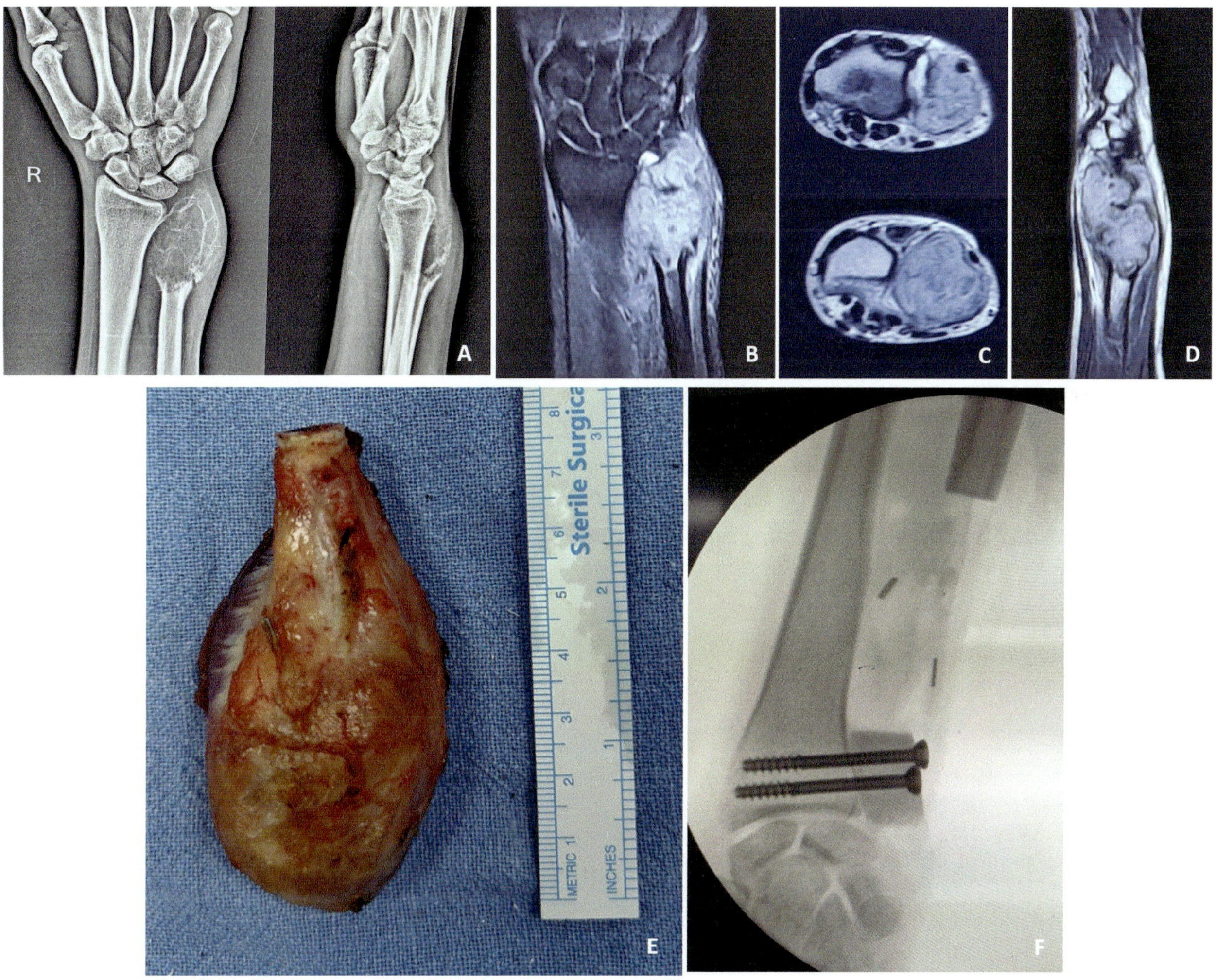

FIGURE 8.4 X-rays (A) and magnetic resonance imaging [coronal (B), axial (C) & sagittal (D) of a patient with Campanacci grade 3 GCTB distal ulna]. En bloc resection was performed (E), followed by Ulnar buttress arthroplasty using a tricortical iliac crest autograft placed adjacent to the carpal–ulnar junction and secured with internal fixation (F).

ALTERNATIVE RECONSTRUCTION TECHNIQUES

- **Allograft reconstruction** with osteoarticular distal ulna segments attempts to restore anatomy and DRUJ congruity, but is limited by risks of nonunion, resorption, and immune rejection [60].
- **Prosthetic replacement** (constrained and non-constrained) may restore anatomy with early mobilization and is sometimes combined with tendon wraps (e.g., brachioradialis) [61, 62]. While short-term outcomes are promising, challenges include bone loss, soft tissue coverage issues, cost, and limited availability. Their long-term durability in oncologic applications remains uncertain, and they are not widely used.

Given these considerations, biologically favorable and technically simpler options—such as ulnar buttress grafting or selective soft tissue stabilization—remain preferred in most centers for distal ulna tumor reconstruction. These methods offer a balance between oncologic safety, functional preservation, and complication minimization.

SUMMARY

- Limb salvage around the wrist requires careful surgical planning to achieve oncological clearance while optimizing functional preservation.
- Total wrist arthrodesis offers reliable structural stability and is preferred in high-demand patients requiring robust load transmission.
- Motion-preserving options, including partial arthrodesis and wrist arthroplasty, are appropriate for selected low-demand individuals, though with higher risk of complications.
- Centralization or translocation of the ulna provides an effective and biologically favorable method for reconstruction following distal radius resection.
- Reconstruction after distal ulna resection can be individualized, with ulnar stump stabilization or ulnar buttress arthroplasty offering improved outcomes in selected cases.

REFERENCES

1. Harness NG, Mankin HJ. Giant-cell tumor of the distal forearm. *J Hand Surg Am.* 2004;29(2):188–193.
2. Khan MT, Gray JM, Carter SR, Grimer RJ, Tillman RM. Management of the giant-cell tumours of the distal radius. *Ann R Coll Surg Engl.* 2004;86(1):18–24.
3. Mavrogenis AF, Galanopoulos J, Vottis C, et al. Osteoarticular allograft reconstruction for an angiosarcoma of the distal radius. *J Long Term Eff Med Implants.* 2016;26(2):79–87.
4. Higuchi T, Yamamoto N, Hayashi K, et al. Successful joint preservation of distal radius osteosarcoma by en bloc tumor excision and reconstruction using a tumor-bearing frozen autograft: a case report. *BMC Surg.* 2018;18(1):12.
5. Ichihara S, Hidalgo-Diaz JJ, Facca S, Liverneaux P. Unicompartmental isoelastic resurfacing prosthesis for malignant tumor of the distal radius: a case report with a 3-year follow-up. *Orthop Traumatol Surg Res.* 2015;101(8):969–971.
6. van de Sande MA, van Geldorp NH, Dijkstra PD, Taminiau AH. Surgical technique: tibia cortical strut autograft interposition arthrodesis after distal radius resection. *Clin Orthop Relat Res.* 2013;471(3):803–813.
7. Wysocki RW, Soni E, Virkus WW, et al. Is intralesional treatment of giant cell tumor of the distal radius comparable to resection with respect to local control and functional outcome? *Clin Orthop Relat Res.* 2015;473(2):706–715.
8. Chadha M, Arora SS, Singh AP, et al. Autogenous non-vascularized fibula for treatment of giant cell tumor of distal end radius. *Arch Orthop Trauma Surg.* 2010;130(11):1467–1473.
9. Liu YP, Li KH, Sun BH. Which treatment is the best for giant cell tumors of the distal radius? A meta-analysis. *Clin Orthop Relat Res.* 2012;470(10):2886–2894.
10. Saini R, Bali K, Bachhal V, et al. En bloc excision and autogenous fibular reconstruction for aggressive giant cell tumor of distal radius: a report of 12 cases and review of literature. *J Orthop Surg Res.* 2011;6:14.
11. Liu W, Wang B, Zhang S, et al. Wrist reconstruction after en bloc resection of bone tumors of the distal radius. *Orthop Surg.* 2021;13(2):376–383.
12. Sargazi N, Philpott M, Malik A, Waseem M. Ulna autograft for wrist arthrodesis: a novel approach in failed wrist arthroplasty. *Open Orthop J.* 2017;11:768–776.
13. Adams BD, Kleinhenz BP, Guan JJ. Wrist arthrodesis for failed total wrist arthroplasty. *J Hand Surg Am.* 2016;41(6):673–679.
14. Grandizio LC, Maschke S. Wrist arthrodesis with femoral head structural allograft after failed total wrist arthroplasty. *Tech Hand Up Extrem Surg.* 2017;21(3):116–120.
15. Bianchi G, Donati D, Staals EL, Mercuri M. Osteoarticular allograft reconstruction of the distal radius after bone tumour resection. *J Hand Surg.* 2005;30(4):369–373.
16. Qu H, Guo W, Li D, et al. Functional results of wrist arthrodesis versus arthroplasty with proximal fibula following giant cell tumour excision of the distal radius. *J Hand Surg Eur.* 2019;44(4):394–401.
17. Clarkson PW, Sandford K, Phillips AE, et al. Functional results following vascularized versus nonvascularized bone grafts for wrist arthrodesis following excision of giant cell tumors. *J Hand Surg.* 2013;38(5):935–940.e1.
18. Wang T, Chan CM, Yu F, et al. Does wrist arthrodesis with structural iliac crest bone graft after wide resection of distal radius giant cell tumor result in satisfactory function and local control? *Clin Orthop Relat Res.* 2017;475(3):767–775.
19. Greenwood HH. Reconstruction of forearm after loss of radius. *Br J Surg.* 1932;20:58–60.
20. Bhagat S, Bansal M, Jandhyala R, Sharma H, Amin P, Pandit JP. Wide excision and ulno-carpal arthrodesis for primary aggressive and recurrent giant cell tumours. *Int Orthop.* 2008;32(5):741–745.
21. Kapoor L, Banjara R, Sahoo B, Kumar VS, Ansari MT, Khan SA. Functional outcomes of centralization of the ulna as a method of reconstruction following resection of Campanacci grade 3 giant cell tumor of the distal radius. *J Hand Surg Am.* 2024;49(1):63.e1–63.e9.
22. Puri A, Gulia A, Agarwal MG, Reddy K. Ulnar translocation after excision of a Campanacci grade-3 giant-cell tumour of the distal radius: an effective method of reconstruction. *J Bone Joint Surg Br.* 2010;92(6):875–879.

23. Chalidis BE, Dimitriou CG. Modified ulnar translocation technique for the reconstruction of giant cell tumor of the distal radius. *Orthopedics*. 2008;31(6):608.
24. Zhang W, Zhong J, Li D, Sun C, Zhao H, Gao Y. Functional outcome of en bloc resection of a giant cell tumour of the distal radius and arthrodesis of the wrist and distal ulna using an ipsilateral double barrel segmental ulna bone graft combined with a modified Sauvé-Kapandji procedure. *J Hand Surg Eur.* 2017;42(4):377–381.
25. Zhu Z, Zhang C, Zhao S, Dong Y, Zeng B. Partial wrist arthrodesis versus arthroplasty for distal radius giant cell tumours. *Int Orthop*. 2013;37(11):2217–2223.
26. Gislason MK, Stansfield B, Bransby-Zachary M, Hems T, Nash DH. Load transfer through the radiocarpal joint and the effects of partial wrist arthrodesis on carpal bone behaviour: a finite element study. *J Hand Surg.* 2012;37(5):871–878.
27. Duan H, Zhang B, Yang HS, et al. Functional outcome of en bloc resection and osteoarticular allograft reconstruction with locking compression plate. *J Orthop Sci.* 2013;18(4):599–604.
28. Scoccianti G, Campanacci DA, Beltrami G, et al. Use of osteoarticular allografts for reconstruction after resection of the distal radius. *J Bone Joint Surg Br.* 2010;92(12):1690–1694.
29. Humail SM, Ghulam MK, Zaidi IH. Reconstruction of the distal radius with non-vascularised fibular graft. *J Orthop Surg*. 2014;22(3):356–359.
30. Chung DW, Han CS, Lee JH, Lee SG. Outcomes of wrist arthroplasty using a free vascularized fibular head graft for Enneking stage II giant cell tumors of the distal radius. *Microsurgery.* 2013;33(2):112–118.
31. Liu Q, Luo W, Zhang C, et al. How to optimize the therapeutic effect of free autogenous fibula graft and wrist arthroplasty for giant cell tumors of distal radius. *Jpn J Clin Oncol.* 2019;49(7):656–663.
32. Yang YF, Wang JW, Huang P, Xu ZH. Distal radius reconstruction with vascularized proximal fibular autograft after en-bloc resection of recurrent giant cell tumor. *BMC Musculoskelet Disord.* 2016;17(1):346.
33. Wang B, Wu Q, Liu J, et al. Functional results and complications of custom unipolar wrist hemiarthroplasty. *Clin Orthop Relat Res.* 2016;474(11):2583–2590.
34. Lu M, Min L, Xiao C, et al. Uncemented 3D-printed prosthetic replacement for distal radius GCT. *Cancer Manag Res.* 2018;10:265–277.
35. Asavamongkolkul A, Waikakul S, Phimolsarnti R, et al. Functional outcome following excision of a tumour and reconstruction of the distal radius. *Int Orthop.* 2009;33(1):203–209.
36. Kocher MS, Gebhardt MC, Mankin HJ. Reconstruction of the distal aspect of the radius with use of an osteoarticular allograft after excision of a skeletal tumor. *J Bone Joint Surg Am.* 1998;80(3):407–419.
37. Li J, Jiao Y, Guo Z, Ji Ch, Wang Z. Comparison of osteoarticular allograft reconstruction with and without the Sauvé-Kapandji procedure following tumour resection in distal radius. *J Plast Reconstr Aesthet Surg.* 2015;68(7):995–1002. doi:10.1016/j.bjps.2015.03.032
38. Innocenti M, Delcroix L, Manfrini M, Ceruso M, Capanna R. Vascularized proximal fibular epiphyseal transfer for distal radial reconstruction. *J Bone Joint Surg Am.* 2005;87(Pt 2):237–246.
39. Qi DW, Wang P, Ye ZM, et al. Clinical and radiographic results of reconstruction with fibular autograft for distal radius giant cell tumor. *Orthop Surg.* 2016;8(2):196–204.
40. Saikia KC, Borgohain M, Bhuyan SK, Goswami S, Bora A, Ahmed F. Resection-reconstruction arthroplasty for giant cell tumor of distal radius. *Indian J Orthop.* 2010;44(3):327–332.
41. Zhang S, Xu MT, Wang XQ, Wang JJ. Functional outcome of en bloc excision and custom prosthetic replacement for giant cell tumor of the distal radius. *J Orthop Sci.* 2015;20(6):1090–1097.
42. Natarajan MV, Chandra Bose J, Viswanath J, Balasubramanian N, Sameer M. Custom prosthetic replacement for distal radial tumours. *Int Orthop.* 2009;33(4):1081–1084.
43. Onoda S, Sakuraba M, Asano T, et al. Use of vascularized free fibular head grafts for upper limb oncologic reconstruction. *Plast Reconstr Surg.* 2011;127(3):1244–1253.
44. Adams BD, Lawler E. Chronic instability of the distal radioulnar joint. *J Am Acad Orthop Surg.* 2007;15(9):571–575.
45. Szabo RM, Anderson KA, Chen JL. Functional outcome of en bloc excision and osteoarticular allograft replacement with the Sauve-Kapandji procedure for Campanacci grade 3 giant-cell tumor of the distal radius. *J Hand Surg Am.* 2006;31(8):1340–1348.
46. Kapoor L, Kumar VS, Ansari MT, Khan SA. Ulnar buttress arthroplasty without ulnar stump stabilization for giant cell tumor of distal ulna. *J Wrist Surg.* 2023;13(3):215–221.
47. Papanastassiou ID, Savvidou OD, Chloros GD, Megaloikonomos PD, Kontogeorgakos VA, Papagelopoulos PJ. Extensor carpi ulnaris tenodesis versus no stabilization after wide resection of distal ulna giant cell tumors. *Hand (N Y).* 2019;14(2):242–248.
48. Dhillon MS, Saini R, Gill SS. Is there a need for reconstruction after excision of the distal ulna for giant-cell tumour? *Acta Orthop Belg.* 2010;76(1):30–37.
49. Naik MA, Sujir P, Rao SK, Tripathy SK. Ulnar buttress arthroplasty after en bloc resection of a giant cell tumor of the distal ulna. *Indian J Orthop.* 2013;47(2):211–214.
50. Goldner JL, Hayes MG. Stabilization of the remaining ulna using one-half of the extensor carpi ulnaris tendon after resection of the distal ulna. *Orthop Trans.* 1979;3:330–331.
51. Kayias EH, Drosos GI, Anagnostopoulou GA. Resection of the distal ulna for tumours and stabilisation of the stump. A case report and literature review. *Acta Orthop Belg.* 2006;72(4):484–491.
52. Gainor BJ. Lasso stabilization of the distal ulna after tumor resection: a report of two cases. *J Hand Surg Am.* 1995;20(2):324–326.
53. Breen TF, Jupiter JB. Extensor carpi ulnaris and flexor carpi ulnaris tenodesis of the unstable distal ulna. *J Hand Surg Am.* 1989;14(4):612–617.
54. Johnson RK. Stabilization of the distal ulna by transfer of the pronator quadratus origin. *Clin Orthop Relat Res.* 1992;(275):130–132.
55. Ferracini R, Masterson EL, Bell RS, Wunder JS. Distal ulnar tumours. Results of management by en bloc resection in nine patients and review of the literature. *J Hand Surg Br.* 1998;23(4):517–521.
56. Wolfe SW, Mih AD, Hotchkiss RN, Culp RW, Keifhaber TR, Nagle DJ. Wide excision of the distal ulna: a multicenter case study. *J Hand Surg Am.* 1998;23(2):222–228.
57. Petersen MS, Adams BD. Biomechanical evaluation of distal radioulnar reconstructions. *J Hand Surg Am.* 1993;18(2):328–334.
58. Sauerbier M, Berger RA, Fujita M, Hahn ME. Radioulnar convergence after distal ulnar resection: mechanical performance of two commonly used soft tissue stabilizing procedures. *Acta Orthop Scand.* 2003;74(4):420–428.

59. Wurapa RK, Whipple R. Distal radioulnar allograft reconstruction after giant cell tumor resection. *Am J Orthop (Belle Mead NJ)*. 2003;32(8):397–400.
60. Burke CS, Gupta A, Buecker P. Distal ulna giant cell tumor resection with reconstruction using distal ulna prosthesis and brachioradialis wrap soft tissue stabilization. *Hand (N Y)*. 2009;4(4):410–414.
61. Gracia I, Proubasta IR, Trullols L, et al. Distal radioulnar joint prosthesis for the treatment of giant cell tumor of the distal ulna: a case report and literature review. *Strategies Trauma Limb Reconstr.* 2011;6(2):103–106.
62. Pirela-Cruz MA, Higgs M, Reddy K, et al. Treatment of a giant cell tumor of the distal ulna with a fully constrained prosthesis. *El Paso Phys Mag*. 2008;31(3):9–13.

Section III

Lower Extremity

9 Proximal Femur Resection and Reconstruction

INTRODUCTION

The proximal femur is a common site for both primary malignant bone tumors—such as osteosarcoma, chondrosarcoma, and Ewing sarcoma—and secondary involvement from metastatic disease, most frequently originating from breast, lung, thyroid, kidney, and prostate carcinomas [1]. Surgical management in this region is challenging due to its critical biomechanical role in weight transmission and mobility, as well as the presence of vital neurovascular structures and key muscle attachments. Preservation or reconstruction of soft tissue stabilizers, particularly the hip capsule and abductor mechanism, is paramount to achieving optimal postoperative stability and function [2]. Preoperative planning must consider the potential for intracapsular tumor extension or skip metastases via the ligamentum teres, which may necessitate intra- or extra-articular resections.

Reconstruction following proximal femoral resection has advanced considerably, with modular endoprosthetic replacement now the standard approach, offering immediate stability and reliable function. Other strategies, including allograft-prosthetic composites and selected biological reconstructions, remain valuable in specific patient populations. This chapter reviews anatomical considerations, surgical approaches, and reconstructive techniques, emphasizing evidence-based selection and functional outcomes.

SURGICAL ANATOMY

The proximal femur is a region of considerable anatomical and functional complexity, and safe oncologic resection demands a thorough understanding of its osseous, capsuloligamentous, muscular, and neurovascular relationships.

OSSEOUS ANATOMY

The proximal femur consists of the femoral head, neck, greater and lesser trochanters, and the proximal metaphyseal–diaphyseal junction. The femoral head articulates with the acetabulum to form the hip joint, with the largely intracapsular neck providing a potential pathway for tumor spread into the joint, particularly in cases of pathologic fracture or aggressive intraosseous lesions. The greater trochanter serves as the insertion site for the gluteus medius and minimus (primary abductors), while the lesser trochanter provides attachment for the iliopsoas tendon (primary hip flexor). Posteriorly, the linea aspera serves as an important muscular origin and a key rotational landmark when native proximal anatomy is lost during reconstruction.

CAPSULE AND LIGAMENTUM TERES

The hip joint capsule attaches from the acetabular rim to the intertrochanteric line anteriorly and the base of the femoral neck posteriorly. Tumor infiltration of the capsule, particularly after fracture, may necessitate en bloc capsular resection or extra-articular hip resection. The ligamentum teres, extending from the femoral head to the acetabular fossa, has oncologic relevance as a rare conduit for transarticular tumor spread, especially in sarcomas, mandating careful preoperative imaging of the acetabulum.

MUSCULAR ATTACHMENTS AND FUNCTION

Hip stability and gait are heavily dependent on the periarticular musculature. The gluteus medius and minimus, inserting on the greater trochanter, are critical abductors; their preservation or reattachment to the prosthesis is essential to prevent Trendelenburg gait. The psoas major, inserting into the lesser trochanter, provides hip flexion and anteromedial stability, and its reattachment helps maintain muscle balance. The gluteus maximus, the primary extensor, is reflected during posterior exposure, while the vastus lateralis is mobilized and advanced proximally for implant coverage. In extra-articular resections, sufficient quadriceps function must be preserved for knee extension. Medial tumor extension may require partial sacrifice of the adductor brevis or magnus, typically with minimal long-term functional deficit.

NEUROVASCULAR ANATOMY

Medially, the femoral artery traverses the femoral triangle before giving rise to the profunda femoris artery—the principal blood supply to the thigh. Tumors with significant medial or posterior soft tissue extension may displace or encase these vessels. Preoperative angiography can delineate vessel involvement and assess collateral flow should vascular sacrifice be required. The femoral vein lies medial to the artery, while the femoral nerve lies lateral and anterior; both are at risk during medial dissection. Posteriorly, the sciatic nerve courses adjacent to the short external rotators and gluteal musculature, making early identification and careful mobilization imperative. Preservation of the sciatic nerve is critical to maintaining distal limb function, especially in ambulatory patients.

A detailed appreciation of these relationships facilitates complete tumor excision while preserving vital structures, optimizing both oncologic safety and postoperative function.

DOI: 10.1201/9780367822002-12

PREOPERATIVE PLANNING

The complexity and anatomical variability of proximal femur tumors demand meticulous preoperative planning, integrating clinical evaluation, imaging, and functional assessment. The objectives are to define the tumor's extent, assess soft tissue, capsular, and neurovascular involvement, plan surgical margins, and select the optimal reconstructive strategy.

Plain radiographs provide an overview of bone destruction, cortical breach, and pathological fractures (Figure 9.1). Magnetic resonance imaging (MRI) is essential for determining intramedullary extent, soft tissue involvement, capsular invasion, and skip lesions (Figure 9.2), while computed tomography (CT) refines cortical assessment and supports 3D planning. CT angiography is particularly useful when medial soft tissue masses may involve major vessels. In hypervascular metastases, such as from renal or thyroid carcinoma, preoperative embolization reduces intraoperative bleeding risk.

Positron emission tomography–CT (PET-CT) assists in evaluating systemic disease, guiding the choice between limb salvage and palliative options. Prosthesis templating is critical, as modular systems require a minimum resection length (≈70 mm). In cases with limited residual bone, custom implants or revision stems may be required, with intraoperative trial reductions ensuring appropriate length and version.

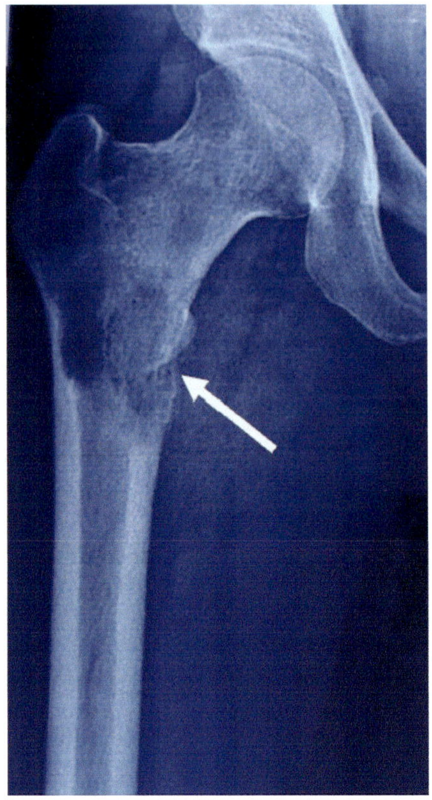

FIGURE 9.1 Plain radiograph shows an ill-defined, lytic lesion involving the proximal femur with cortical destruction (arrow) and extension into the soft tissues.

SURGICAL TECHNIQUE OF PROXIMAL FEMUR RESECTION

Patient Positioning and Exposure

Proximal femur resections are most commonly performed with the patient in the **lateral decubitus position**, which offers optimal access to both anterior and posterior compartments of the hip and proximal thigh. The pelvis and contralateral limb are securely stabilized, with meticulous padding of pressure points. A long, extensile lateral incision is made, extending from several centimeters above the greater trochanter distally along the lateral thigh (Figure 9.3). In cases of medial or proximal tumor extension, an **ilioinguinal extension** can be incorporated to expose the femoral triangle and medial soft tissues.

Following incision of the fascia lata, the **gluteus maximus** is split along its fibers to expose the retrogluteal space, short external rotators, posterior capsule, and sciatic nerve. The sciatic nerve is identified early and mobilized if distorted by a posterior soft tissue mass (Figure 9.4).

The **gluteus medius and minimus** are visualized, and if oncologically feasible, a **trochanteric osteotomy** is performed to preserve the abductor mechanism as a composite unit; otherwise, their tendinous insertions are divided and tagged for later reattachment. Anteriorly, the **tensor fascia lata** is elevated, the **rectus femoris** is identified, and the **vastus lateralis** is reflected from its femoral origin after ligating posterior perforators. The vastus lateralis is preserved for later prosthetic coverage.

AUTHORS' PREFERRED ANTERIOR APPROACH (FIGURE 9.5)

In selected cases—especially with anterior or medial soft tissue extension—an **anterior approach** is favored. This approach provides early control of the **superficial femoral vessels**, minimizes disruption of posterior musculature, and allows precise prosthetic placement.

With the patient supine on a radiolucent table, a skin incision extends from the anterior iliac crest to the anterior superior iliac spine (ASIS), then curves inferomedially toward the lateral patella, depending on resection length (Figure 9.5B). Care is taken to preserve the **lateral femoral cutaneous nerve (LFCN)** to avoid postoperative dysesthesia or neuroma.

The superficial internervous plane is developed between the **sartorius** (femoral nerve) medially and **tensor fascia lata** (superior gluteal nerve) laterally (Figure 9.5C). The **ascending branch of the lateral femoral circumflex artery** is identified and ligated. If required, the sartorius is detached proximally for improved exposure and later reattached for anterior prosthetic coverage.

The deep internervous plane lies between the **rectus femoris** (femoral nerve) and **gluteus medius** (superior gluteal nerve; Figure 9.5D). The rectus femoris is detached from both heads, and the iliopsoas is retracted medially (Figure 9.5E).

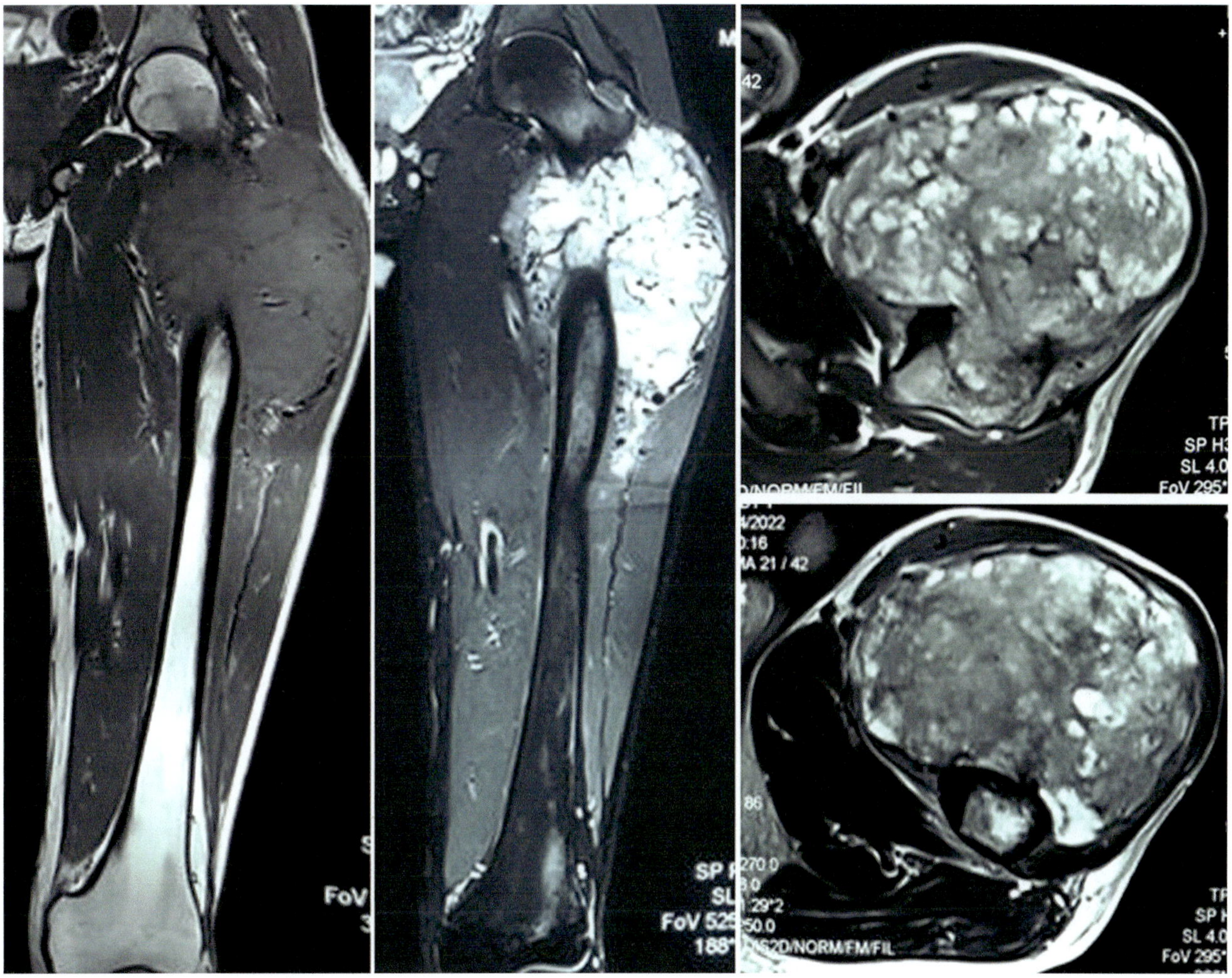

FIGURE 9.2 MRI images demonstrate a large, heterogeneous intramedullary lesion with cortical breach and extensive soft tissue extension. The tumor shows areas of necrosis and mineralization with heterogeneous contrast enhancement. MRI clearly delineates the extent of marrow involvement, soft tissue spread, and relation to surrounding neurovascular structures, which is crucial for surgical planning.

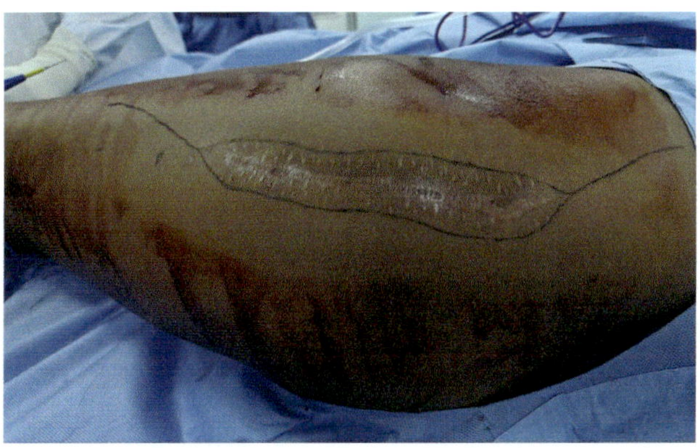

FIGURE 9.3 Lateral incision extending from above the greater trochanter, extending distally along the lateral thigh, incorporating the previous scar, in a case of Ewing sarcoma of the proximal femur.

The gluteus medius is retracted laterally to expose the anterior capsule and proximal femur. Capsulotomy, performed longitudinally or in a T-shape, is followed by gentle dislocation of the hip (Figure 9.5F, G).

SOFT TISSUE DISSECTION AND NEUROVASCULAR MANAGEMENT

Medially, the **psoas tendon** is divided at the lesser trochanter, with detachment of adductor brevis and magnus as required. The **profunda femoris artery** may be sacrificed if tumor-encased, provided that superficial femoral artery patency is confirmed preoperatively. The **femoral nerve** is preserved unless directly invaded.

Posteriorly, the sciatic nerve remains protected throughout. Dissection is guided by preoperative imaging, with angiography recommended for lesions near major vessels.

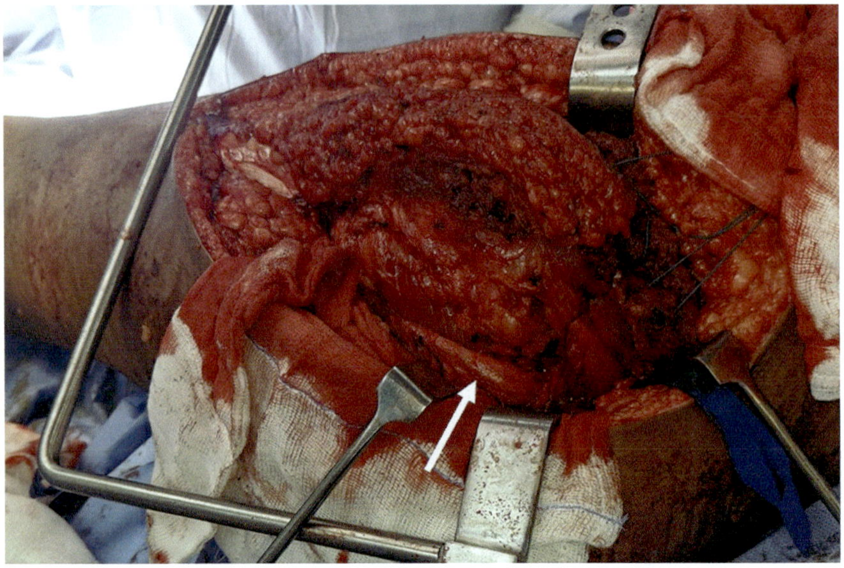

FIGURE 9.4 Intra-operative picture showing the sciatic nerve (white arrow) identified early and mobilized.

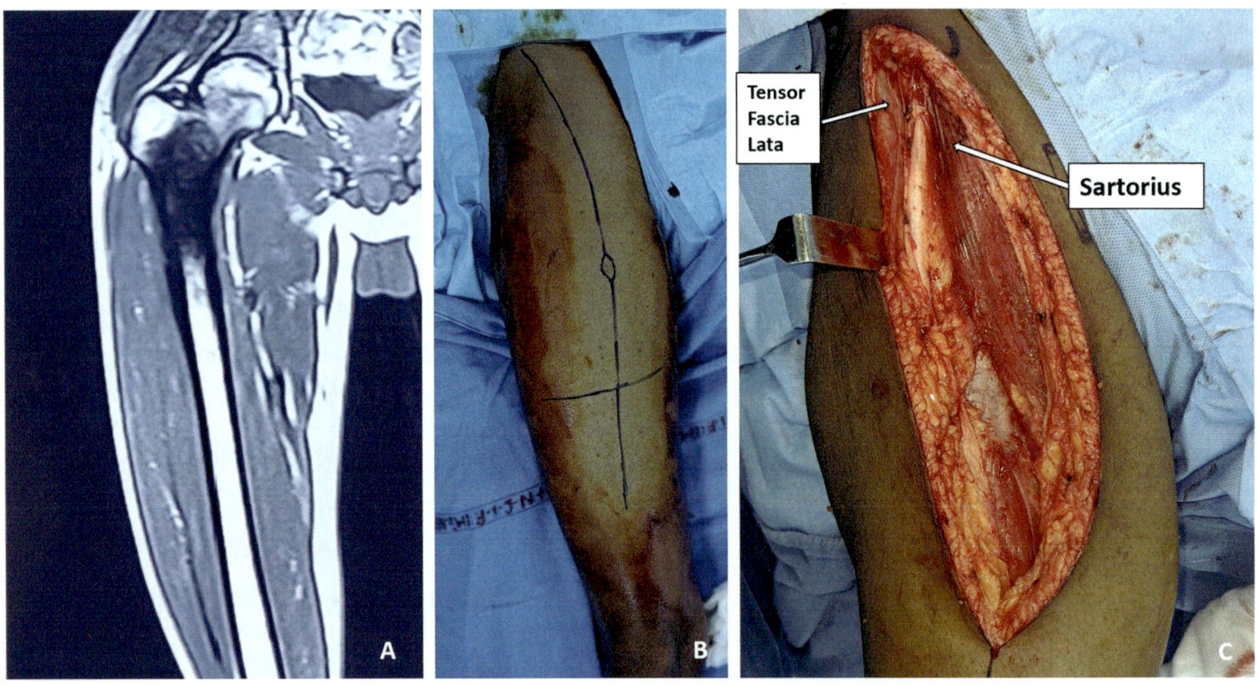

FIGURE 9.5 (A) MRI of a 19-year-old male with Ewing sarcoma of the proximal femur. (B) Skin incision starting from the anterior iliac crest to the anterior superior iliac spine, and extending distally over the anterior proximal thigh towards the lateral patella. (C) The superficial plane is developed between the sartorius medially and tensor fascia lata laterally.

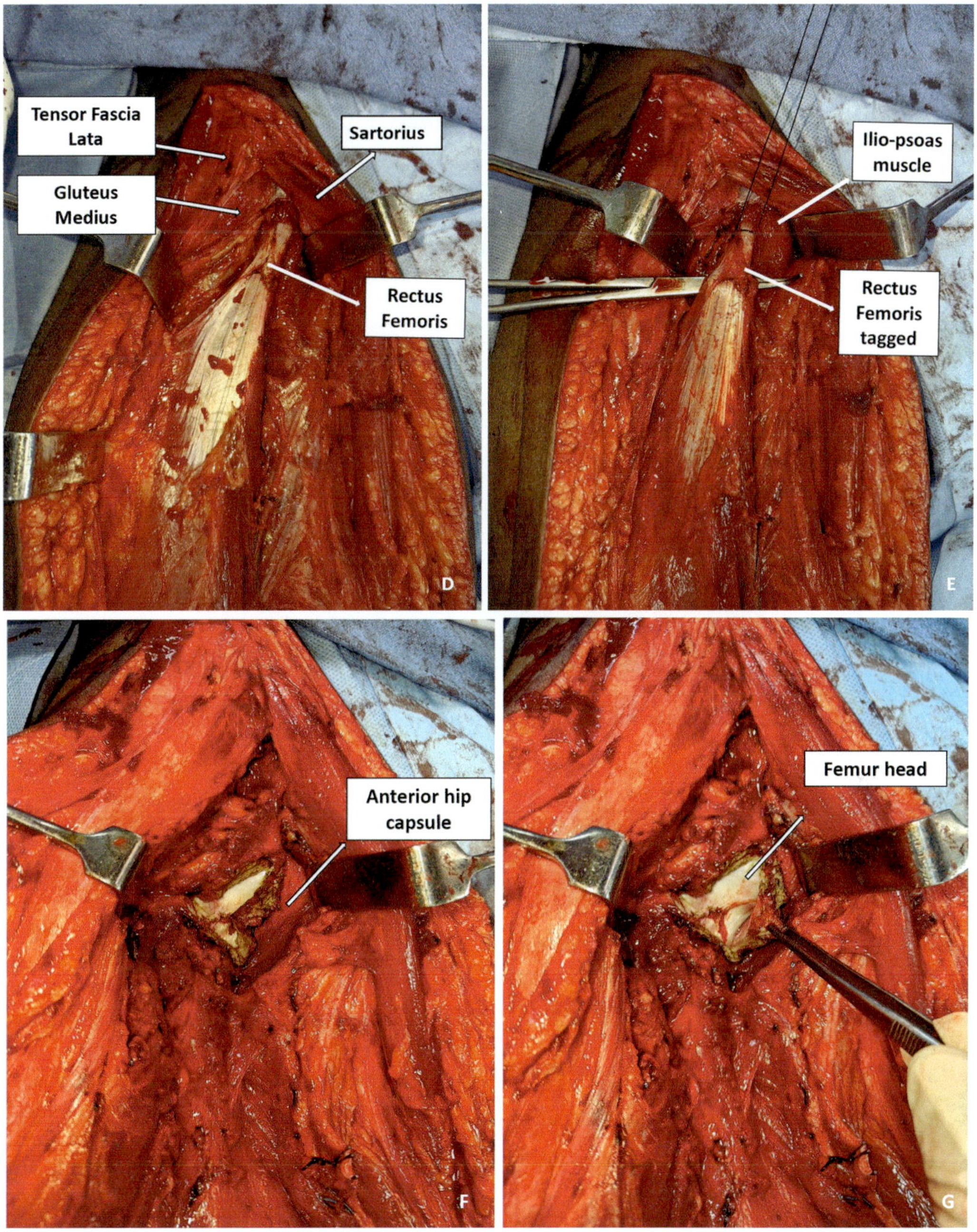

FIGURE 9.5 (Continued) (D) The deep plane is developed between the rectus femoris and gluteus medius. (E) The rectus femoris is detached from both heads, and the iliopsoas is retracted medially. (F) Exposure of the anterior hip capsule. The capsule is incised in a T-shape manner. (G) Incision of the hip capsule exposes the femoral head.

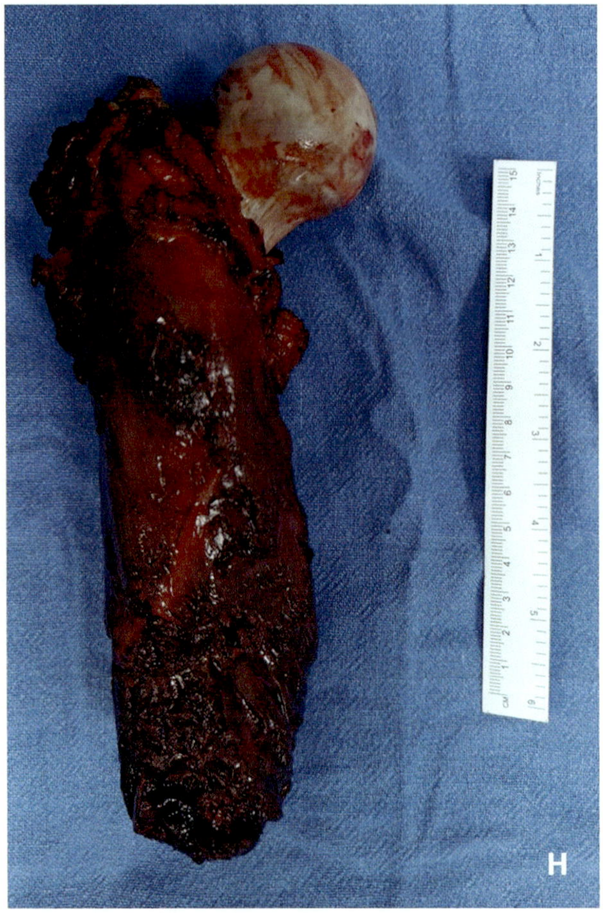

FIGURE 9.5 (Continued) (H) Resected tumor specimen.

DETERMINATION OF RESECTION LEVEL AND OSTEOTOMY

Osteotomy level is dictated by MRI and radiographic margins: **3–5 cm beyond tumor** for high-grade sarcomas, and **1–2 cm** for low-grade or metastatic lesions. An oscillating saw is used with medial retractor protection. Excessive limb distraction post-osteotomy is avoided to protect the sciatic nerve and femoral vessels.

The specimen is removed en bloc, labeled, and oriented for pathology (Figure 9.5H). Frozen sections from the medullary canal may confirm clear margins before reconstruction.

PREPARATION FOR RECONSTRUCTION

Residual tendinous and muscular structures—including the abductors, psoas, and adductors—are tagged for reattachment. If the greater trochanter is preserved, it may be reattached to the prosthetic shoulder with cables or screws to restore the **abductor lever arm**, thereby improving postoperative gait mechanics.

RECONSTRUCTION OPTIONS

Proximal Femur Endoprosthesis

Endoprosthetic replacement remains the most widely adopted method of reconstruction following proximal femoral tumor resection, offering immediate structural stability, restoration of limb length and alignment, and the potential for early mobilization. Its versatility is largely attributed to advances in **modular prosthetic systems**, which allow intraoperative customization of implant length, version, and head configuration, thereby accommodating a broad spectrum of resection lengths and patient anatomies. This adaptability is particularly valuable in oncologic surgery, where resection margins may vary depending on intraoperative findings. The technique can be divided into several key stages.

Implant Selection

Implant selection begins with a comprehensive preoperative imaging review to determine the anticipated resection length, residual canal diameter, and likely hip joint configuration—whether a bipolar or total hip design is more suitable, and whether a constrained liner is required. Templating allows estimation of the stem diameter and length and ensures that adequate residual femur will remain to accommodate a standard stem; in cases with insufficient length, a **custom stem** or even total femoral replacement may be necessary. Following tumor resection, the excised segment length, femoral head size, and distal canal diameter are measured to guide final implant selection.

Canal Preparation

Preparation of the femoral canal is tailored to bone quality and oncologic context. For patients with metastatic disease or osteoporotic bone, **cemented fixation** is preferred, allowing immediate full weight-bearing and reducing the risk of early loosening. Here, the largest feasible stem is selected, with a 1-mm circumferential cement mantle achieved by reaming the canal approximately 2 mm larger than the stem diameter. Conversely, **uncemented porous-coated or fluted stems** are often used in younger patients with good diaphyseal bone stock to promote long-term biological fixation [3]. The distal osteotomy is fashioned perpendicular to the femoral axis to provide flat cortical apposition, facilitating optimal stem seating and load transfer. Canal clearance is confirmed to prevent malalignment or rotational errors during implantation.

Trial Assembly and Limb Reconstruction

A **trial assembly** is then performed using modular components to reproduce the planned limb length, offset, and anteversion. In older patients or those with deficient abductor function, a bipolar hemiarthroplasty is often preferred, whereas younger patients with preserved acetabular cartilage and abductor mechanism may benefit from total hip replacement. Trial reduction allows assessment of stability in flexion, adduction, and internal rotation, with soft tissue tension and distal pulses checked to ensure adequate limb perfusion and alignment. Discrepancies in leg length can be addressed by adjusting neck lengths or adding modular spacers, with the use of intraoperative fluoroscopy to verify component alignment.

Measures to Ensure Rotational Alignment

Rotational alignment remains a technical challenge after proximal femoral resection because native anatomic references, such as the femoral neck or greater trochanter, are absent. While the linea aspera can provide a posterior reference, its orientation is variable and unreliable in isolation. Optimal anteversion is approximately 10°–15° relative to the knee flexion axis. In cemented stems, trial components may lack rotational stability, complicating anteversion assessment before final fixation. In uncemented stems, insertion before determining anteversion may preclude subsequent adjustment. Some surgeons confirm alignment by ensuring the stem points anteriorly when the knee is flexed to 90°, which restores physiological rotation and reduces the risk of dislocation.

Prosthesis Implantation

Definitive implantation follows thorough canal lavage and preparation. Cemented stems are inserted after placement of a distal cement restrictor, allowing adequate cement pressurization and uniform distribution. Uncemented stems are inserted with a line-to-line fit to achieve primary stability. Continuous verification of implant rotation and alignment during cement curing is essential to avoid malposition. For hemiarthroplasty, the prosthetic head is articulated with the native acetabulum; for total hip arthroplasty, the acetabulum is prepared and fitted with a press-fit or cemented cup, often with constrained liners in cases of abductor deficiency or capsular loss [4].

Acetabular Considerations

Acetabular considerations are dictated by patient age, tumor involvement, and anticipated longevity. In elderly patients with intact acetabular cartilage, bipolar hemiarthroplasty is generally adequate, although it carries a long-term risk of acetabular erosion. In younger patients or those with pre-existing arthritis, total hip arthroplasty with either cemented or uncemented cups may be preferable. Constrained liners may be indicated in the presence of deficient capsular support or absent abductors.

Soft Tissue Reattachment and Stability Restoration

Soft tissue reconstruction is critical to stability and function, as resection frequently sacrifices the joint capsule and abductor mechanism. Dislocation is the most common early complication after proximal femur endoprosthetic replacement, with reported rates ranging from 2% to 8%. Many modern prostheses incorporate dedicated abductor attachment devices such as suture holes, porous-coated cones, or trochanteric plates to facilitate reattachment. When the greater trochanter is preserved, it can be re-secured to the prosthetic shoulder with cables or screws to restore the abductor lever arm. In cases with only tendinous remnants, the gluteus medius and minimus are reattached to the prosthesis using nonabsorbable sutures passed through suture holes or porous-coated areas. Posterolateral stability can be reinforced by suturing the external rotators proximally, while anterior stability is aided by psoas tenodesis to the capsule.

Reconstruction of the hip capsule is often attempted to reduce dislocation risk. Techniques include purse-string repair with heavy suture or synthetic materials such as Dacron tape, Trevira tubes, or Prolene mesh. Bickels et al. [5] reported only one dislocation using Dacron capsulorrhaphy in 36 patients, although two cases of deep infection occurred. Gosheger et al. [6] reported two dislocations and three late infections using a Trevira tube in 38 cases. Some authors advocate wrapping the prosthesis with mesh or synthetic sleeves to promote soft tissue ingrowth and provide a stable interface [7, 8]. The present authors prefer a Prolene mesh construct anchored circumferentially to the remaining capsule and acetabular labrum with No. 5 Ethibond sutures, then wrapped around the prosthesis to create a reinforced sleeve to which the abductors are reattached (Figures 9.6A–9.6E).

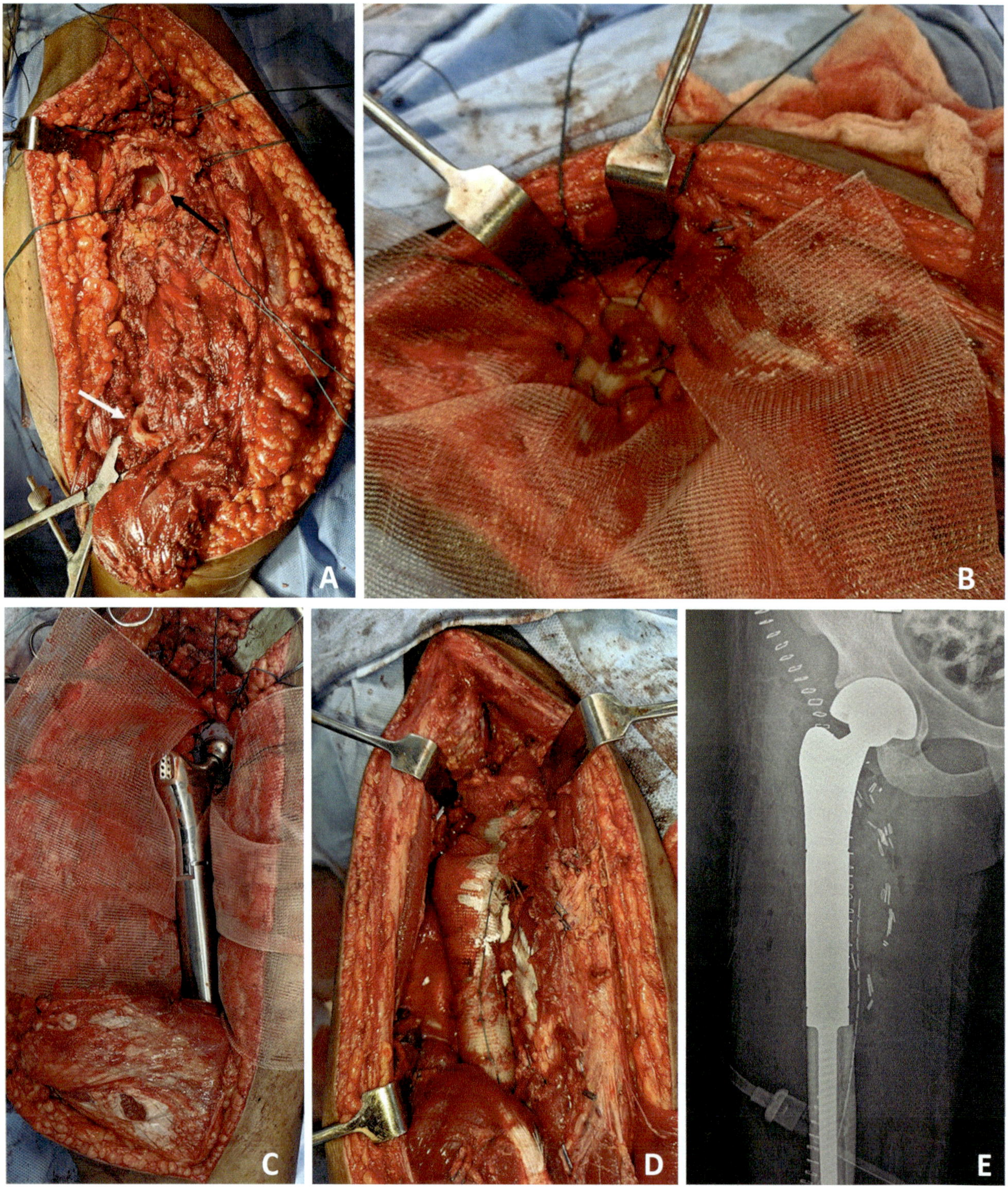

FIGURE 9.6 (A) Intra-operative picture of the surgical bed after tumor resection showing the acetabulum (black arrow) and the residual femur (white arrow). (B) Prolene mesh construct anchored circumferentially to the remaining capsule and acetabular labrum with No. 5 Ethibond sutures. (C) Reconstruction of the defect with implantation of the proximal femur endoprosthesis. (D) Mesh is then wrapped around the prosthesis to create a reinforced sleeve to which the abductors and residual muscles are reattached. (E) Post-operative radiographs following reconstruction with proximal femur endoprosthesis.

Wound Closure and Postoperative Protocol

Wound closure is performed in layers, ensuring robust muscular coverage over the prosthesis. Drains are routinely placed, and antibiotic prophylaxis is continued per institutional protocol. Weight-bearing is generally permitted immediately for cemented stems, whereas uncemented stems require protected loading for six to eight weeks. Abduction orthoses are selectively used in patients with compromised soft tissue reconstructions during the first postoperative month. Physiotherapy begins on the first postoperative day, emphasizing gait training, hip range of motion, and progressive abductor strengthening.

Outcomes of proximal femoral endoprostheses are generally favorable in oncologic reconstruction. Functional recovery is satisfactory, with most studies reporting **Musculoskeletal Tumor Society (MSTS)** scores of 20–25/30. Li et al. [1], in a meta-analysis of 265 patients across nine studies, reported a pooled mean MSTS score of 22.5. Implant survival is excellent in the short-to-medium term, with pooled survival rates of 98% at one year, 88% at five years, and 73% at ten years. Dislocation remains the leading early complication, whereas deep infection (3%–7%) and aseptic loosening (3%–6%) account for most late failures. Periprosthetic fractures occur in 1%–3% of cases, and local recurrence rates of approximately 7% have been reported in high-grade sarcoma cohorts. Revision rates increase with time, reaching 21% at 10 years and up to 47% at 20 years, most often for mechanical loosening or infection.

Acetabular wear after hemiarthroplasty remains a potential late concern, particularly in younger, more active patients. Short-term studies, such as that of Stevenson et al. [9], found minimal acetabular migration and no conversions to total hip arthroplasty in a series of 100 oncologic proximal femur resection (PFR) patients over a median 3.6-year follow-up. In contrast, longer-term studies have shown conversion rates of up to 4.6% [10], with some reporting greater migration over a decade [11], though often without the need for revision. In metastatic or elderly patients, this complication is rarely clinically significant, but in younger patients with anticipated long survival, primary total hip arthroplasty or vigilant radiographic surveillance is advisable.

Proximal femur endoprosthetic reconstruction remains the gold standard for restoring form and function following oncologic resection in this region. Success depends on meticulous preoperative planning, precise restoration of limb biomechanics, secure fixation, and robust soft tissue reconstruction to optimize stability and longevity while minimizing complications.

COMPOSITE RECONSTRUCTIONS

Composite reconstruction strategies integrate the immediate mechanical stability of an endoprosthesis with the biological benefits of bone grafts, aiming to improve soft tissue reattachment, enhance hip stability, and promote long-term durability. These techniques are particularly valuable in younger patients and in cases where restoration of soft tissue continuity is critical. They are broadly classified into **allograft-prosthesis composites (APCs)** and **autograft-prosthesis composites (AuPCs)**.

ALLOGRAFT-PROSTHESIS COMPOSITE

In APC reconstruction, a size-matched cadaveric proximal femur is prepared to accept a prosthetic stem, typically cemented within the allograft. The composite is implanted into the host femoral canal, with the host–graft junction stabilized using plates, cerclage wires, or intramedullary fixation. Soft tissue attachments, including the capsule and abductors, are reattached directly to the allograft, providing a biological envelope that aids in joint stability and prosthesis longevity.

The biological incorporation potential and capacity for robust soft tissue fixation are key advantages. However, complications such as nonunion at the host–graft junction, graft fracture, and infection are not uncommon. In a systematic review, Janssen et al. reported a 19% revision rate, with structural failure in 8.3% and infection in 6.5% of cases. Five- and ten-year survival rates ranged from 84% to 100% and 81% to 86%, respectively, with MSTS functional scores of 58%–93%, comparable to those of endoprosthetic replacements alone. Notably, soft tissue failure was rare due to the biological surface available for reattachment [2].

AUTOGRAFT-PROSTHESIS COMPOSITE (AUPC)

AuPCs use the patient's resected tumor-bearing bone after sterilization by extracorporeal irradiation, pasteurization, or liquid nitrogen freezing. The segment is reamed for a prosthetic stem, which is cemented proximally into the graft and fixed distally into the host femur.Chen et al. [12] achieved union in 85% of cases using extracorporeally irradiated autografts with porous-coated long stems, reporting satisfactory function. Xu et al. [13] reported a mean MSTS score of 26.4 (88%) with frozen AuPCs, 100% survival at five years, and 50% at ten years. Complications occurred in 26% of patients, including deep infection, acetabular wear, and prosthesis removal, but no cases of loosening, graft resorption, or limb length discrepancy.

Advantages include anatomical preservation, immunologic safety, and cost-effectiveness; limitations involve risks of delayed union, devitalized graft fracture, and reduced mechanical integrity after sterilization.

CLINICAL CONSIDERATIONS

Compared with standalone endoprostheses, composites offer superior opportunities for soft tissue reconstruction and stability but carry greater technical demands and complication risks. Endoprostheses remain mechanically reliable and less morbid but may lack secure abductor reattachment options. Selection should be individualized, considering patient age, oncologic prognosis, and reconstructive goals.

SUMMARY

- Proximal femur tumor resection poses unique surgical challenges due to complex anatomy and the need to preserve joint function and stability.
- Proximal femur endoprosthetic reconstruction offers durable, functionally effective, and reproducible outcomes.

- Technical precision in prosthetic alignment, cementation strategy, and soft tissue reconstruction is crucial to prevent complications such as dislocation, loosening, or limb length discrepancy.
- Potential for complications—particularly dislocation, infection, and long-term mechanical failure—necessitates careful patient selection, meticulous soft tissue handling, and vigilant postoperative surveillance with endoprosthesis reconstruction.
- Composite reconstructions, including APCs and AuPCs, enable biological integration and soft tissue reattachment but carry higher risks of nonunion and infection.
- Reconstruction choice should be individualized based on patient age, pathology, soft tissue status, and resource availability to optimize both oncological and functional outcomes.

REFERENCES

1. Li B, Yu Y, Bao Y, Song J. Proximal femoral tumor resection followed by joint prosthesis replacement: a systematic review and meta-analysis. *BMC Musculoskelet Disord.* 2023;24(1):779. doi:10.1186/s12891-023-06913-w
2. Janssen SJ, Langerhuizen DWG, Schwab JH, Bramer JAM. Outcome after reconstruction of proximal femoral tumors: A systematic review. *J Surg Oncol.* 2019;119(1): 120–129. doi:10.1002/jso.25297
3. Bruns J, Delling G, Gruber H, Lohmann CH, Habermann CR. Cementless fixation of megaprostheses using a conical fluted stem in the treatment of bone tumours. *J Bone Joint Surg Br.* 2007;89(8):1084–1087. doi:10.1302/0301-620X.89B8.19236
4. Henderson ER, Jennings JM, Marulanda GA, Palumbo BT, Cheong D, Letson GD. Purse-string capsule repair to reduce proximal femoral arthroplasty dislocation for tumor--a novel technique with results. *J Arthroplasty.* 2010;25(4):654–657. doi:10.1016/j.arth.2009.11.002
5. Bickels J, Meller I, Henshaw RM, Malawer MM. Reconstruction of hip stability after proximal and total femur resections. *Clin Orthop Relat Res.* 2000;375: 218–230. doi:10.1097/00003086-200006000-00027
6. Gosheger G, Hillmann A, Lindner N, et al. Soft tissue reconstruction of megaprostheses using a trevira tube. *Clin Orthop Relat Res.* 2001;393:264–271. doi:10.1097/00003086-200112000-00030
7. Henderson ER, Jennings JM, Marulanda GA, Groundland JS, Cheong D, Letson GD. Enhancing soft tissue ingrowth in proximal femoral arthroplasty with aortograft sleeve: a novel technique and early results. *J Arthroplasty.* 2011;26(1): 161–163. doi:10.1016/j.arth.2010.07.006
8. Henderson ER, Keeney BJ, Pala E, et al. The stability of the hip after the use of a proximal femoral endoprosthesis for oncological indications: analysis of variables relating to the patient and the surgical technique. *Bone Joint J.* 2017;99-B(4):531–537. doi:10.1302/0301-620X.99B4.BJJ-2016-0960.R1
9. Stevenson JD, Kumar VS, Cribb GL, Cool P. Hemiarthroplasty proximal femoral endoprostheses following tumour reconstruction: is acetabular replacement necessary?. *Bone Joint J.* 2018;100-B(1):101–108. doi:10.1302/0301-620X.100B1.BJJ-2017-0005.R1
10. Drexler M, Gortzak Y, Sternheim A, Kollender Y, Amar E, Bickels J. The radiological evaluation of the hip joint after prosthetic arthroplasty of the proximal femur in patients with a tumour using a bipolar femoral head. *Bone Joint J.* 2015; 97-B(12):1704–1709. doi:10.1302/0301-620X.97B12.36366
11. Cannon CP, Lin PP, Lewis VO, Yasko AW. Acetabular outcome after hip hemiarthroplasty in patients with tumors. *Clin Orthop Relat Res.* 2007;457:183–187. doi:10.1097/BLO.0b013e31802dc4e7
12. Chen CF, Chen WM, Cheng YC, Chiang CC, Huang CK, Chen TH. Extracorporeally irradiated autograft-prosthetic composite arthroplasty using AML extensively porous-coated stem for proximal femur reconstruction: a clinical analysis of 14 patients. *J Surg Oncol.* 2009;100(5):418–422. doi:10.1002/jso.21351
13. Xu G, Miwa S, Yamamoto N, et al. Pedicle frozen autograft-prosthesis composite reconstructions for malignant bone tumors of the proximal femur. *BMC Musculoskelet Disord.* 2020;21(1):81. doi:10.1186/s12891-020-3112-0

10 Distal Femur Resection and Reconstruction

INTRODUCTION

Primary bone malignancies such as osteosarcoma and Ewing sarcoma frequently involve the distal femur. Historically, above-knee amputation was the mainstay of treatment; however, advances in chemotherapy, imaging, prosthetic design, and surgical techniques have shifted practice toward limb-sparing surgery with reconstruction, now considered standard care [1]. This approach offers superior functional outcomes compared with amputation, without compromising survival, and carries a low risk of local recurrence [2, 3]. Furthermore, limb salvage is more cost-effective [4].

The primary objective is complete oncologic resection while preserving adequate musculature to achieve a painless, functional limb. In distal femoral osteosarcoma treated with neoadjuvant chemotherapy, oncologic resection, and endoprosthetic reconstruction, reported local recurrence rates range from 5% to 10% [5, 6]. Adequate surgical margins and a favorable histologic response to chemotherapy are key determinants in minimizing recurrence [7].

Reconstruction most commonly utilizes modular endoprosthetic systems or allograft–prosthetic composites. Distal femoral resection with these reconstructive techniques should be considered when anticipated oncologic and functional outcomes exceed those of above-knee amputation or rotationplasty. This chapter outlines perioperative considerations, reconstructive options, and functional and oncologic outcomes following distal femoral resection and reconstruction.

ANATOMIC CONSIDERATIONS

Knee Joint

In tumor surgery involving the knee, it is essential to determine whether the joint is involved or at risk. Potential sites of tumor invasion include the suprapatellar pouch, cruciate ligaments, articular surface, and collateral ligaments. Magnetic resonance imaging (MRI) abnormalities in these regions should alert the surgeon to possible intra-articular extension. True joint invasion is rare but may be suggested by effusion; in such cases, aspiration with histologic evaluation is indicated. Hemarthrosis usually signifies synovial involvement.

Knee joint contamination may occur via tumor spread along cruciate ligaments, biopsy-related capsular breach, or pathological fractures involving articular cartilage. The extensive joint capsule, extending beyond the articular margins, is vulnerable to improper biopsy placement. The capsule is thinnest at the suprapatellar pouch, which may extend well proximal to the patella and bulge medially and laterally into the paracondylar gutters. Consequently, biopsy of a distal femoral metaphyseal tumor must be planned using detailed imaging to avoid capsular violation.

Sartorial (Adductor) Canal

The adductor magnus attaches to the adductor tubercle via a strong tendon. The sartorial canal, between the vastus medialis, sartorius, and adductor magnus, extends from the adductor hiatus to the femoral triangle. It contains the superficial femoral artery and vein, the saphenous nerve, and the motor branch to the vastus medialis obliquus. Near the adductor hiatus, vessels are bound tightly by thick fascia. Large soft tissue tumors may compress this fascia, increasing intraluminal tension and compressing canal contents.

Surgical exposure of the adductor canal in such cases requires meticulous dissection to avoid vascular or tumor capsule injury. Division of the adductor magnus tendon may relieve pressure from tumor compression. The vein is particularly at risk; blunt dissection is preferred. The vessels should be mobilized from the canal and released through the hiatus into the popliteal fossa, permitting safe displacement during tumor dissection. Tethering of vessels at the hiatus may hinder mobilization and increase the risk of injury when separating them from tumor extensions into the popliteal space.

Popliteal Vessels and Nerves

Anatomically, the popliteal fossa is approached medially for vascular structures and laterally for nerves. The tibial and common peroneal branches of the sciatic nerve traverse the fossa within a thin areolar fascia. The common peroneal nerve passes laterally beneath the biceps tendon, over the lateral gastrocnemius. It can be identified by sharp dissection above the biceps tendon, about 10 cm proximal to its fibular head insertion. An interval between the fascia lata ridge inserting into the Gerdy tubercle and the biceps tendon provides lateral access. The nerve lies parallel to the biceps belly; dividing and retracting the biceps tendon posteriorly exposes the fossa and popliteal nerve.

Medial exposure of the popliteal vessels involves separating the upper border of the sartorius, gracilis, and semitendinosus tendons from the medial intermuscular septum and vastus medialis, then retracting them posteriorly. Division of their distal pes anserinus attachment allows

DOI: 10.1201/9780367822002-13

greater mobilization. The medial gastrocnemius head is then divided from its femoral origin, revealing the popliteal artery and vein. These vessels pass distally beneath the fossa, giving off branches to the vastus medialis and profunda femoris network, including genicular vessels, which must be ligated to free the vessels.

In large posteriorly extending tumors, these vascular branches may tether the artery and vein to the femur, complicating mobilization and increasing hemorrhage risk if avulsed. Careful ligation and controlled division are therefore essential to minimize intraoperative bleeding and maintain oncologic safety.

PREOPERATIVE CONSIDERATIONS

Imaging

Plain Radiographs

Biplanar radiographs of the entire femur are essential for assessing cortical destruction, periosteal reaction, and new bone formation (Figure 10.1). As plain films require ≥30% bone loss for lytic lesion detection, subtle disease may be missed. Long-leg standing anteroposterior views aid in evaluating mechanical alignment and limb deformity. 1:1 magnification radiographs are critical for accurate templating of the distal femur, proximal tibia, and intramedullary canal to select appropriate stem dimensions. This is particularly important when non-standard implant sizes are anticipated and require preordering.

Magnetic Resonance Imaging

MRI provides superior soft tissue contrast, crucial for knee tumors due to the proximity of the popliteal neurovascular bundle. High-quality multiplanar imaging delineates dissection planes and assesses intra-articular extension via the suprapatellar pouch, cruciate ligaments, subarticular bone, and collateral ligaments (Figure 10.2). Effusions suggesting joint involvement are readily detected. Whole-femur MRI best identifies intramedullary tumor spread and skip metastases, which must be addressed during surgery.

Angiography

Vascular imaging is indicated when popliteal artery involvement is suspected, particularly with large soft tissue masses or proximal extension affecting the superficial femoral artery. Computed tomography (CT) or MR angiography, preferred over conventional angiography, defines vessel–tumor relationships (Figure 10.3). In hypervascular metastases (renal, thyroid, myeloma), angiography guides preoperative embolization to minimize intraoperative hemorrhage.

Computed Tomography

CT complements MRI by evaluating cortical and trabecular bone quality at the planned resection level and quantifying bone loss from tumor, fracture, or periprosthetic lysis. Multiplanar and 3D reconstructions aid spatial planning for reconstruction, including the need for bulk allografts or segmental megaprostheses. Advanced software allows

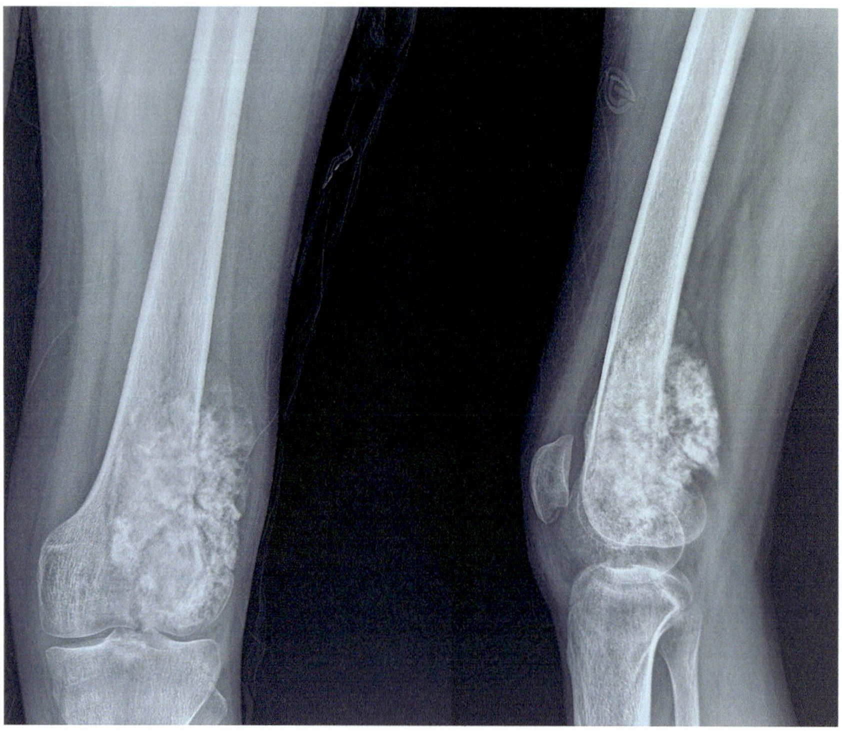

FIGURE 10.1 Plain radiographs of the distal femur in a 19-year-old male with osteosarcoma. The images reveal a mixed lytic–sclerotic lesion with ill-defined margins, cortical breach, and extension into surrounding soft tissues. Dense, cloud-like osteoid matrix mineralization is characteristic of high-grade osteosarcoma.

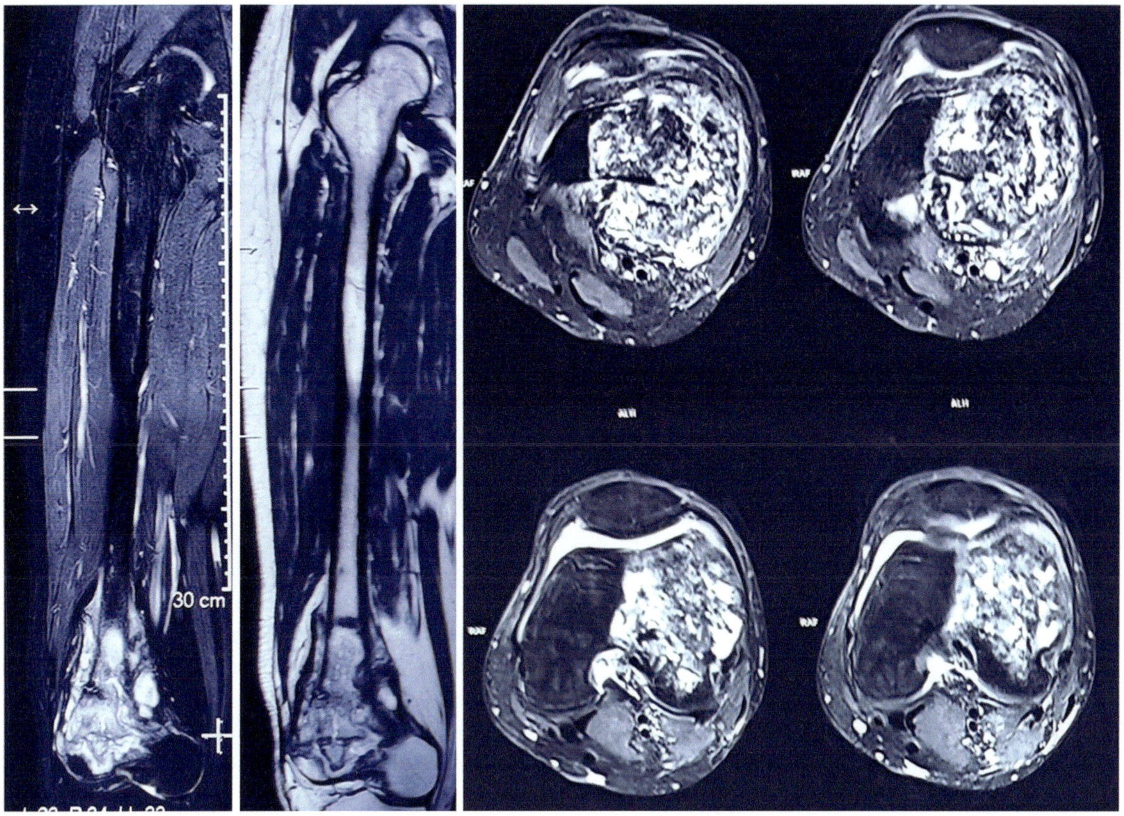

FIGURE 10.2 MRI of the distal femur in a case of osteosarcoma. Coronal and sagittal images demonstrate a heterogeneous intramedullary lesion with cortical breach and soft tissue extension. Axial sections reveal irregular margins with areas of necrosis and tumor infiltration into surrounding soft tissues, characteristic of aggressive osteosarcoma.

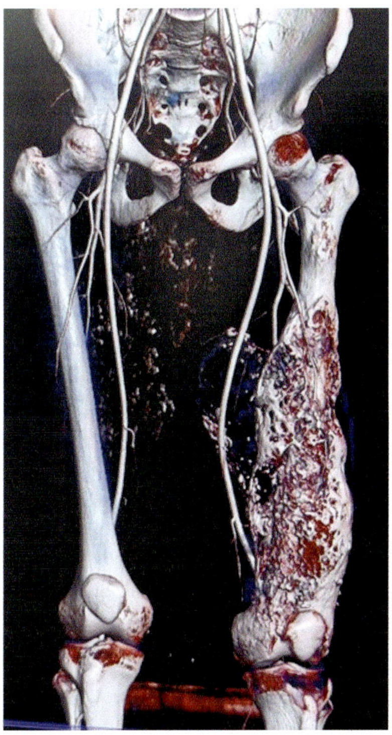

FIGURE 10.3 CT angiography of a patient with Osteosarcoma femur, with a large medial soft tissue extension, showing the superficial femoral vessel and tumor relationship.

metal artifact reduction and prosthesis subtraction, improving visualization of periprosthetic bone loss.

Nuclear Scintigraphy

Bone scintigraphy detects increased turnover earlier than radiographs, highlighting metabolically active lesions for targeted biopsy. Co-registration with multislice CT enhances specificity. Tracers such as thallium and glucose-6-phosphate identify malignant activity and enable assessment of treatment response by comparing uptake pre- and post-chemotherapy or radiotherapy, helping define surgical margins.

Collectively, these imaging modalities guide decisions on tumor extent, resectability, biopsy targeting, surgical type, incision placement, intra- versus extra-articular resection, and femoral osteotomy level.

SURGICAL MANAGEMENT

Timing of Limb-Sparing Procedures

Appropriate timing is critical, particularly for patients receiving preoperative chemotherapy or radiotherapy (e.g., Ewing sarcoma). Surgery is generally performed 2–3 weeks after completion of treatment, ensuring recovery of white blood cell and platelet counts and resolution of radiation-induced skin erythema.

Surgical Preparation and Positioning

The patient is positioned supine on a radiolucent table to permit fluoroscopic imaging. After anesthesia, intravenous antibiotics are administered, and a urinary catheter is placed. The entire limb is prepared and draped. A tourniquet may be used if resection length permits. Given the potential need for transfusion, especially post-chemotherapy, adequate peripheral, or central access is established and type–crossmatch confirmed.

Incision

Approach may be lateral, anterior, or medial, modified to incorporate any biopsy or prior surgical scars to excise potentially contaminated tissue. The preferred anterior incision begins proximal to the planned resection, curves distally along the anteromedial knee, and extends just medial to the tibial tubercle (Figure 10.4).

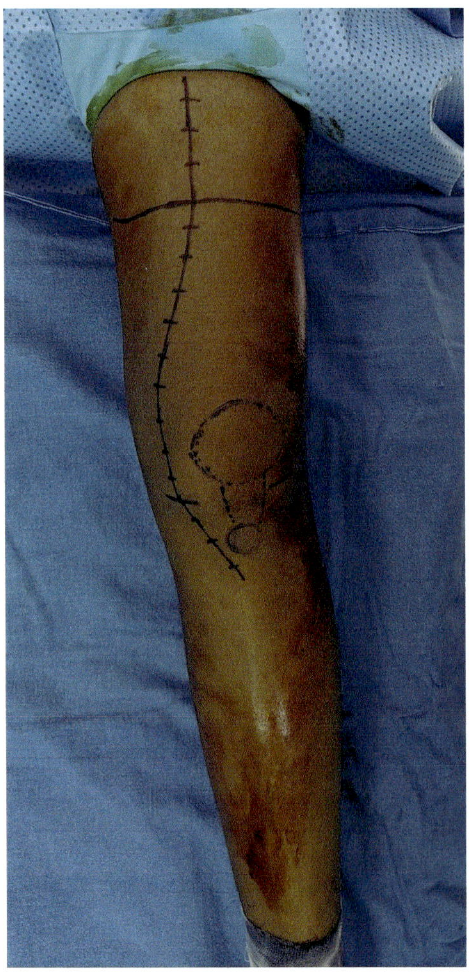

FIGURE 10.4 Anterior skin incision beginning proximal to the planned resection, curving distally along the anteromedial knee, and extending just medial to the tibial tubercle.

Surgical Resection

Medial and lateral skin flaps of adequate thickness are raised. A medial parapatellar arthrotomy is performed, preserving a cuff of medial retinaculum for extensor repair. The rectus femoris is incised longitudinally, and the patella is everted laterally with careful protection of the patellar tendon. The joint is inspected; signs of hemorrhage or contamination may warrant extra-articular resection.

The vastus intermedius is usually excised as a margin over the tumor; further quadriceps may be removed if required. The vastus medialis is retracted medially, and the medial collateral ligament is transected proximal to the medial meniscus. Medial gastrocnemius origin and adductor insertions are released, aided by knee flexion.

Along the adductor canal, care is taken to avoid injury to tethered femoral vessels (Figure 10.5A–10.5C). The femoral vein, often with multiple draining branches from the tumor, is ligated to mobilize the neurovascular bundle posteriorly. The medial intermuscular septum is incised to access the distal posterior femur. Popliteal artery and vein branches to the intercondylar notch are ligated before proceeding proximally.

The lateral quadriceps and most of the rectus femoris are retracted laterally with the patella. The lateral patellofemoral ligament and lateral collateral ligament are transected proximal to the lateral meniscus. The lateral intermuscular septum is divided to enter the posterior compartment, and the lateral gastrocnemius origin is released. Dissection continues proximally to the planned osteotomy level with circumferential subperiosteal exposure. The mid-anterior femoral cortex is marked proximally for later rotational alignment.

FEMORAL OSTEOTOMY AND MARGIN ASSESSMENT

Osteotomy is performed 2–3 cm proximal to the most cranial tumor extent on MRI, using a power saw perpendicular to the femur with posterior protection by a malleable retractor (Figure 10.6). Alternatively, some surgeons disarticulate at the knee before proximal transection. A frozen section from the proximal marrow margin is obtained, and bone wax is applied to both cut ends to prevent tumor spillage. The distal femur is elevated with a clamp, and residual posterior attachments are released. Frozen section analysis guides any additional bone resection before reconstruction.

Knee Disarticulation

The ACL and PCL are sharply divided at their tibial insertions (Figure 10.7), followed by division of the posterior capsule under the protection of the popliteal vessels.

The specimen is removed, and the resection length is measured from the proximal cut to the medial joint line (Figure 10.8A and 10.8B).

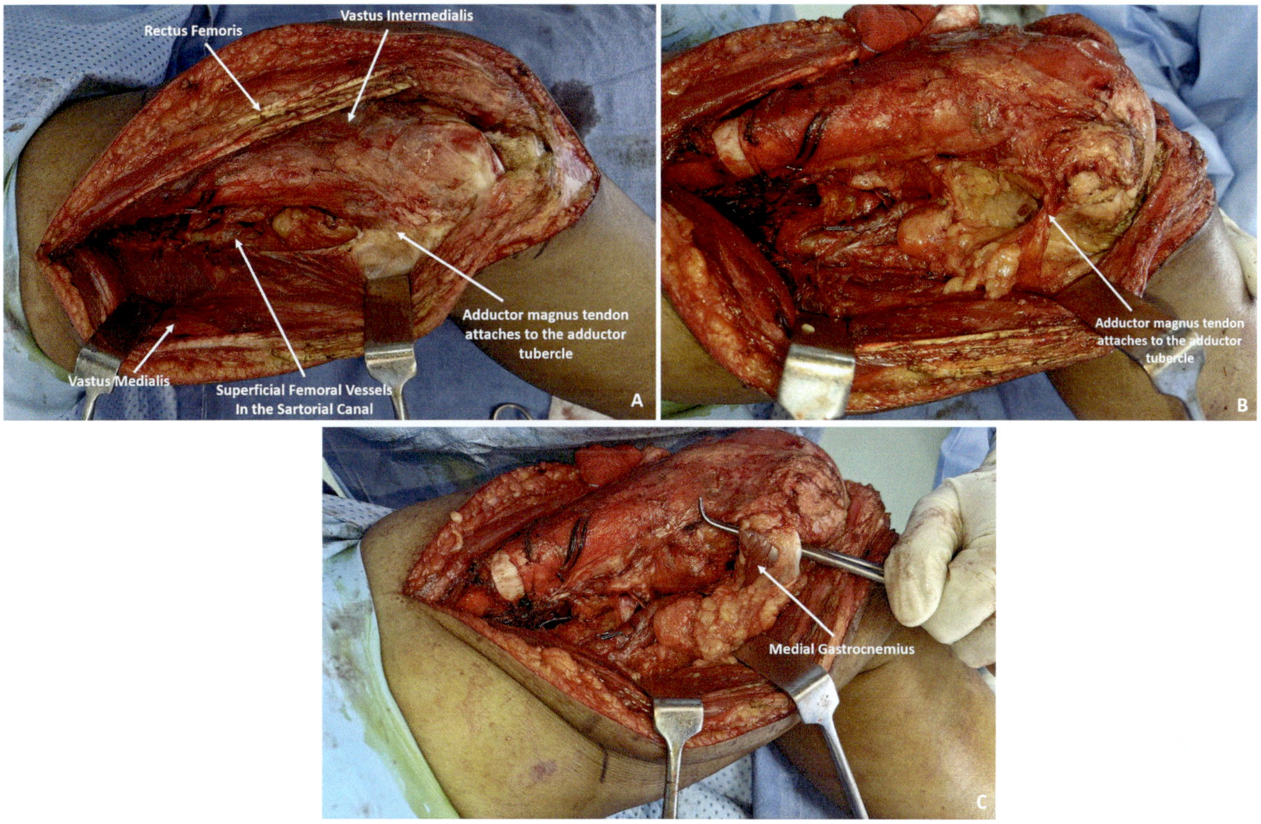

FIGURE 10.5 Intra-operative picture showing the medial dissection. (A) Superficial femoral vessels course through the sartorial canal, formed by the vastus medialis (retracted medially), sartorius, and (B) adductor magnus (attached to the adductor tubercle). The vastus intermedius is excised as a margin over the tumor. (C) Medial gastrocnemius origin and adductor insertions are released, revealing the popliteal vessels, passing distally beneath the popliteal fossa, giving off branches, including genicular vessels, which must be ligated to free the vessels.

HAEMOSTASIS AND FIELD PREPARATION FOR RECONSTRUCTION

If a tourniquet was used, it is deflated gradually. Bleeding points are coagulated or ligated, and the wound is irrigated with pulsed saline lavage. To reduce contamination risk, gowns, gloves, instruments, suction devices, light handles, electrocautery equipment, and superficial drapes are changed before reconstruction.

RECONSTRUCTION OF SKELETAL DEFECT – ENDOPROSTHESIS RECONSTRUCTION

Femoral Preparation

- **Cemented Stem** – Flexible reamers enlarge the canal to ~2 mm beyond the planned stem diameter, selecting the largest size that avoids excessive endosteal removal (Figure 10.9). Reaming extends 2–3 cm proximal to the stem to allow a cement restrictor and extra cement beyond the tip.
- **Uncemented Stem** – Straight reamers are used for line-to-line preparation. The cut surface is chamfered with a facing reamer for optimal fit.
- **Trial Stem** – Insert and check fit, then remove and pack the canal to limit blood loss. Standard stems are ~120 mm long and available in straight or curved versions, with or without porous or hydroxyapatite coating.

Tibial Preparation

- Remaining menisci are excised (Figure 10.10A). The patellar tendon may be subperiosteally elevated to expose the anterior tibia; in contracted revision cases, tibial tubercle osteotomy or extensor lengthening may be necessary. A portion of the fat pad may be removed at the surgeon's discretion.
- **Canal Identification and Alignment** – A drill identifies the canal anterior to the ACL insertion; a T-handled finder confirms alignment. Intramedullary or external alignment guides may be used.
- **Tibial Cutting** – External alignment guides align with the ankle or second metatarsal. The cutting guide is positioned perpendicular to the tibial axis to create a surface neutral to the tibial axis in all planes, with no or slight posterior slope; anterior slope is avoided to prevent flexion contracture (Figure 10.10B). A

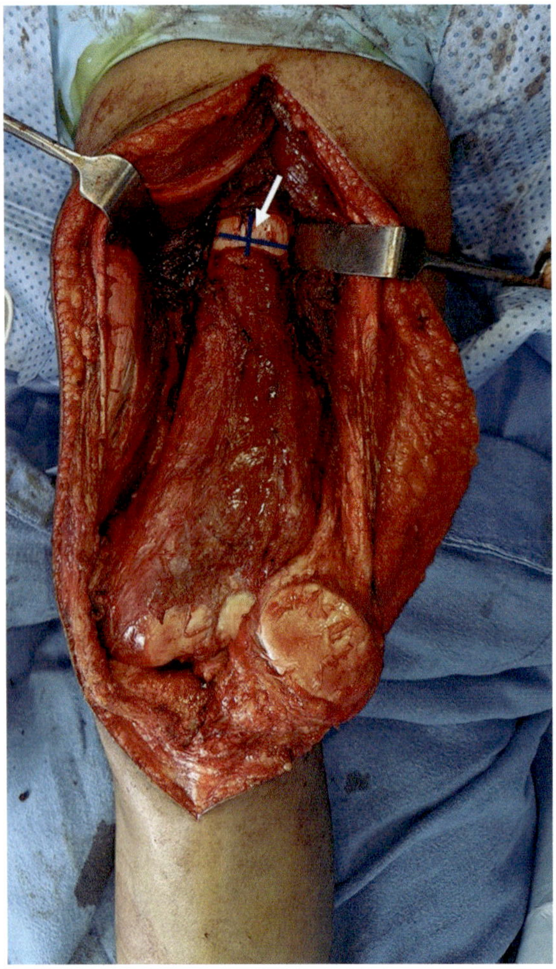

FIGURE 10.6 Planned osteotomy perpendicular to the femur.

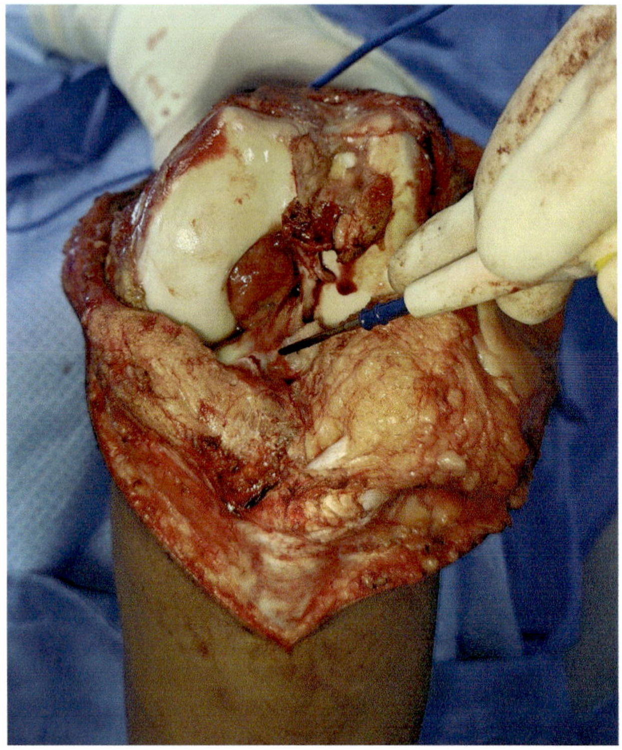

FIGURE 10.7 Intra-articular resection: The cruciate ligaments are sharply divided at their tibial insertions.

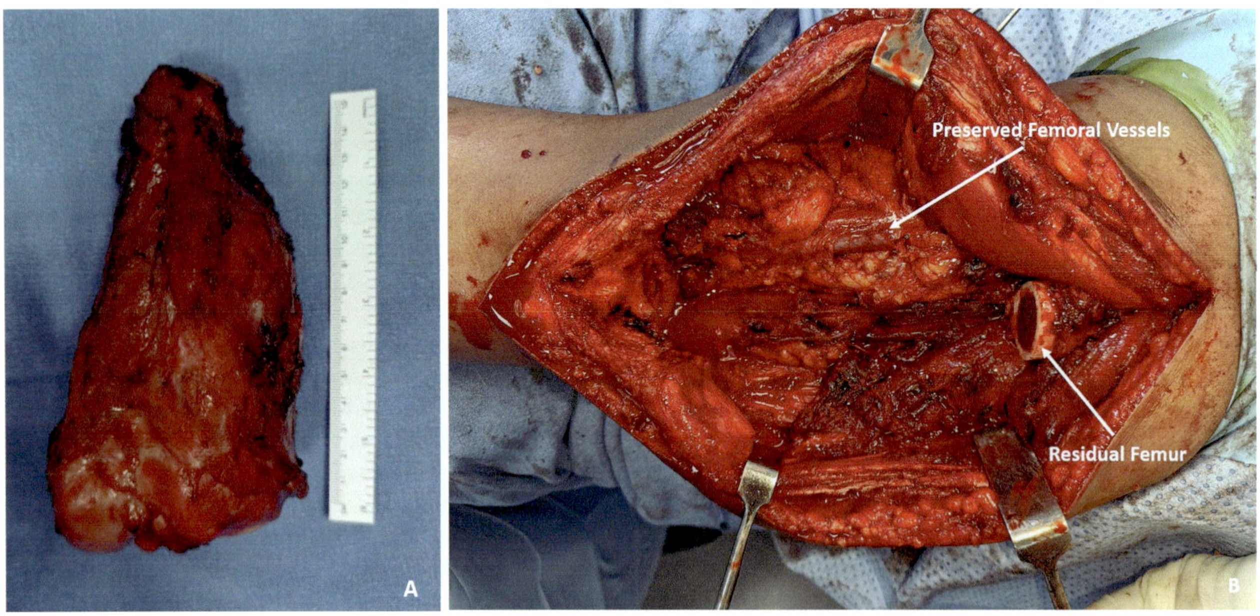

FIGURE 10.8 (A) Resected tumor specimen. (B) Surgical bed post tumor resection, showing preserved vascular bundle and residual femur.

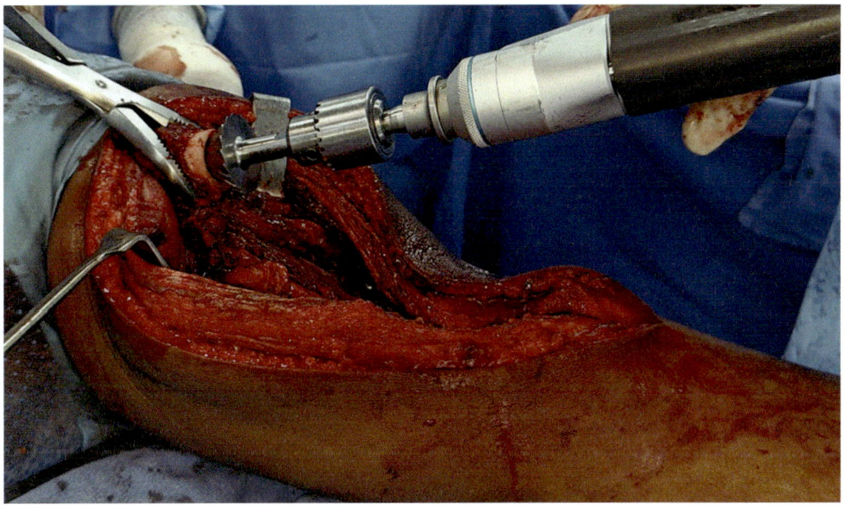

FIGURE 10.9 Femoral preparation: The residual femur is reamed using flexible reamers to enlarge the canal to ~2 mm beyond the planned stem diameter, selecting the largest size that avoids excessive endosteal removal. Reaming extends 2–3 cm proximal to the stem to allow a cement restrictor and extra cement beyond the tip.

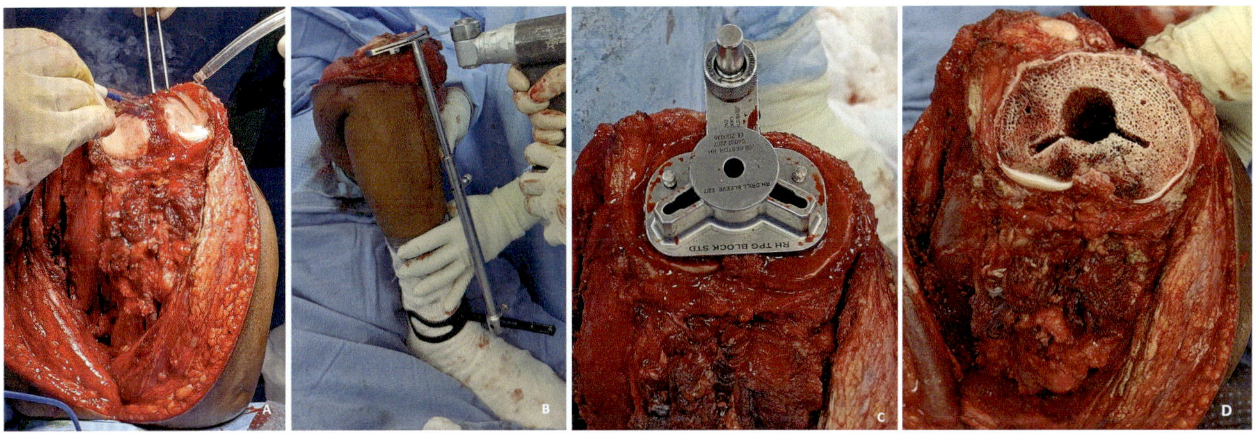

FIGURE 10.10 (A) Remaining menisci are excised. (B) The cutting guide is positioned perpendicular to the tibial axis, to create a surface neutral to the tibial axis in all planes, with no or slight posterior slope. (C and D) The tibial baseplate is placed on the cut tibial surface, aligning with the medial one-third of the tibial tubercle, avoiding overhang and medialization. Baseplate is secured with pins; reamers and punches are used to prepare for the stem and tibial surface.

malleable retractor protects posterior neurovascular structures while the proximal tibial cut is made using a power saw. The tibial baseplate is placed on the cut tibial surface, aligning with the medial one-third of the tibial tubercle, avoiding overhang and medialization. Baseplate is secured with pins; reamers and punches are used to prepare for the stem and tibial surface (Figure 10.10C and 10.10D).

TRIAL PLACEMENT AND ADJUSTMENTS

- **Femoral and Tibial Trial** – Modular components are selected to match the total bone resected from the femur and tibia. Rotational alignment follows the anterior femoral cortex mark made during resection. The tibial trial component is inserted and reduced with the femoral trial component (Figure 10.11).
- **Joint Line and Length** – Normal joint line must be recreated for patellar function. Overlengthening is avoided to prevent peroneal/sciatic nerve palsy. Neurovascular structures are palpated in extension to check for tension; distal pulses are verified.
- **Function Testing** – Aim for smooth flexion–extension of 110–120°. Ensure patella tracks centrally without subluxation; perform lateral release if required, particularly in scarred revision cases.

Patellar Resurfacing – Performed if indicated, freehand or with a guide. Excessive bone removal, especially laterally/inferiorly, is avoided. Thickness should be measured with a caliper before trial component placement.

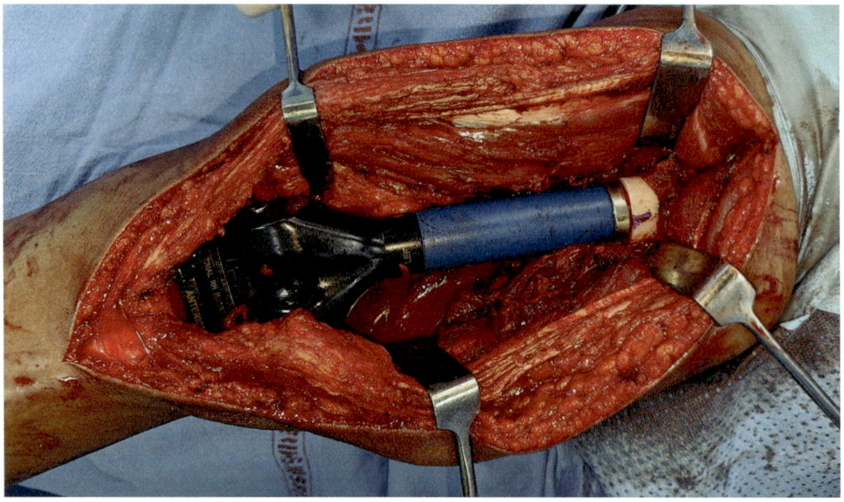

FIGURE 10.11 Trial placement and adjustment.

FINAL PREPARATION AND CEMENTING OF COMPONENTS

- **Irrigation and Cement Restrictor Placement** – The femoral canal is pulse-lavaged. For cemented stems, a restrictor is placed 1–2 cm beyond the planned tip; trial stem confirms placement. The canal is packed while cement is mixed.
- **Tibial Canal** – Lavaged and packed; a restrictor is placed if cemented fixation is chosen.
- **Tibial Component Cementation** – With the limb elevated and tourniquet inflated, antibiotic-loaded cement is inserted using a cement gun. The tibial (and patellar if resurfaced) component is implanted in one step with sustained pressure until curing to prevent lift-off.
- **Femoral Component Cementation** – Components are assembled on the table. Cement is injected into the canal while fluid, ensuring pressurization for interdigitation. The stem is inserted slowly to reduce fat embolism risk, avoiding rotation after placement. Steady alignment and pressure are maintained until curing. For uncemented stems, the implant is impacted for a tight canal fit.

FINAL ASSEMBLY AND ASSESSMENT

After the cement hardens and excess is removed, the tourniquet is deflated. Articulating elements (axle, bumper, tibial rotating component) are inserted (Figures 10.12 and 10.13). Full ROM and patellar tracking are reassessed; neurovascular status is verified in extension.

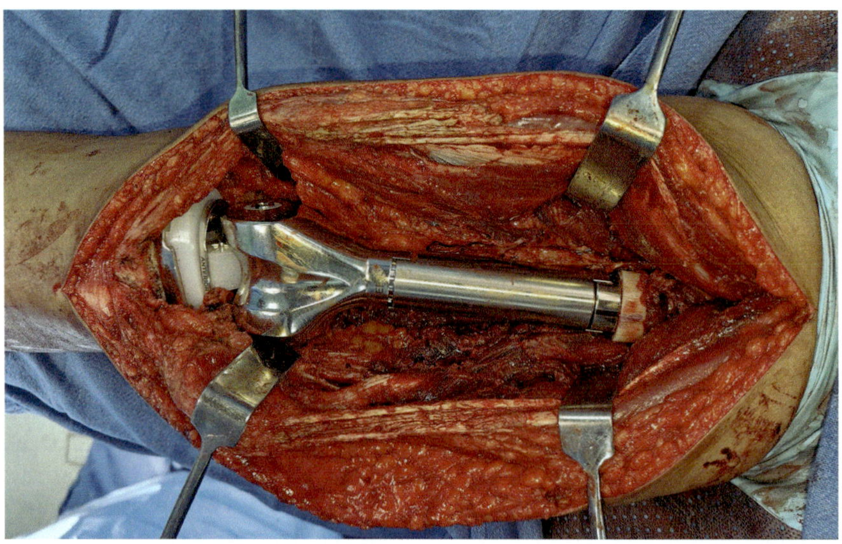

FIGURE 10.12 Final implantation and assembly.

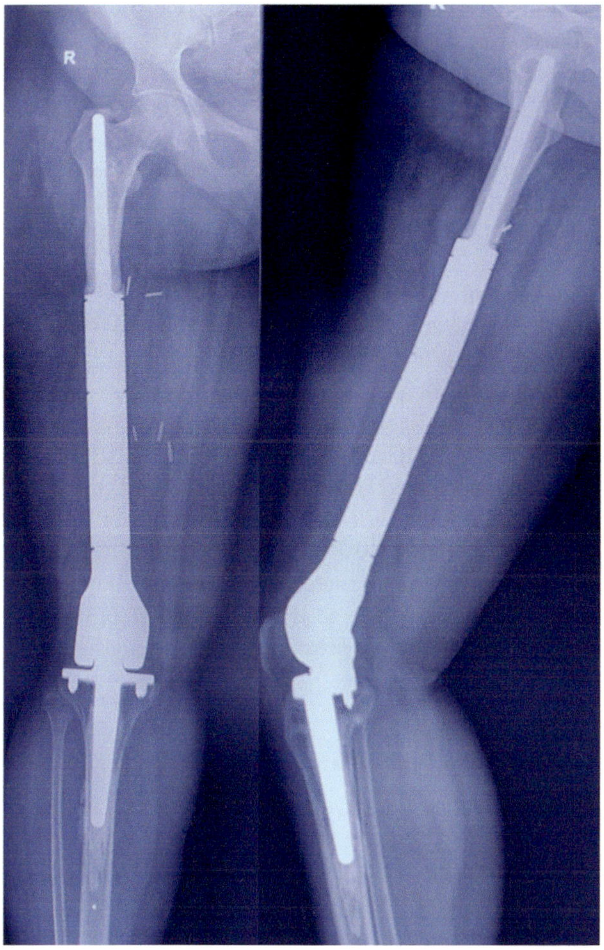

FIGURE 10.13 Post-operative radiographs following reconstruction with a distal femur endoprosthesis.

CLOSURE

Hemostasis is secured, and the wound is thoroughly irrigated. Deep drains are placed, exiting in line with the incision. Closure is layered, with meticulous repair of the extensor mechanism around the patella reinforced with heavy sutures. The repair is tested by flexing to 90° before subcutaneous closure. Skin is closed with staples, particularly where the incision crosses anteriorly over the knee. A sterile dressing is applied, avoiding peroneal nerve compression.

STEM FIXATION TECHNIQUES FOR FEMORAL PROSTHESES

- **Types of Fixation** – Options include cemented stems, uncemented press-fit stems, and compression-based press-fit stems.
- **Cemented Stems** – Provide immediate weight bearing and initial strength but lack bony ingrowth, making long-term aseptic loosening a major failure mode.
- **Uncemented Press-Fit Stems** – Permit osseointegration but require a protected period of 6–12 weeks to allow bony ingrowth.
- **Compression-Based Press-Fit Stems** – The *Compress* system applies axial compression at the bone–prosthesis interface to enhance bone mass and strength. It is useful in revision cases with poor bone quality or short proximal femoral remnants. Implantation involves an Anchor Plug with crossed pins and a Spindle at the interface.

Comparative data show five- and ten-year survival rates for conventional press-fit stems of 85% and 71%, respectively, with aseptic loosening the main late failure cause [8]. Smaller stems (<13.5 mm) and high diaphyseal/stem coefficient (>2.5 mm) correlated with reduced survival. Compression-based stems demonstrated slightly better five-year survival (88%), with early failures due to fixation loss or fracture; no failures occurred beyond the first year, and functional outcomes were similar for survivors.

Implant Coatings – Silver-coated endoprostheses have been linked to lower infection rates, likely due to higher local silver ion concentration [9]. Iodine-coated implants show promising infection prevention and treatment potential, particularly in immunocompromised patients [10].

Selection should balance biomechanical needs, patient activity level, compliance, and infection risk to optimize long-term function.

COMPLICATIONS

Infection

Prosthetic infection remains a major concern, particularly in immunocompromised patients, those with prior prosthetic infection, or poor soft tissue coverage. Reported superficial infection rates are ~7%, while deep infection rates range from 0% to 14.5% in large series [11–16]. A systematic review reported a 9% weighted mean for deep infections after lower extremity endoprosthetic reconstruction [17]. In 428 distal femoral resections with prosthetic reconstruction, deep infection occurred in 9.6% at 13 months [15]. Rigorous perioperative infection prevention is essential in distal femoral prosthetic reconstruction.

Hardware Failure

All prosthetic components are subject to fatigue. Modern designs incorporate extramedullary porous coating, modularity, and forged metals to improve durability.

- **Femoral Stem Fractures** – Early custom-cast stems showed 9% fracture rates versus 1.2% in modular forged stems [11]. Fixed-hinge implants fracture in ~0.6% compared with 3.5% in modular designs [15].
- **Bushing/Axle Failure** – More common, often not requiring revision. Fixed-hinge designs show 28% failure versus 6% in modular implants at 11 years [15]. Schwartz et al. reported 11.8% incidence at 160 months [11].

Neurovascular Injury

Occurs in 0%–12.5% of cases [11, 14, 18, 19]. Risk is highest in skeletally immature patients with expandable prostheses undergoing repeated lengthening. Overlengthening in chemotherapy patients increases stretch-related nerve injury.

Periprosthetic Fracture

In 154 *Compress* uncemented prostheses, periprosthetic fracture occurred in 3.9% [20].

Aseptic Loosening

The leading long-term failure mode (Figure 10.14). Rates range from 0%–8.4% at 52–90 months [12, 14, 16]. Myers et al. reported cemented prosthesis survival of 77%, 58%, and 50% at 10, 20, and 25 years, respectively, with modular designs outperforming older customs (94% vs. 52% at 15 years), and only 3.5% loosening in modular stems [15]. Stem diameter relative to diaphyseal width predicts loosening risk; canal-filling stems improve longevity [21].

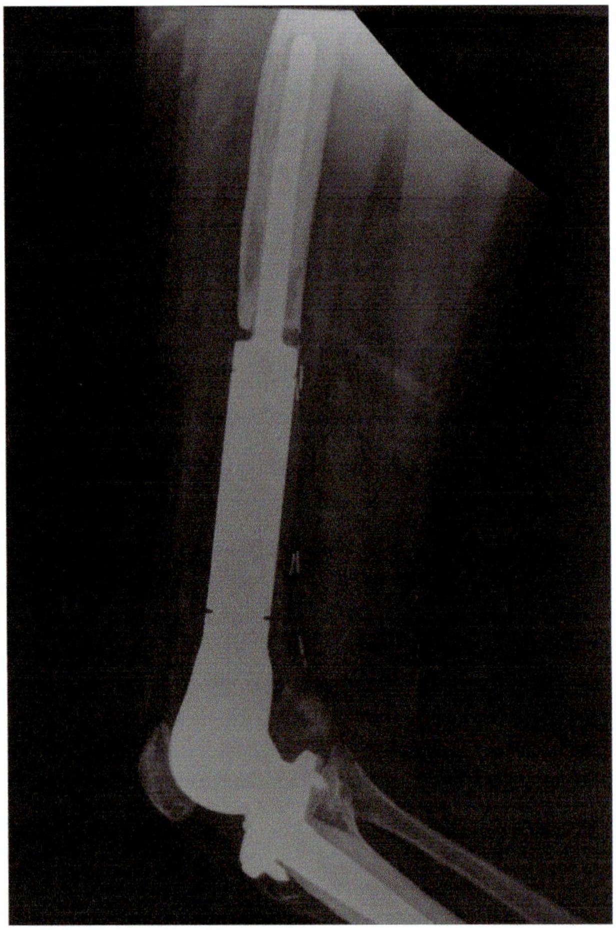

FIGURE 10.14 Radiological images of aseptic loosening of a distal femur endoprosthesis. Radiographs show radiolucent lines at the bone–prosthesis interface with evidence of stem subsidence and cortical thinning, consistent with loss of fixation in the absence of infective changes.

Modern cemented stems often incorporate porous-coated collars to encourage extracortical bone bridging, reducing stress shielding and particle migration. In 335 cases, aseptic loosening occurred in 35% of fixed hinge but in none of the modular rotating-hinge designs with hydroxyapatite collars at 10 years [11]. Reported cemented DFR survival is ~85% at five years and 55%–79% at ten years [12, 16, 22]. Cross-pin fixation for short proximal femoral segments showed no loosening in 20 patients at >2 years [23].

Uncemented Stems – Developed to reduce loosening rates. Capanna et al. [24] found no loosening in 95 modular uncemented DFRs at 52 months, though bushing failure occurred in 42% at 64 months, and stem fracture in 6% (linked to narrow stems). Infection rates were 5% (primary) and 6% (revision). Griffin et al. [25] reported 2.7% loosening in 74 uncemented DFRs, with smaller diameters predisposing to fracture. In 117 cementless reconstructions, resections exceeding 40% of femoral length correlated with higher failure [26]. Biomechanical studies show modern uncemented stems have acceptable initial stability; cylindrical reaming provides greater torsional strength than flexible reaming [27].

Patellar Complications

Patellar problems are frequent after DFR [11, 28, 29]. Schwab et al. [29] reported a 63% incidence in 43 cases, most commonly patella baja and impingement, the latter often due to joint line malposition leading to contact with the tibial component.

REHABILITATION AND FUNCTIONAL RESULTS

Following cemented megaprosthetic reconstruction, early weight bearing is typically permitted, using assistive devices until quadriceps strength allows an unassisted straight leg raise. Uncemented stems require protected weight bearing for 6–12 weeks. Use of continuous passive motion (CPM) devices postoperatively is debated; some employ CPM during inpatient recovery until 90° passive knee flexion is achieved, after which patients continue quadriceps strengthening, gait training, and knee range of motion exercises.

FUNCTIONAL RESULTS AFTER DISTAL FEMORAL PROSTHETIC RECONSTRUCTION

Schwartz et al. reported a mean Musculoskeletal Tumor Society (MSTS) score of 86.7% and mean knee flexion of 110° in 160 patients after distal femur endoprosthetic reconstruction, with flexion contracture in 4% (mean 10°) [11]. Most patients resume unrestricted activities, except for limitations in kneeling, running, and contact sports. No significant difference in Toronto Extremity Salvage Score (TESS) was found between rotating-hinge and fixed-hinge designs [30].

Malo et al. compared 31 uncemented with 25 cemented hinged prostheses and found significantly better MSTS 1993 and TESS scores in the cemented group at ≥1-year follow-up [31]. Functional outcomes correlate with quadriceps preservation, with greater resection associated with poorer results [24].

SUMMARY

- Limb-sparing distal femur resection with endoprosthetic or composite reconstruction offers superior functional outcomes and comparable survival to amputation when oncologic margins are achieved.
- Detailed preoperative imaging—particularly MRI and angiography—guides surgical planning, margin assessment, and preservation of vital neurovascular structures.
- Meticulous surgical technique with appropriate timing, exposure, and reconstruction choice (cemented, uncemented, or compression-based stems) is essential for durable fixation and function.
- Complications include infection, aseptic loosening, hardware failure, and patellar maltracking, with stem diameter, fixation method, and joint line restoration influencing long-term outcomes.
- Most patients achieve high functional scores and a satisfactory range of motion, with quadriceps preservation and accurate joint line restoration critical for optimal results.

REFERENCES

1. DiCaprio MR, Friedlaender GE. Malignant bone tumors: limb sparing versus amputation. *J Am Acad Orthop Surg.* 2003;11(1):25–37.
2. Aksnes LH, Bauer HC, Jebsen NL, et al. Limb-sparing surgery preserves more function than amputation: a Scandinavian sarcoma group study of 118 patients. *J Bone Joint Surg Br.* 2008;90(6):786–794.
3. Sluga M, Windhager R, Lang S, Heinzl H, Bielack S, Kotz R. Local and systemic control after ablative and limb sparing surgery in patients with osteosarcoma. *Clin Orthop Relat Res.* 1999;358:120–127.
4. Grimer RJ, Carter SR, Pynsent PB. The cost-effectiveness of limb salvage for bone tumours. *J Bone Joint Surg Br.* 1997;79(4):558–561.
5. Bickels J, Wittig JC, Kollender Y, et al. Distal femur resection with endoprosthetic reconstruction: a long-term followup study. *Clin Orthop Relat Res.* 2002;400:225–235.
6. Katagiri H, Cannon S, Briggs T, Cobb J, Witt J, Pringle J. Local recurrence of osteosarcoma: survival rate and management. *Orthop Procs.* 2003;85-B(SUPP_I):50.
7. Bacci G, Longhi A, Fagioli F, Briccoli A, Versari M, Picci P. Adjuvant and neoadjuvant chemotherapy for osteosarcoma of the extremities: 27 year experience at Rizzoli Institute, *Italy. Eur J Cancer.* 2005;41(18):2836–2845.
8. Farfalli GL, Boland PJ, Morris CD, Athanasian EA, Healey JH. Early equivalence of uncemented press-fit and Compress femoral fixation. *Clin Orthop Relat Res.* 2009;467(11):2792–2799. doi:10.1007/s11999-009-0912-9
9. Hussmann B, Johann I, Kauther MD, Landgraeber S, Jäger M, Lendemans S. Measurement of the silver ion concentration in wound fluids after implantation of silver-coated megaprostheses: correlation with the clinical outcome. *Biomed Res Int.* 2013;2013:763096. doi:10.1155/2013/763096
10. Tsuchiya H, Shirai T, Nishida H, et al. Innovative antimicrobial coating of titanium implants with iodine. *J Orthop Sci.* 2012;17(5):595–604. doi:10.1007/s00776-012-0247-3
11. Schwartz AJ, Kabo M, Eilber FC, et al. Cemented distal femoral endoprostheses for musculoskeletal tumor: improved survival of modular versus custom implants. *Clin Orthop Relat Res.* 2010;468:2198–2210.
12. Bickels J, Wittig JC, Kollender Y, et al. Distal femur resection with endoprosthetic reconstruction: a long-term follow-up study. *Clin Orthop Relat Res.* 2001;400:125–135.
13. Capanna R, Morris HG, Campanacci D, et al. Modular uncemented prosthetic reconstruction after resection of tumors of the distal femur. *J Bone Joint Surg.* 1994;76:178–186.
14. Frink SJ, Rutledge J, Lewis VO, et al. Favorable long-term results of prosthetic arthroplasty of the knee for distal femur neoplasms. *Clin Orthop Relat Res.* 2005;438:65–70.
15. Myers GJ, Abudu AT, Carter SR, et al. Endoprosthetic replacement of the distal femur for bone tumors: long-term results. *J Bone Joint Surg Br.* 2007;89:521–526.
16. Sharma S, Turcotte RE, Isler MH, et al. Cemented rotating-hinge endoprosthesis for limb salvage of distal femur tumors. *Clin Orthop Relat Res.* 2006;450:28–32.
17. Racano A, Pazionis T, Farrokhyar F, Deheshi B, Ghert M: High infection rate outcomes in long-bone tumor surgery with endoprosthetic reconstruction in adults: A systematic review. *Clin Orthop Relat Res* 2013;471(6):2017–2027.
18. Akiyama A, Viola DC, Menis CD, et al. Coaxial extendible knee equalizes limb length in children with osteogenic sarcoma. *Clin Orthop Relat Res.* 2001;459:60–65.
19. Eckardt JJ, Kabo JM, Kelley CM, et al. Expandable endoprosthesis reconstruction in skeletally immature patients with tumors. *Clin Orthop Relat Res.* 2000;373:51–61.
20. Tyler WK, Healey JH, Morris CD, et al. Periprosthetic fracture of the distal femur after endoprosthetic replacement. *Clin Orthop Relat Res.* 2009;467:178–185.
21. Bergin PF, Noveau JB, Jelinek JS, Henshaw RM. Aseptic loosening rates in distal femoral endoprostheses: does stem size matter?. *Clin Orthop Relat Res.* 2012;470(3):743–750. doi:10.1007/s11999-011-2081-x
22. Biau D, Faure F, Katsahian S, et al Survival of total knee replacement with megaprostheses after bone tumor resection. *J Bone Joint Surg Am.* 2006;88:1285–1293.
23. Cannon CP, Eckardt JJ, Kabo JM, et al. Custom cross-pin fixation of 32 tumor endoprosthetic stems. *Clin Orthop Relat Res.* 2003;417:285–292.
24. Capanna R, Morris HG, Campanacci D, Del Ben M, Campanacci M. Modular uncemented prosthetic reconstruction after resection of tumours of the distal femur. *J Bone Joint Surg Br.* 1994;76(2):178–186.
25. Griffin AM, Parsons JA, Davis AM, et al. Uncemented tumor endoprostheses at the knee: root causes of failure. *Clin Orthop Relat Res.* 2005;438:71–79.
26. Song WS, Kong CB, Jeon DG, et al. The impact of amount of bone resection on uncemented prosthesis failure in patients with a distal femoral tumor. *J Surg Oncol.* 2011;104(2):192–197. doi:10.1002/jso.21924
27. Ferguson PC, Zdero R, Schemitsch EH, Deheshi BM, Bell RS, Wunder JS. A biomechanical evaluation of press-fit stem constructs for tumor endoprosthetic reconstruction of the distal femur. *J Arthroplasty.* 2011;26(8):1373–1379. doi:10.1016/j.arth.2010.12.005

28. Springer BD, Hanssen AD, Sim FH, Lewallen DG. The kinematic rotating hinge prosthesis for complex knee arthroplasty. *Clin Orthop Relat Res.* 2001;392: 283–291. doi:10.1097/00003086-200111000-00037
29. Schwab JH, Agarwal P, Boland PJ, Kennedy JG, Healey JH. Patellar complications following distal femoral replacement after bone tumor resection. *J Bone Joint Surg Am* 2006;88(10):2225–2230. doi:10.2106/JBJS.E.01279
30. Jones KB, Griffin AM, Chandrasekar CR, et al: Patient-oriented functional results of total femoral endoprosthetic reconstruction following oncologic resection. *J Surg Oncol* 2011;104(6):561–565.
31. Malo M, Davis AM, Wunder J, et al. Functional evaluation in distal femoral endoprosthetic replacement for bone sarcoma. *Clin Orthop Relat Res.* 2001;(389):173–180. doi:10.1097/00003086-200108000-00024

11 Proximal Tibia Resection and Reconstruction

INTRODUCTION

The proximal tibia is the second most common site for primary bone sarcomas after the distal femur. Limb salvage surgery in this region is technically demanding due to its intricate anatomical and functional considerations. While oncologic cure remains the foremost objective in musculoskeletal oncology, advances in chemotherapy and surgical techniques have increasingly allowed limb-sparing procedures without compromising survival. Historically, above-knee amputation was the standard approach, given the difficulty in achieving wide margins while preserving vital neurovascular structures and functional capacity.

Tumor resection in the proximal tibia presents unique reconstructive challenges arising from its superficial location, limited soft tissue envelope on the anteromedial aspect, and inevitable disruption of the extensor mechanism. These factors contribute to higher complication rates and relatively inferior functional outcomes compared with resections at other sites.

Reconstruction options include endoprosthetic replacement, osteoarticular or intercalary allografts, and arthrodesis. Endoprosthetic reconstruction is generally favored for its lower risk of nonunion, reduced infection rates, and superior mobility. Critical determinants of success include restoration of the extensor mechanism, adequate soft tissue coverage—often achieved using a medial gastrocnemius rotational flap—and meticulous infection prevention, making limb salvage a viable and functionally acceptable option for most patients [1].

This chapter outlines the indications, preoperative planning, surgical technique, reconstruction strategies, and complications associated with proximal tibia tumor resections.

ANATOMIC CONSIDERATIONS

Surgical management of proximal tibial tumors demands precise knowledge of the region's complex anatomy. Although tumors often lie close to the knee joint, direct intra-articular invasion is uncommon and typically occurs secondary to pathological fractures, biopsy tract contamination, or tumor spread along the cruciate ligaments. Hemarthrosis should prompt suspicion of such involvement. MRI is the most reliable preoperative tool for assessing cruciate ligament extension, though confirmation is frequently made intraoperatively. When nodular deposits are identified on cruciate ligaments, extra-articular resection—removing the proximal tibia, joint capsule, and femoral condyles en bloc—may be necessary to achieve oncologically safe margins.

The tibial tuberosity, a critical attachment for the extensor mechanism, is invariably resected during proximal tibial tumor surgery. Its preservation or reconstruction is essential for restoring active knee extension and functional mobility. Posteriorly, the popliteal artery bifurcates beneath the popliteus muscle, first giving rise to the anterior tibial artery—often sacrificed during resection—followed by the tibioperoneal trunk, which divides into posterior tibial and peroneal arteries. Although this is the most common branching pattern of the popliteal artery, anatomical variations are not uncommon, and orthopedic oncologists must recognize these to prevent catastrophic iatrogenic vascular injuries during proximal tumor resections (Table 11.1).

The popliteus muscle serves as a protective barrier between the tumor and neurovascular bundle, an advantage absent in distal femoral resections. The proximal tibiofibular joint, located posterolaterally, may be involved in high-grade sarcomas via direct extension. Extra-articular excision of this joint is necessary in such cases to avoid local recurrence.

The subcutaneous medial tibial surface poses reconstructive challenges after resection, as its limited soft tissue coverage increases the risk of wound breakdown and deep infection—historically a major cause of secondary amputation. An established solution is anterior transfer of the medial gastrocnemius muscle, providing robust vascularized coverage for the prosthesis and aiding extensor mechanism reconstruction. This flap reduces infection risk, improves wound healing, and enhances functional outcomes by contributing to knee extension.

A thorough understanding of these anatomic relationships underpins safe resection, optimal reconstruction, and complication prevention in proximal tibial tumor surgery.

PREOPERATIVE CONSIDERATIONS

Successful resection of proximal tibial tumors requires meticulous preoperative planning based on comprehensive imaging. Initial staging includes plain radiographs of the entire tibia to assess bone involvement (Figure 11.1). Long-leg weight-bearing anteroposterior views are useful for evaluating mechanical alignment and detecting femoral or tibial deformities.

MRI is indispensable for assessing cortical destruction, proximal tibiofibular and knee joint involvement, intramedullary tumor extent, soft tissue invasion, skip lesions, and the tumor's relationship to the extensor mechanism and neurovascular bundle (Figure 11.2). The distal resection

DOI: 10.1201/9780367822002-14

TABLE 11.1

Variations in Terminal Branches of the Popliteal Artery

Type/Subtype	Description	Key Features
Type I – Normal Branching		
Type IA	Usual branching pattern	Anterior tibial artery arises first; tibioperoneal trunk bifurcates into posterior tibial and peroneal arteries
Type IB	Trifurcation pattern	Anterior tibial, posterior tibial, and peroneal arteries arise within 0.5 cm; no tibioperoneal trunk
Type IC	Anterior tibioperoneal trunk	Posterior tibial artery arises first; common trunk bifurcates into anterior tibial and peroneal arteries
Type II – High Division		
Type IIA1	High origin of anterior tibial artery	Origin above knee; normal posterior course behind popliteus
Type IIA2	High origin of anterior tibial artery	Origin above knee; medial course anterior to popliteus
Type IIB	High origin of posterior tibial artery	Posterior tibial arises first above knee; common trunk for anterior tibial and peroneal arteries
Type IIC	High origin of peroneal artery	Peroneal artery is the first branch above knee
Type III – Hypoplasia/Aplasia		
Type IIIA	Hypoplastic/aplastic posterior tibial artery	Peroneal artery enlarged and continues distally as posterior tibial artery
Type IIIB	Hypoplastic/aplastic anterior tibial artery	Peroneal artery enlarged and substitutes distally as dorsalis pedis artery
Type IIIC	Hypoplastic/aplastic anterior and posterior tibial arteries	Peroneal artery replaces both dorsalis pedis and posterior tibial arteries

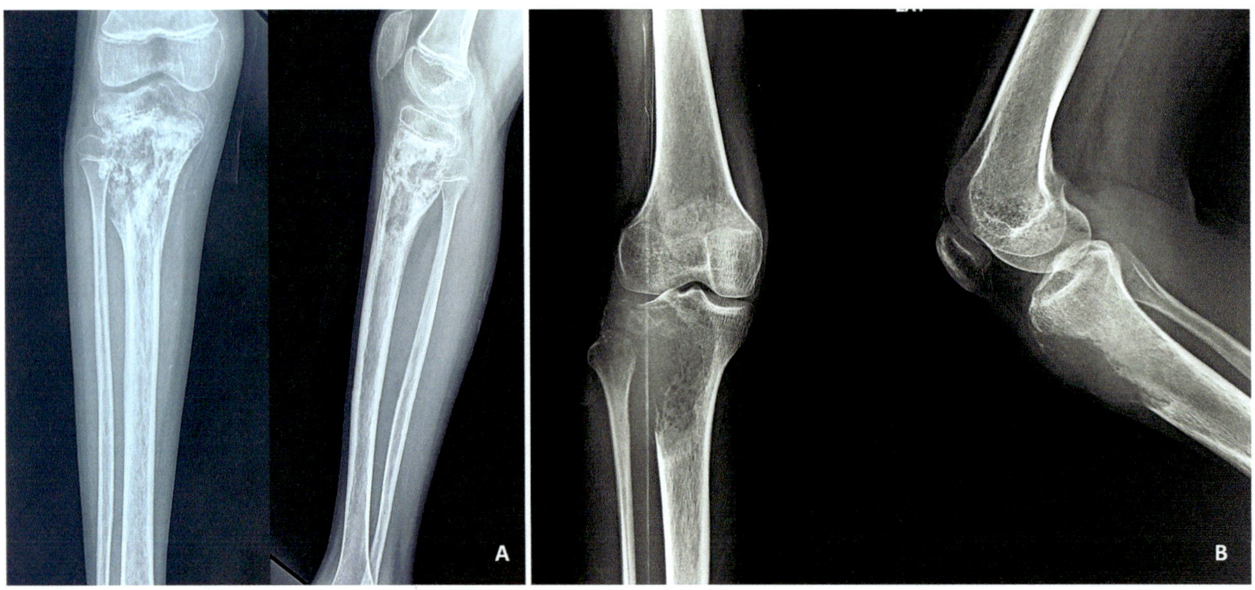

FIGURE 11.1 (A) Radiographs of osteosarcoma of the proximal tibia showing a mixed lytic–sclerotic lesion with aggressive periosteal reaction, cortical destruction, and soft tissue extension. The lesion demonstrates poorly defined margins with a sunburst-type pattern, typical of high-grade osteosarcoma. (B) Radiographs of a giant cell tumor of the proximal tibia depicting a purely lytic, expansile, and eccentric lesion extending up to the subarticular region. The lesion has well-defined but non-sclerotic margins, without periosteal reaction, consistent with the benign but locally aggressive nature of giant cell tumor.

level is generally planned 2–3 cm beyond the most distal intramedullary involvement.

When posterior soft tissue extension is suspected, CT angiography is used to evaluate the popliteal bifurcation and define tumor-vessel relationships (Figure 11.3). These imaging studies guide the selection of biopsy sites, incision placement, decision-making regarding intra- versus extra-articular resection, and the planned level of tibial osteotomy, ensuring oncologic safety while optimizing functional reconstruction.

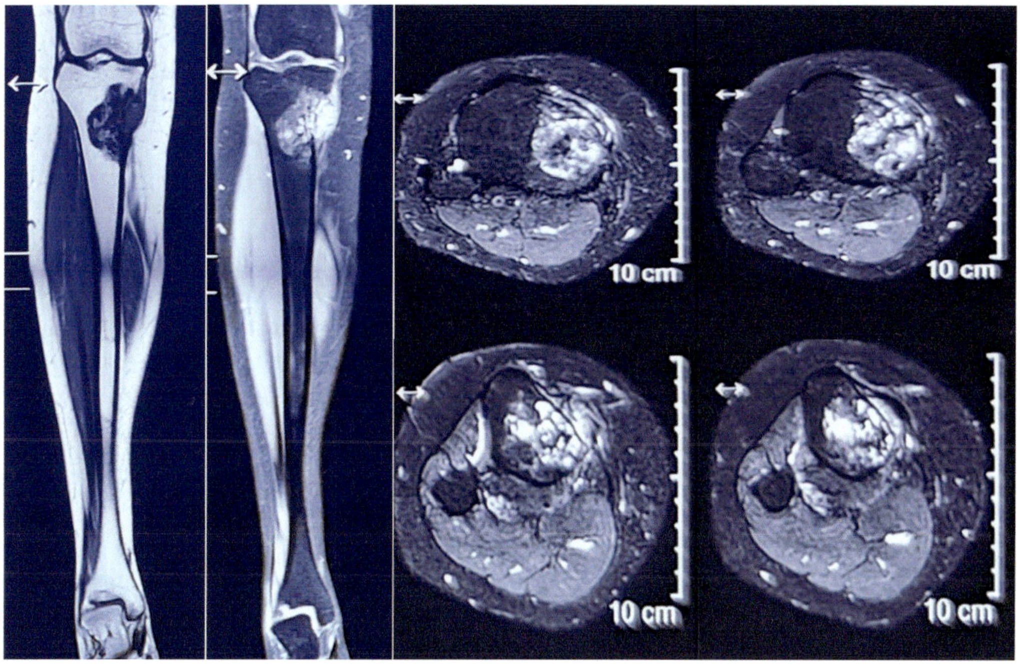

FIGURE 11.2 MRI of osteosarcoma of the proximal tibia. Coronal (left) and axial (right) sequences demonstrate a heterogeneous lesion with mixed solid and cystic areas, arising from the metaphysis of the proximal tibia. The mass shows cortical breach with an associated large soft tissue component extending into the surrounding musculature. Areas of necrosis and hemorrhage are interspersed within the lesion, while heterogeneous post-contrast enhancement is evident. The tumor extends close to the epiphysis, but the articular surface appears preserved. MRI delineates intraosseous extent, extraosseous soft tissue involvement, and the relationship with adjacent neurovascular structures, aiding in surgical planning.

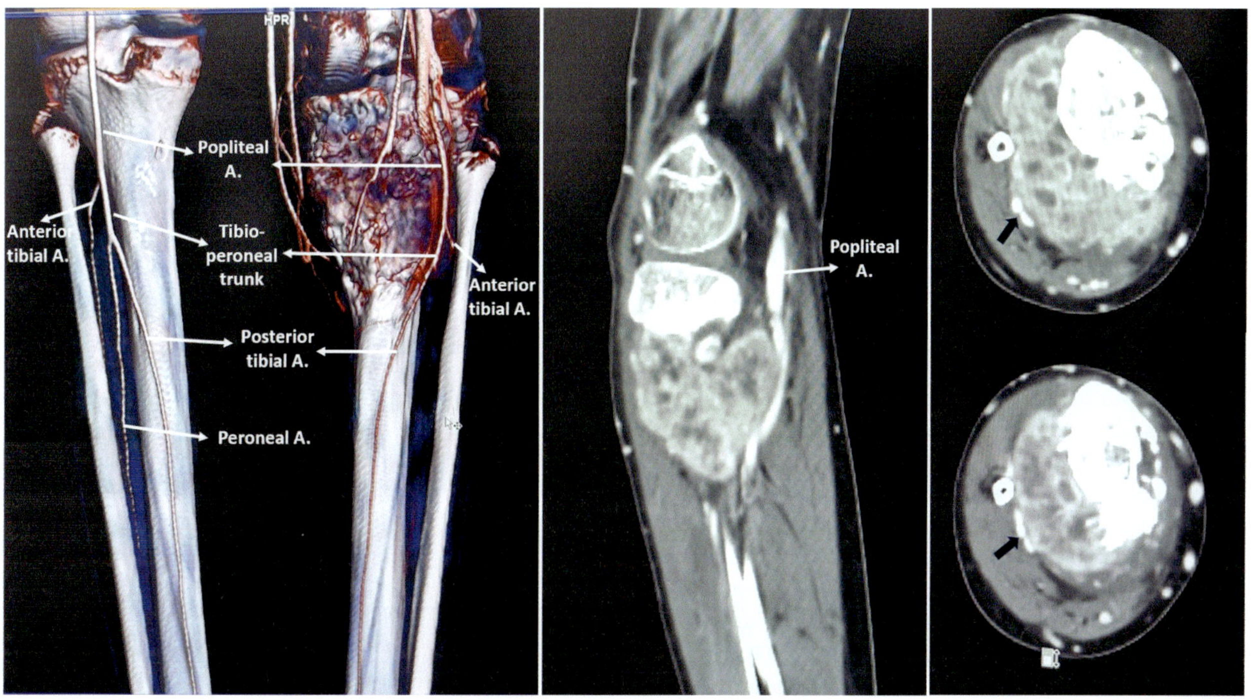

FIGURE 11.3 CT angiography images of osteosarcoma of the proximal tibia. (Left) Three-dimensional reconstructed angiographic images showing the relationship of the tumor with the popliteal artery and its major branches, including the anterior tibial, posterior tibial, peroneal arteries, and the tibioperoneal trunk. (Center) Sagittal reconstruction depicting the proximity of the tumor mass to the popliteal artery. (Right) Axial sections demonstrate the tumor closely abutting the vascular bundle (black arrows), emphasizing the importance of angiographic evaluation in preoperative surgical planning.

SURGICAL MANAGEMENT

The surgical management of proximal tibial tumors involves three critical components:

1. En bloc tumor resection with oncologically safe margins
2. Skeletal and knee joint reconstruction
3. Extensor mechanism and soft tissue reconstruction, typically using a medial gastrocnemius flap

POSITIONING AND PREPARATION

The patient is positioned supine under general anesthesia, with perioperative intravenous antibiotics administered. Adequate peripheral or central venous access is secured, and urinary catheterization is performed. Blood products are cross-matched in anticipation of potential intraoperative transfusion.

A pneumatic tourniquet is applied to the proximal thigh but inflated only after gravity-assisted exsanguination; elastic bandages are avoided to prevent tumor manipulation. The entire limb is prepared and draped to allow unrestricted intraoperative maneuvering.

INCISION AND SURGICAL APPROACH

A longitudinal anteromedial incision is made, extending from the distal third of the thigh to the proximal leg, according to the planned resection length. The biopsy tract is incorporated with at least a 1–2 cm margin to avoid contamination. Medial and lateral fasciocutaneous flaps of adequate thickness are developed to reduce ischemia and necrosis. Early arthrotomy allows inspection for intra-articular tumor spread.

EXPLORATION OF THE POPLITEAL FOSSA

The medial hamstrings (sartorius, gracilis, semitendinosus) are divided 2–3 cm from their tibial insertions (Figure 11.4A). The medial gastrocnemius is partially mobilized (Figure 11.4B), and the soleus is split to expose the neurovascular bundle (Figure 11.4C).

The popliteal artery is identified proximally and followed distally to the popliteal trifurcation. The anterior tibial artery is ligated after careful isolation, allowing the entire neurovascular bundle to fall away from the tumor; the peroneal artery may also be ligated in large posterior tumors. The posterior tibial artery is preserved unless directly involved. The inferior geniculate vessels are ligated to facilitate further mobilization of the neurovascular bundle, which is then dissected distally to a level that permits safe osteotomy (Figure 11.4D).

TUMOR RESECTION

Circumferential capsulotomy is performed 1–2 cm from the tibial insertion. The patellar tendon is divided 1–2 cm proximal to the tibial tubercle. Cruciate ligaments, collateral ligaments, and the joint capsule are divided close to their femoral origins, with menisci retained on the resected tibia.

The popliteus muscle is routinely sacrificed to ensure a safe posterior margin (Figure 11.5). Posterior capsule dissection is performed only after the neurovascular bundle is fully mobilized. The proximal tibiofibular joint is resected en bloc in high-grade tumors; preservation is acceptable in uninvolved joints to retain lateral collateral ligament function. The peroneal nerve is identified and protected throughout fibular head dissection.

DETERMINING RESECTION MARGINS AND OSTEOTOMY

Margins are determined by preoperative MRI and intraoperative palpation, aiming for 2–3 cm of normal bone distal to the tumor. All contaminated tissues, including the biopsy tract, involved synovium, and joint capsule, are excised with the specimen. The interosseous membrane and posterior attachments are released under direct vision, ensuring the tumor remains covered by uninvolved tissue to prevent seeding.

The tibial osteotomy is performed under direct visualization, and frozen section analysis of the distal medullary margin is recommended.

INTRA-ARTICULAR VS. EXTRA-ARTICULAR RESECTION

- **Intra-articular resection** is appropriate if the joint fluid is clear and there is no evidence of tumor contamination.
- **Extra-articular resection** is indicated in cruciate ligament invasion, biopsy tract contamination into the joint, or pathological fracture with synovial breach. This may necessitate removal of the femoral condyles and occasionally the patella, preserving the extensor apparatus via coronal osteotomy of the patella if oncologically safe.

MEDIAL GASTROCNEMIUS FLAP PREPARATION

The medial head of the gastrocnemius is preferred for flap creation due to its robust vascular supply, proximity, and reliable arc of rotation. The muscle is carefully dissected free from the underlying soleus while preserving its vascular pedicle.

Proximal identification is aided by locating the medial sural cutaneous nerve between the two gastrocnemius heads. The median raphe is released longitudinally using electrocautery. Distal release occurs just proximal to the musculo-tendinous junction, freeing the flap while maintaining perfusion. The mobilized flap is wrapped in saline-soaked gauze until it is transposed anteriorly for coverage (Figures 11.6 and 11.7).

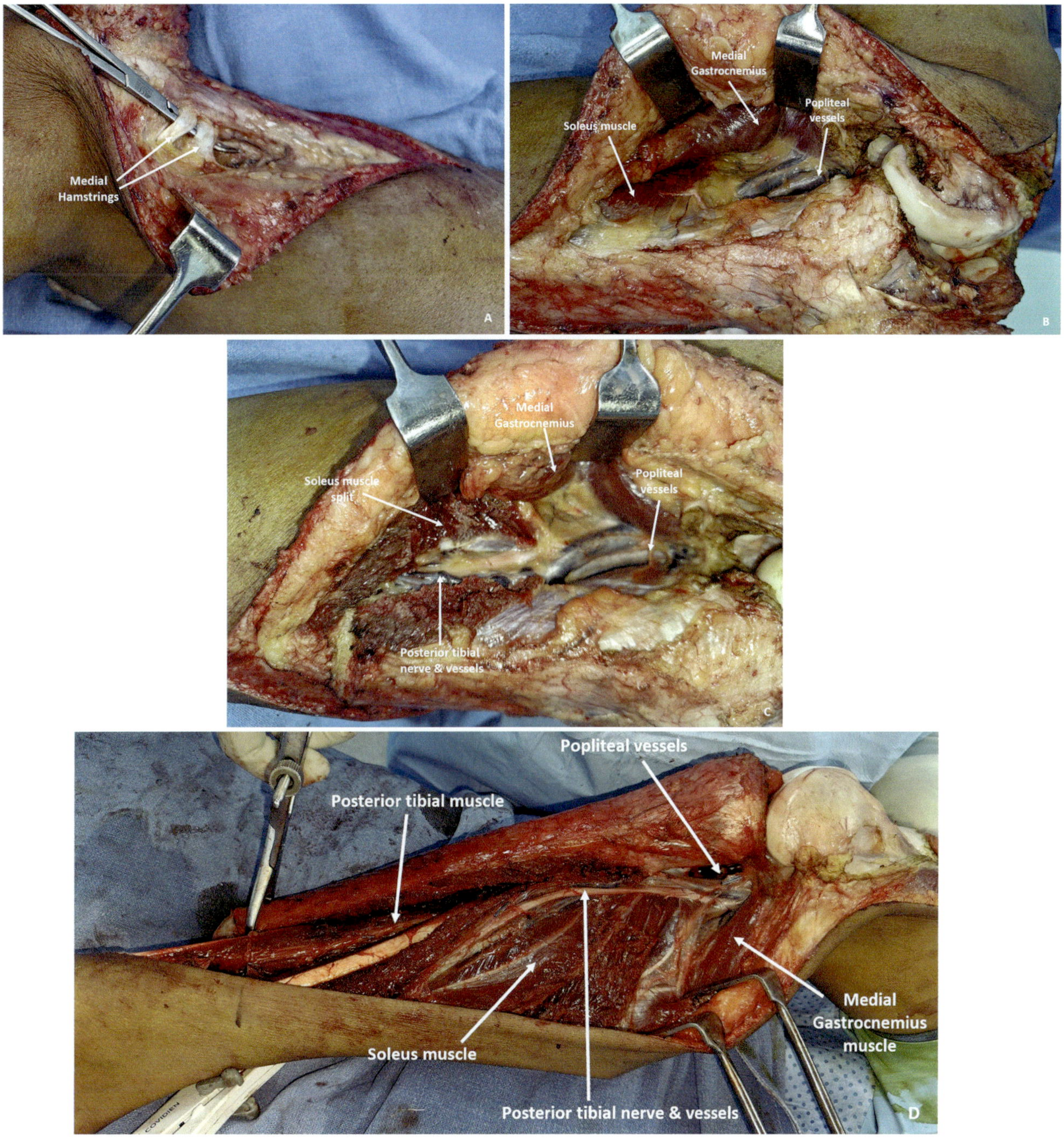

FIGURE 11.4 Intraoperative dissection of critical neurovascular structures during proximal tibia tumor resection. (A) The medial hamstrings' insertions are identified and divided from their tibial insertions to facilitate exposure. (B) Mobilization of the medial gastrocnemius and exposure of the popliteal vessels, along with the underlying soleus muscle. (C) Splitting of the soleus to identify the posterior tibial nerve and vessels, with further delineation of the popliteal vessels. (D) The popliteal artery identified proximally and traced to its trifurcation; the anterior tibial artery ligated, allowing mobilization of the neurovascular bundle. The peroneal artery may also be ligated in large posterior tumors. Inferior geniculate vessels are ligated to enhance mobilization, with preservation of the posterior tibial artery unless directly involved, permitting safe osteotomy and resection.

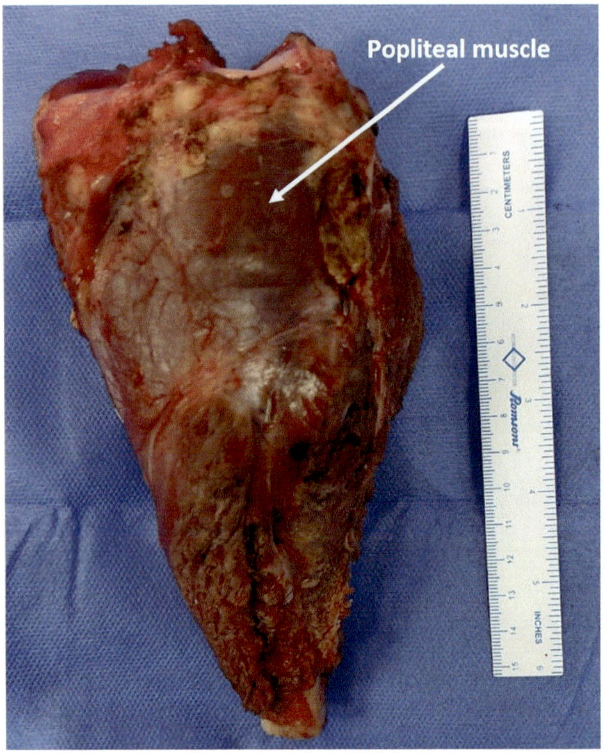

FIGURE 11.5 Posterior view of the resected proximal tibia osteosarcoma. The popliteus muscle is sacrificed, serving as the safe posterior margin.

PREVENTION OF FLAP NECROSIS

The medial gastrocnemius receives its blood supply from the medial sural artery, a 2–3 mm branch of the popliteal artery, accompanied by 1–2 sizable veins. This proximal pedicle allows safe distal detachment and anterior rotation.

Flap necrosis may occur if the pedicle is injured during dissection between the gastrocnemius heads or at the proximal release. Preservation of the vascular pedicle is critical; blunt midline dissection should be avoided.

Meticulous surgical technique—respecting oncologic margins, preserving vital neurovascular structures, and ensuring robust soft tissue coverage—remains essential to optimizing outcomes in proximal tibial tumor resection. The medial gastrocnemius flap is integral to both extensor mechanism restoration and prosthesis protection, significantly reducing postoperative wound complications.

RECONSTRUCTION OF SKELETAL DEFECT: ENDOPROSTHESIS RECONSTRUCTION

Endoprosthetic reconstruction is the current standard for skeletal restoration following proximal tibial tumor resection, particularly in adolescents and young adults with primary bone sarcomas. Compared to biological options such as osteoarticular allografts, endoprostheses offer predictable mechanical performance, modular customization, and ease of intraoperative application.

Modern proximal tibial tumor prostheses incorporate features aimed at optimizing fixation, soft tissue integration, and joint stability. These include modularity for intraoperative adaptability, porous coatings for osseointegration and soft tissue attachment, suture holes for muscular reattachment, and an anterior metal loop to secure the patellar tendon. Rotating-hinge mechanisms are preferred over fixed hinges, as they dissipate torsional forces at the bone-implant interface, reducing the risk of aseptic loosening [2].

Fixation may be achieved via uncemented press-fit stems—favored in younger patients for biological integration—or cemented stems, preferred in metastatic lesions or elderly patients [3]. Porous coatings on the stem and body encourage bone and fibrous tissue ingrowth, enhancing stability, soft tissue anchorage, and minimizing periprosthetic dead space.

TIBIAL PREPARATION

Cemented Stem Technique

- Ream the tibial canal with flexible reamers to a diameter 2 mm larger than the planned stem.
- Select the largest stem that avoids unnecessary endosteal removal.
- Extend reaming 2–3 cm distal to the stem tip for cement restrictor placement and adequate cement mantle.
- Chamfer the resection surface using a facing reamer for optimal stem–bone interface.
- Insert and remove a trial stem to confirm fit, then pack the canal to reduce bleeding.

Femoral Preparation

- Identify the femoral canal just anterior and medial to the posterior cruciate ligament insertion using a drill, followed by a T-handled canal finder.
- Perform femoral cutting with appropriate guides, protecting posterior neurovascular structures with a malleable retractor.

Trial Placement and Alignment

- Use modular tibial segments to match resected length.
- Assemble trial femoral and tibial components, ensuring reconstruction length matches the bone removed.
- Align the tibial component with premarked rotational reference on the anterior cortex.
- Recreate the normal joint line for optimal patellar tracking.
- Avoid overlengthening to prevent peroneal nerve stretch injury.
- Palpate neurovascular structures in extension and confirm distal pulses.
- Confirm smooth flexion–extension arc (110°–120°) and normal patellar tracking without maltracking or subluxation.

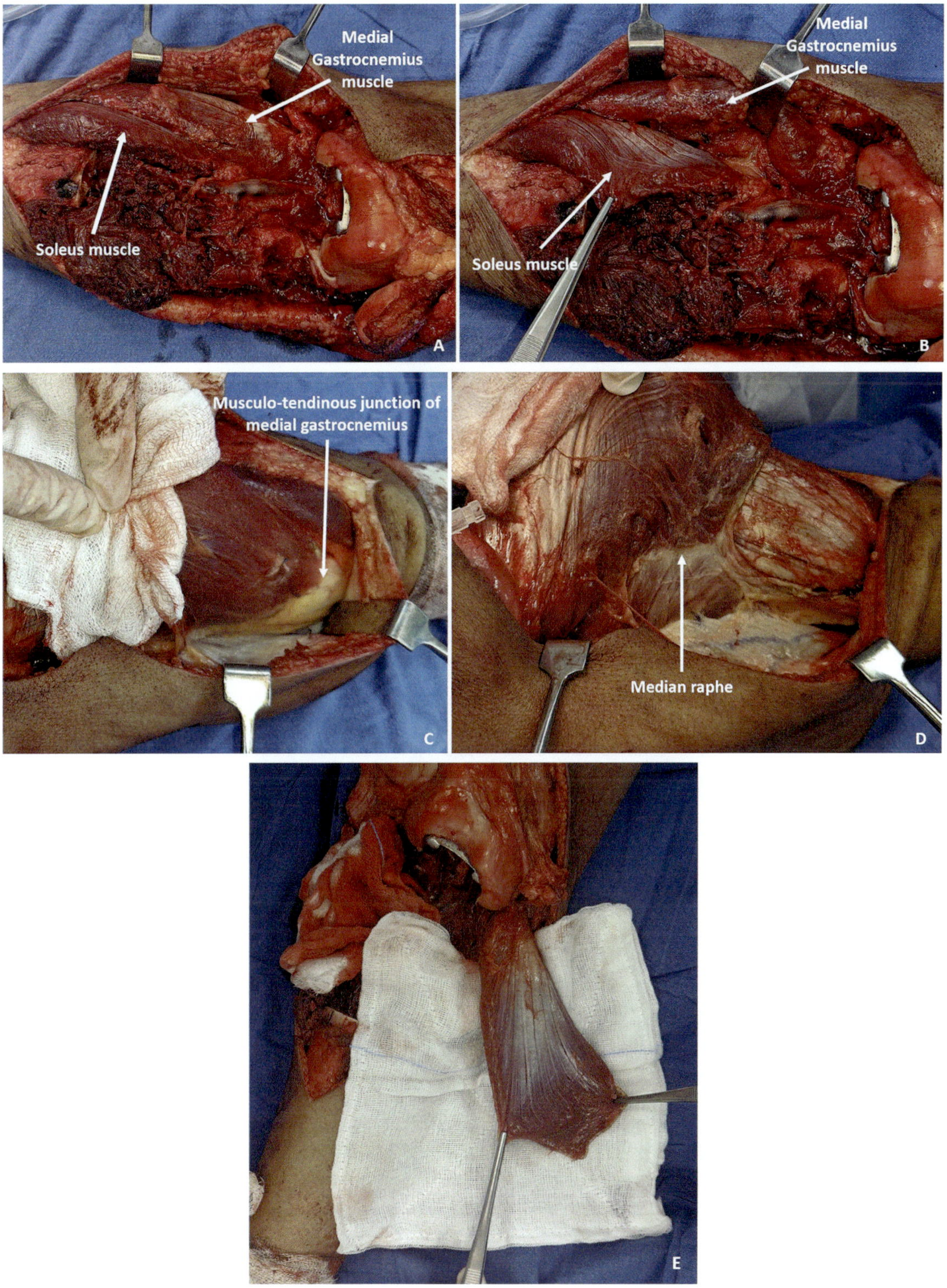

FIGURE 11.6 Intraoperative steps of medial gastrocnemius muscle flap harvest. (A, B) The medial gastrocnemius muscle is dissected free from the underlying soleus while preserving its vascular pedicle. Proximal identification is aided by locating the medial sural cutaneous nerve between the two heads of gastrocnemius. (C) The muscle is released distally just proximal to the musculo-tendinous junction, ensuring flap perfusion while allowing adequate mobilization for coverage. (D) The median raphe is released longitudinally using electrocautery to mobilize the flap. (E) The harvested medial gastrocnemius flap serves as a vascular cover for the endoprosthesis.

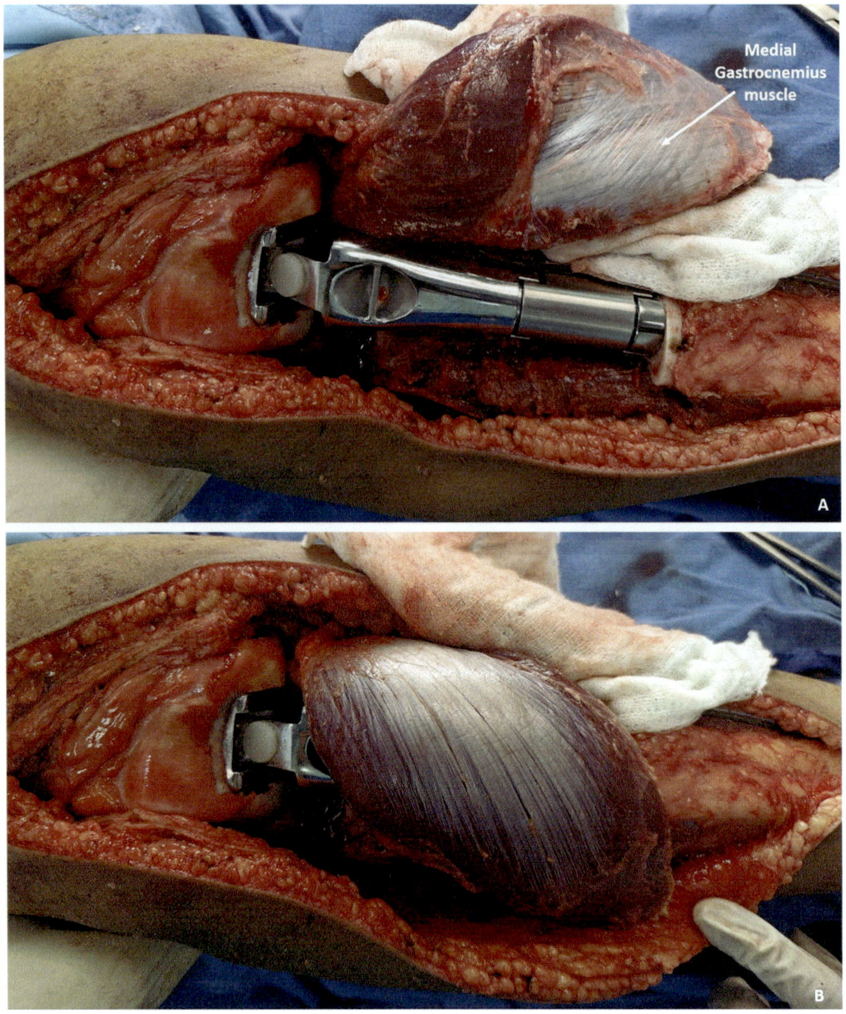

FIGURE 11.7 The proximal tibia endoprosthesis (A) is covered with the medial gastrocnemius flap (B) rotated anteriorly over the prosthesis.

FINAL PREPARATION AND CEMENTING

Irrigation and Restrictor Placement

- Irrigate both canals with pulse lavage.
- For cemented stems, place a cement restrictor 1–2 cm beyond the stem tip.
- Re-check with the trial stem to ensure the restrictor position is satisfactory.

Femoral Component Cementation

- Elevate the limb and inflate the tourniquet.
- Use antibiotic-impregnated cement applied with a cement gun.
- Insert the component under sustained pressure until cement cures to avoid lift-off.

Tibial Component Cementation

- Assemble tibial components on the table.
- Inject cement into the canal while still in a low-viscosity state, pressurizing for better penetration.
- Insert the stem slowly to avoid fat embolism; once positioned, maintain alignment without rotation until the cement hardens.
- For uncemented stems, achieve a press-fit using an impactor.

Final Assembly

- Remove excess cement and deflate the tourniquet.
- Assemble articulating components (axle, bumper).
- Reassess range of motion, patellar tracking, and neurovascular integrity.

EXTENSOR MECHANISM RECONSTRUCTION—*AUTHORS' PREFERRED TECHNIQUE*

Restoration of the extensor mechanism is critical for functional recovery. The authors utilize a multi-layered Prolene mesh (Ethicon, Johnson & Johnson) tube, 1.5–2 cm in width, rolled into six layers and secured with sutures or staples to provide high tensile strength [4] (Figure 11.8A and 11.8B).

- **Proximal fixation**: Mesh anchored to medial parapatellar tissues and the residual patellar tendon using No. 5 Ethibond sutures (Figure 11.8C).
- **Distal fixation**: Mesh passed through the prosthetic anterior slot simulating the native tibial tubercle, then secured back to the proximal mesh and medial tissues with the knee in 15°–20° flexion (Figure 11.8D and 11.8E).

SOFT TISSUE COVERAGE

Meticulous soft tissue coverage is essential for implant protection and infection prevention.

- **Medial Gastrocnemius Flap**: Rotated anteriorly to cover the proximal prosthesis and mesh.
- **Soleus Muscle Mobilization**: Advanced anteriorly to cover the middle third of the implant, adding vascularized bulk.
- The gastrocnemius is sutured to anterior compartment muscles and the patellar tendon, completing a circumferential, vascularized envelope around the implant (Figure 11.8F and 11.8G).

HEMOSTASIS AND CLOSURE

- Achieve meticulous hemostasis and irrigate thoroughly.
- Place deep suction drains close to the incision line.
- Perform layered closure, avoiding dead space beneath the flap.

POSTOPERATIVE CARE AND REHABILITATION

- **Immobilization**: Limb maintained in extension or 15–20° flexion with a knee immobilizer or plaster slab for six weeks to protect the extensor mechanism.
- **Antibiotics**: IV first-generation cephalosporin until drain removal.
- **Mobilization**: After six weeks, initiate gradual passive and active flexion alongside quadriceps strengthening.
- **Weight-Bearing**: Begin as tolerated, progressing gradually.
- **Flexion Progression**: Delay full flexion until active extension is achieved to ensure optimal functional recovery.

EXTENSOR MECHANISM RECONSTRUCTION CONSIDERATIONS

Reconstruction of the extensor mechanism after proximal tibial resection remains one of the most technically demanding steps in limb salvage surgery. Conventional techniques—direct patellar tendon fixation to the prosthesis using sutures or loops—often produce inconsistent outcomes, primarily due to poor healing potential over polished metal and the frequent presence of a short residual tendon. Over-tensioning in such cases risks shortening the extensor apparatus and limiting flexion.

Multiple reconstruction strategies have been described (Table 11.2). Jentzsch et al. reported patella alta in 69% and extension lag >10° in over 60% of patients with traditional repair [18], while Dominkus et al. observed a mean lag of 25° using LARS ligaments [12]. Alternatives such as porous-coated prostheses, autologous bone grafting, and synthetic materials (Trevira tubes, Dacron, Goretex) have been used, though often complicated by synovitis, infection, or prosthetic loosening. More complex constructs, such as mesh fixation with bone tunnels (Ichikawa et al. [7]), show promise but lack standardization.

The authors' preferred method employs a cylindrical Prolene mesh tube anchored to the medial patellar retinaculum and residual tendon, passed through a prosthetic slot, and tensioned. In 30 patients, this achieved a mean lag of 2.33°, mean flexion of 95°, and no deep infections, offering a reproducible and durable solution [4].

COMPLICATIONS AND OUTCOMES OF ENDOPROSTHESIS RECONSTRUCTION

Proximal tibial endoprosthetic reconstruction carries higher complication rates than other anatomic sites due to procedural complexity and limited soft tissue coverage. Major complications include flap ischemia, deep infection, wound dehiscence, limb edema, extensor mechanism dysfunction, polyethylene wear, and aseptic loosening.

Infection remains one of the most serious concerns. While historical rates approached 40%, the use of medial gastrocnemius flaps, perioperative antibiotics, and meticulous wound care has reduced incidence to 12%–18% in recent series. Nevertheless, late hematogenous infections can delay adjuvant therapy, cause implant failure, and occasionally require amputation.

Mechanical failure is multifactorial: early failures stem from design flaws, soft tissue imbalance, or technical error; late failures often result from polyethylene wear, stem fracture, or aseptic loosening—frequently associated with osteolysis. Modern advances, including porous collars, compressive osseointegration, and rotating-hinge designs, have improved durability.

Extensor mechanism impairment remains a common functional limitation, and flap necrosis increases risk of

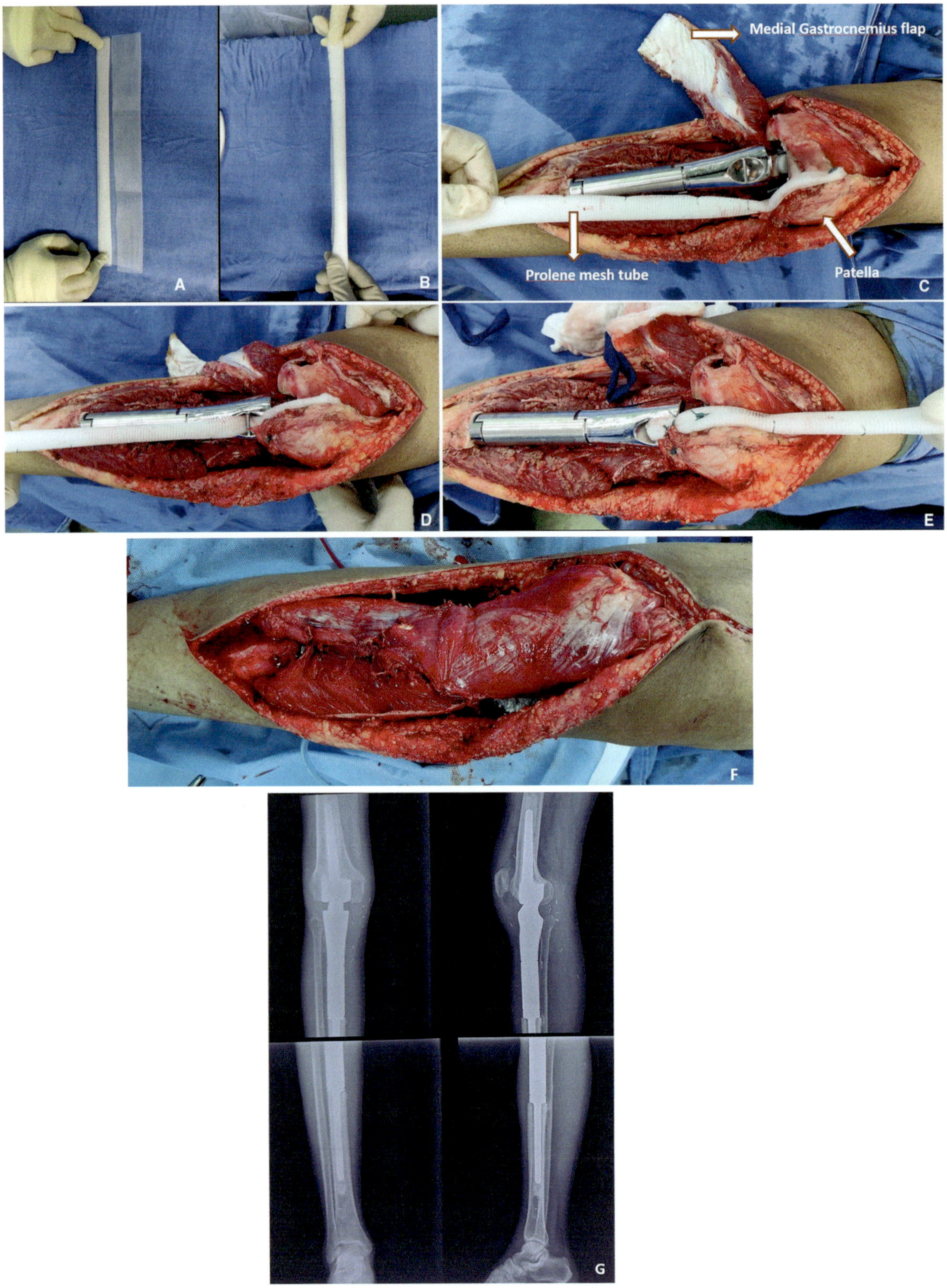

FIGURE 11.8 (A & B) Prolene mesh is rolled over itself to a breadth of ~1.5 to 2 cm into a tube (6–8 layers in cross section) and secured with sutures or staples. (C) Prolene mesh tube sutured proximally to the medial para-patellar tissues and to the remaining patellar tendon using Ethibond No. 5. This provides a larger area of interface b/w the mesh and extensor apparatus. (D & E) The distal part of the tube is then passed through a slot on the anterior surface of the proximal part of the prosthesis. (F) Medial gastrocnemius flap rotated anteriorly to cover the prosthesis and the mesh. Complete coverage of the mesh is ensured. (G) Post-operative radiographs following reconstruction with proximal tibia endoprosthesis.

TABLE 11.2
Review of Literature for Extensor Mechanism Reconstruction Techniques Following Proximal Tibia Tumor Resection

Study	Cases (n)	Type of Reconstruction	Surgical Technique	Mean ROM/ Extension Lag	Follow-Up (Months)	Functional Outcomes	Complications
Ebeid and Hassan (2023) [5]	55	Endoprosthesis	Ethibond sutures + medial gastrocnemius flap	(a) 72.63°, (b) 15.09°	71.69 (49.76)	MSTS 26.5	Superficial infection (5), Deep infection (1)
Liu et al. (2019) [6]	14	Endoprosthesis + mesh	Synthetic mesh (Bard) + medial gastrocnemius flap	(a) 105°, (b) 1.57°	23.50 (14 to 37)	MSTS 23.57	N/A
Ichikawa et al. (2015) [7]	9	Endoprosthesis	Mesh + medial gastrocnemius flap	(a) 97.5°, (b) 5°	33 (20 to 50)	ISOLS 21	Infection in one case (amputation)
Titus and Clayer (2008) [8]	10	Endoprosthesis	Cerclage wire	(a) 96°, (b) 4° to 20°	48 (24 to 89)	MSTS 82.1%, TESS 90.5%	Nerve palsy, Infection, Adhesions
Biau et al. (2007) [9]	26	Allograft-prosthetic composite	Medial gastrocnemius flap	(a) 80.96°, (b) 7.7°	128 (6 to 195)	N/A	Extensor mechanism rupture (23%)
Ayerza et al. (2006) [10]	34	Allograft	N/A	(a) 110°, (b) 6.5°	52 (24 to 136)	MSTS 26.6	N/A
Biau et al. (2006) [11]	35	Endoprosthesis	Medial gastrocnemius flap + ligament augmentation	N/A	62 (6 to 343)	TESS 81.8	Extensor mechanism rupture (26%)
Dominkus et al. (2006) [12]	11	Endoprosthesis	LARS ligament + medial gastrocnemius flap	Lag 25°	44 (8 to 67)	Enneking 83.3	Extensor mechanism rupture (27%)
Shimose et al. (2005) [13]	7	Endoprosthesis	Medial gastrocnemius flap + ligament augmentation	Lag 15.5°	32.1 (8 to 33)	N/A	Extensor mechanism rupture (42%)
Kollender et al. (2004) [14]	7	Endoprosthesis	Medial gastrocnemius flap + Goretex	Lag < 20°	58 (29 to 83)	MSTS 29	N/A
Gosheger et al. (2003) [15]	7	Endoprosthesis	Medial gastrocnemius flap + Trevira tube	Knee flexion 85.5°, lag 7.5°	31.6 (9 to 78)	MSTS 78.2%	N/A
Grimer et al. (2000) [16]	50	Endoprosthesis	N/A	Flexion 104°, lag 30°	N/A	MSTS 77%	N/A
Salunke et al. (2024) [17]	15	Endoprosthesis + ipsilateral hamstring tendon	Medial gastrocnemius flap + eq. ligament augmentation	Active knee flexion 92°, lag 4.6°	19 (13 to 24)	MSTS 24	Wound infection (3 cases)
Kapoor et al. (2022) [4]	30	Endoprosthesis	Medial gastrocnemius flap + Prolene Mesh tube	Mean active flexion 95°, lag 2.33°	16.43 (6 to 30 mo)	N/A	Aseptic wound dehiscence/necrosis (5 patients)

implant exposure and infection. With optimized technique and design, 10-year survival rates of 75%–86% are achievable, supporting limb salvage as a reliable strategy [2, 19].

ALTERNATE MODES OF RECONSTRUCTION OF SKELETAL DEFECT

Osteoarticular Allograft Reconstruction

Osteoarticular allograft (OAA) reconstruction provides a biological means of restoring proximal tibial defects after tumor resection, allowing reconstitution of bone stock and anatomic reattachment of the extensor mechanism. It is best suited for young, active patients with long-term survival prospects. In a large series by Muscolo et al. [20], 5- and 10-year allograft survival rates were 65%, with limb preservation in 91% and a mean MSTS score of 26. Complications included infection (22%), articular collapse (19%), and graft fracture (5%). Retained grafts yielded good function with minimal extensor lag. Compared with endoprostheses, OAAs offer superior extensor function but require delayed rehabilitation—full weight-bearing is usually deferred until union—and depend on bone bank availability. Albergo et al. [21] found similar failure and amputation rates for OAA and endoprosthetic reconstructions, but OAAs achieved better extensor performance (mean lag 2.4° vs. 13.5°).

Allograft/Autograft-Prosthetic Composite (APC)

APC reconstruction combines the biological benefit of robust patellar tendon attachment to an allograft or sterilized autograft with the mechanical stability of a rotating-hinge prosthesis. The prosthetic stem is cemented into the graft, while host fixation may be cemented or press-fit. Avoiding cement at the graft-host junction is critical to reduce nonunion risk. Fixation options include compression plating or long-stem prostheses spanning the graft. The extensor mechanism is reattached in full extension and covered with a medial gastrocnemius flap. Postoperative care involves immobilization in extension for six weeks, gradual flexion, and delayed weight-bearing until radiologic union. Despite functional benefits, nonunion (20%–27%) and infection (8%–24%) rates remain substantial, warranting meticulous surgical planning and patient selection [22, 23].

SUMMARY

- **Proximal tibia tumor resections** are technically complex due to limited soft tissue coverage, proximity to neurovascular structures, and resection of the extensor mechanism.
- **Comprehensive preoperative imaging** (MRI, CT, angiography) is essential for accurate assessment and surgical planning.
- **Reconstruction options** include:
  - **Endoprostheses**: allow early weight-bearing but have a risk of mechanical failure.
  - **Osteoarticular allografts**: restore bone stock and extensor continuity but require prolonged rehabilitation and bone bank availability.
  - **APC**: combine the advantages of both biological and mechanical reconstruction.
- The **medial gastrocnemius flap** is vital for both soft tissue coverage and extensor mechanism reconstruction.
- **Complications** such as deep infection, prosthetic loosening, flap necrosis, and extension lag remain frequent.
- **Structured rehabilitation** including immobilization, gradual knee flexion, and quadriceps strengthening is critical for functional recovery.
- **Reconstruction choice** should be individualized, considering patient age, tumor biology, and long-term functional demands.

REFERENCES

1. Malawer MM, Sugarbaker HS. *Musculoskeletal Cancer Surgery*. Dordrecht, The Netherlands: Kluwer Academic Publishers; 2001.
2. Myers GJ, Abudu AT, Carter SR, Tillman RM, Grimer RJ. The long-term results of endoprosthetic replacement of the proximal tibia for bone tumours. *J Bone Joint Surg Br.* 2007;89(12):1632–1637.
3. Bickels J, Wittig JC, Kollender Y, et al. Reconstruction of the extensor mechanism after proximal tibia endoprosthetic replacement. *J Arthroplasty.* 2001;16:856–862.
4. Kapoor L, Banjara R, Khan SA, Majeed A. Extensor apparatus reconstruction using prolene mesh tube and medial gastrocnemius flap following proximal tibial endoprosthetic reconstruction. *Tech Orthop.* 2022;37(1):65–69.
5. Ebeid WA, Hassan ME. Functional outcome following proximal tibial osteosarcoma resection and reconstruction by modular endoprosthesis. *Ann Surg Oncol.* 2023;30(3):1914–1925.
6. Liu B, Tan JC, Wang HL, Wu Z, Yuan ZC, Wei CY. The role of mesh technology with tumor prosthesis reconstruction to reconstruct the extensor mechanism of knee joint after resection of proximal tibial tumors. *J Orthop Surg Res.* 2019;14(1):64.
7. Ichikawa J, Matsumoto S, Shimoji T, Ae K, Tanizawa T, Gokita T. A new technique using mesh for extensor reconstruction after proximal tibial resection. *Knee.* 2015;22(6):659–663.
8. Titus V, Clayer M. Protecting a patellar ligament reconstruction after proximal tibial resection: a simplified approach. *Clin Orthop Relat Res.* 2008;466(7):1749–1754.
9. Biau DJ, Dumaine V, Babinet A, Tomeno B, Anract P. Allograft prosthesis composites after bone tumor resection at the proximal tibia. *Clin Orthop Relat Res.* 2007;456:211–217.
10. Ayerza MA, Aponte-Tinao LA, Abalo E, Muscolo DL. Continuity and function of patellar tendon host-donor suture in tibial allograft. *Clin Orthop Relat Res.* 2006;450:33–38.
11. Biau D, Faure F, Katsahian S, Jeanrot C, Tomeno B, Anract P. Survival of total knee replacement with a megaprosthesis after bone tumor resection. *J Bone Joint Surg Am.* 2006;88(6):1285–1293.
12. Dominkus M, Sabeti M, Toma C, Abdolvahab F, Trieb K, Kotz RI. Reconstructing the extensor apparatus with a new polyester ligament. *Clin Orthop Relat Res.* 2006;453:328–334.
13. Shimose S, Sugita T, Kubo T, Matsuo T, Ochi M. Reconstructed patellar tendon length after proximal tibia prosthetic replacement. *Clin Orthop Relat Res.* 2005;439:176–180.
14. Kollender Y, Bender B, Weinbroum AA, Nirkin A, Meller I, Bickels J. Secondary reconstruction of the extensor mechanism using part of the quadriceps tendon, patellar retinaculum, and Gore-Tex strips after proximal tibial resection. *J Arthroplasty.* 2004;19(3):354–360.
15. Gosheger G, Hillmann A, Lindner N, et al. Soft tissue reconstruction of megaprostheses using a trevira tube. *Clin Orthop Relat Res.* 2001;393:264–271.
16. Grimer RJ, Carter SR, Tillman RM, et al. Endoprosthetic replacement of the proximal tibia. *J Bone Joint Surg Br.* 1999;81(3):488–494.
17. Salunke AA, Bharwani N, Patel D, et al. Salunke's GCRI surgical technique for neopatellar ligament reconstruction using hamstring tendon in proximal tibia tumour megaprosthesis. *Bone Jt Open.* 2025;6(3):342–351.
18. Jentzsch T, Erschbamer M, Seeli F, et al. Extensor function after medial gastrocnemius flap reconstruction of the proximal tibia. *Clin Orthop Relat Res.* 2013;471:2333–2339.
19. Schwartz AJ, Kabo JM, Eilber FC, Eilber FR, Eckardt JJ. Cemented endoprosthetic reconstruction of the proximal tibia: How long do they last? *Clin Orthop Relat Res.* 2010;468(11):2875–2884.

20. Muscolo DL, Ayerza MA, Farfalli G, Aponte-Tinao LA. Proximal tibia osteoarticular allografts in tumor limb salvage surgery. *Clin Orthop Relat Res.* 2010;468(5):1396–1404.
21. Albergo JI, Gaston CL, Aponte-Tinao LA, et al. Proximal tibia reconstruction after bone tumor resection: Are survivorship and outcomes of endoprosthetic replacement and osteoarticular allograft similar? *Clin Orthop Relat Res.* 2017;475(3):676–682.
22. Gilbert NF, Yasko AW, Oates SD, Lewis VO, Cannon CP, Lin PP. Allograft-prosthetic composite reconstruction of the proximal part of the tibia: An analysis of the early results. *J Bone Joint Surg Am.* 2009;91(7):1646–1656.
23. Kim JD, Lee GW, Chung SH. Reconstruction with extracorporeal irradiated autograft in osteosarcoma around the knee. *J Surg Oncol.* 2011;104(2):187–191.

12 Distal Tibia Resection and Reconstruction

INTRODUCTION

Primary malignant bone tumors of the distal tibia are uncommon, representing less than 2%–3% of all bone sarcomas, with osteosarcoma and Ewing's sarcoma being the predominant histological subtypes [1]. Historically, below-knee amputation was the standard treatment, given the difficulty of achieving wide margins and reconstructing the weight-bearing ankle. Advances in chemotherapy, imaging, surgical techniques, and reconstruction have now made limb salvage the preferred approach in most cases [2].

The distal tibia's subcutaneous location, limited soft tissue envelope, and proximity to neurovascular structures pose significant challenges for oncologically safe resection while preserving limb function [1, 3]. Additionally, the short residual tibial segment and small talar surface complicate stable reconstruction, particularly with prosthetic devices [1].

Reconstructive strategies range from biological methods—such as autografts, allografts, and distraction osteogenesis—to nonbiological options using custom prostheses [4–6]. Vascularized fibular grafts have shown particular promise for their biological incorporation and durability [4, 7].

This chapter reviews the principles, surgical techniques, and outcomes of distal tibia tumor resection and reconstruction, synthesizing literature evidence, and clinical experience to guide management in this complex anatomical region.

SURGICAL ANATOMY AND PREOPERATIVE PLANNING

Surgical Anatomy

A precise understanding of the distal tibial anatomy is critical for safe tumor resection and successful reconstruction. The distal third of the leg is one of the narrowest segments of the lower limb, where bone, tendons, and neurovascular structures are concentrated within a limited soft tissue envelope. This close proximity increases the risk of inadvertent injury and restricts options for soft tissue coverage after resection.

Bony Landmarks

The distal tibia articulates inferiorly with the talus at the tibiotalar joint, while the distal fibula contributes laterally via the tibiofibular syndesmosis. The medial malleolus is subcutaneous and serves as a palpable surgical landmark. The tibial plafond bears the body's axial load, making its preservation important in joint-sparing procedures. The talus, although vital to ankle biomechanics, offers a small surface area for prosthetic fixation or graft fusion, complicating reconstruction.

Soft Tissue Relationships

Anteriorly, from medial to lateral, are the tibialis anterior tendon, extensor hallucis longus tendon, anterior tibial artery with the deep peroneal nerve, extensor digitorum longus tendons, and peroneus tertius. Posteriorly, the tibialis posterior and flexor hallucis longus tendons separate the tibia from the posterior tibial artery and tibial nerve, which pass behind the medial malleolus.

Medially, the tibia lies directly beneath the skin, making it susceptible to wound breakdown.Laterally, the distal fibula and peroneal tendons lie behind the lateral malleolus. Dense fascial and retinacular structures limit tissue mobility, and tumor extension into these compartments may cause neurovascular compression.

Vascular Considerations

The anterior tibial artery runs along the interosseous membrane, continuing as the dorsalis pedis artery at the ankle, while the posterior tibial artery passes behind the medial malleolus to supply the plantar foot. Dominance in the pedal arch by either vessel must be determined preoperatively, as arterial sacrifice may severely impair distal perfusion. Bypass procedures at this level have higher failure rates, making vessel preservation a priority.

Neurological Structures

The superficial and deep peroneal nerves supply anterior and lateral sensation, while the tibial nerve supplies the posterior and plantar aspects of the foot. Injury can result in sensory loss over weight-bearing areas, impairing postoperative protection and healing.

Joint and Ligamentous Anatomy

The ankle mortise is formed by the medial and lateral malleoli and the tibial plafond, with stability reinforced by the deltoid ligament medially and the anterior/posterior talofibular and calcaneofibular ligaments laterally. The syndesmosis confers axial and rotational stability. The ankle capsule, thin anteriorly and posteriorly, may be breached by tumors only a few centimeters proximal to the joint. Its extension toward the interosseous tibiofibular ligament must be appreciated during intra-articular resections.

DOI: 10.1201/9780367822002-15

Preoperative Planning

Successful management of distal tibial tumors requires a multidisciplinary approach involving orthopedic oncology, radiology, reconstructive surgery, and vascular surgery. The aim is to achieve oncologically safe resection while maximizing functional preservation.

Imaging

- **Plain Radiographs**: Antero-posterior (AP) and lateral radiographs of the tibia assess lesion characteristics and guide osteotomy levels. Full-length views help evaluate alignment and plan implant sizing.
- **MRI**: Essential for mapping intra- and extraosseous tumor spread, joint or syndesmotic involvement, and neurovascular encasement. Determines resectability and margin planning (Figure 12.1).
- **CT**: Offers detailed cortical anatomy for surgical planning, especially for metastatic disease or custom implant design. 3D reconstructions aid in templating allografts.
- **PET-CT/Bone Scintigraphy**: Used for staging and detecting skip lesions. PET-CT also assists in biopsy targeting.

Biopsy

Biopsy planning is crucial to ensure the tract can be excised en bloc with the tumor. A longitudinal incision along the subcutaneous anteromedial tibial surface is preferred to preserve reconstructive options. Transverse incisions or medial approaches are avoided.

SURGICAL MARGIN PLANNING

Margins are determined by tumor type, grade, soft tissue extension, joint involvement, and patient factors. Intra-articular resection is necessary if subchondral bone or articular cartilage is involved. Joint-sparing resections are possible if the tumor is ≥3 cm from the articular surface.

Reconstructive Considerations

- **Residual Bone Length**: Adequate length is required for secure implant fixation or graft incorporation.
- **Host Bone Quality**: Osteoporotic bone may limit fixation options.
- **Soft Tissue Status**: Preexisting scars, irradiation, or infection risk influence flap choice.
- **Coverage**: Local fasciocutaneous flaps, gastrocnemius rotational flaps, or free microvascular flaps are selected based on defect size and location.

Careful preoperative mapping of tumor margins, vascular anatomy, and nerve course, combined with appropriate reconstructive planning, is essential to optimize oncologic safety and functional outcomes in distal tibia tumor surgery.

SURGICAL TECHNIQUE

Surgical resection of distal tibial tumors requires strict adherence to oncologic principles to achieve tumor-free margins while preserving optimal function. The operative plan must integrate biopsy tract excision, careful soft tissue handling, neurovascular preservation, and reconstruction preparation.

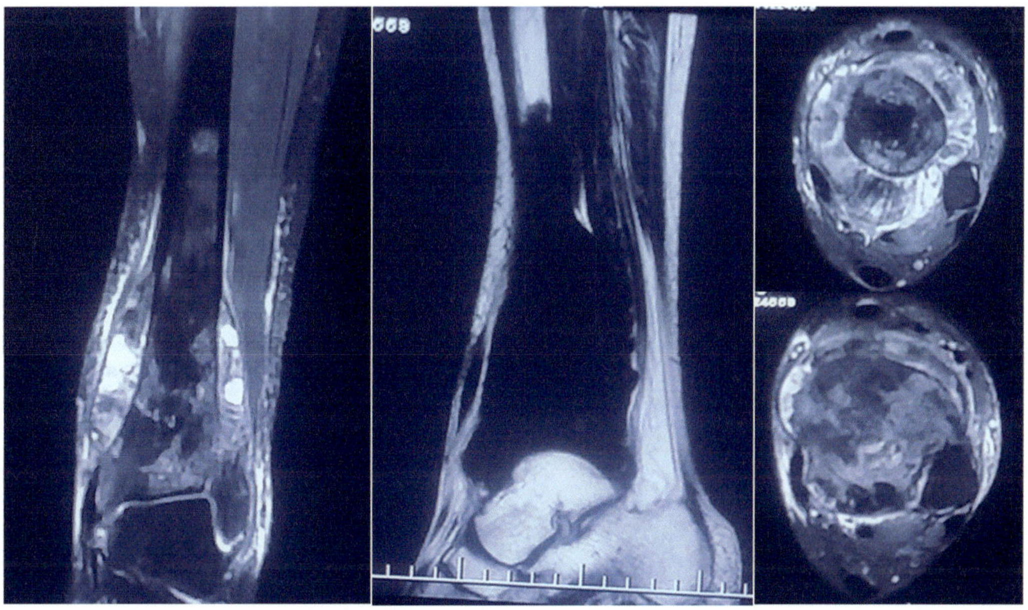

FIGURE 12.1 MRI of osteosarcoma of the distal tibia. Coronal, sagittal, and axial sections demonstrate a large, heterogeneous intramedullary lesion involving the distal tibia, extending up to the metaphysis and epiphysis. The tumor shows cortical destruction with breach and extension into adjacent soft tissues. Areas of necrosis and heterogeneous contrast enhancement are evident, along with perilesional edema. MRI clearly outlines the intramedullary extent, soft tissue involvement, and relationship with adjacent neurovascular structures, which are critical for preoperative planning.

PATIENT POSITIONING

The patient is positioned supine to allow optimal access to the anterior and medial compartments of the distal leg and ankle. A sandbag beneath the ipsilateral hip provides slight internal rotation, improving visualization of the anterior tibial crest. The limb is prepared circumferentially and draped free from mid-thigh to foot to permit manipulation.

A tourniquet may be applied to minimize blood loss; however, many oncologic surgeons avoid its use to facilitate detection of vascular compromise and ensure meticulous hemostasis. If used, it should be deflated prior to closure for final hemostatic control.

INCISION AND APPROACH

A longitudinal anterior incision, incorporating the previous biopsy tract en bloc, is preferred. It is placed over the subcutaneous border of the tibia and extended proximally to the planned osteotomy site. Distally, it may be carried over the ankle joint for talar resection or arthrodesis. If required, the incision can be curved to enhance exposure or extended over the dorsum of the foot for joint access.

SOFT TISSUE DISSECTION

Fasciocutaneous flaps are elevated with care to preserve vascularity, particularly distally, where soft tissue is minimal.

- **Anterior dissection**: The compartment fascia is opened in line with the incision. The tibialis anterior, extensor hallucis longus, and extensor digitorum longus tendons are sequentially identified, with the anterior tibial artery and deep peroneal nerve protected. In cases with anterior soft tissue involvement, dissection proceeds outside the pseudocapsule to avoid tumor violation.
- **Posterior dissection**: The posterior tibial neurovascular bundle, located between the tibialis posterior and flexor hallucis longus, is exposed and safeguarded. Dissection is maintained extraperiosteally along the tibial shaft to ensure oncologic clearance.

BONE RESECTION

The proximal osteotomy is performed 2–3 cm above the most proximal tumor margin (as per MRI), ensuring adequate clearance for high-grade sarcomas.

- **Joint-sparing intercalary resection**: Possible if the tumor is ≥3 cm from the articular surface.
- **Intra-articular resection**: Required if tumor proximity is <3 cm.
- **Extra-articular resection**: Involves en bloc removal of the distal tibial plafond, talus, and, if necessary, distal fibula.

Osteotomies are executed using an oscillating saw; the interosseous membrane is divided, and the fibula osteotomized when indicated. The specimen is removed en bloc, with margins assessed intraoperatively; frozen sections may be employed selectively.

PREPARATION FOR RECONSTRUCTION

Following resection, the defect is measured, and bone ends are prepared according to the planned reconstruction. The proximal medullary canal is reamed, and talar surfaces contoured for graft or prosthetic seating. For ankle arthrodesis, the talar dome is burred to accept the fusion interface.

SOFT TISSUE MANAGEMENT

Tendons such as the extensor hallucis longus or peroneus longus can be mobilized to enhance soft tissue coverage over implants or grafts. The surgical field is evaluated for the need for flap coverage—options include gastrocnemius muscle flaps, fasciocutaneous rotational flaps, or free microvascular flaps, coordinated with reconstructive surgery when primary closure is not feasible.

RECONSTRUCTION OPTIONS

Allograft Reconstructions

Massive allograft reconstruction remains a well-recognized biological method for managing defects after distal tibial tumor resection. It entails transplantation of a size-matched cadaveric bone segment to restore anatomical contour and mechanical function, and is particularly indicated in younger patients where preservation of bone stock is a priority.

Following wide en bloc tumor resection, the allograft is typically fixed using intramedullary nails, plates, or a combination. Xu et al. described the use of a retrograde intramedullary nail for tibiotalocalcaneal arthrodesis, which provided robust stability and permitted early mobilization [8]. Secure compression and fixation at the graft–host junctions are critical for osteointegration, although delayed union is a well-recognized drawback.

The key advantages of allografts include the ability to restore the native anatomy precisely and their ready availability in institutions with established bone banks, thus avoiding donor site morbidity. However, union is typically protracted because allografts are avascular and heal via creeping substitution; Zhao et al. reported mean union times of 17.2 months proximally and 16.2 months distally, compared with 11.1 and 9.5 months for autografts, respectively [1]. Complication rates are high: a meta-analysis by Zhao et al. documented a 55% overall complication rate, with infection and graft fracture each occurring in 27% of cases [1]. Immunogenicity and the risk of disease transmission are rare with modern sterilization but remain theoretical concerns.

Despite these limitations, functional outcomes are acceptable in selected patients. Xu et al. reported a mean MSTS score of 74.3% following retrograde nailing with allograft [8], while Zhao et al. noted slightly lower MSTS scores with allografts (67%) compared to autografts (81%) [1]. Common complications include graft fracture due to incomplete incorporation, infection (especially in immunocompromised patients), nonunion at the junctions, and ankle instability or deformity if arthrodesis is insufficiently stabilized. Careful patient selection, precise surgical technique, and long-term follow-up are critical for success.

Fibular Autograft Reconstructions

The fibula, owing to its cortical strength, length, and relative expendability, is a versatile autologous graft source for distal tibial reconstruction. This is especially relevant in settings with limited access to allografts or prostheses. Reconstruction can be performed with nonvascularized (pedicled) or vascularized fibular grafts.

Ipsilateral Nonvascularized Fibular Autograft (Fibular Centralization)

Also known as tibialization of the fibula, this technique mobilizes the ipsilateral fibula medially to bridge the post-resection defect. The pedicled fibula, retaining its muscular and vascular attachments at one end, is osteotomized and transposed into the defect. The proximal end is inserted into the tibial canal, and the distal end is secured into a talar notch to achieve tibiotalar fusion. The construct is supported with a plate, and the fixation may be supplemented with Kirschner wires or cortical screws (Figure 12.2).

This technique is technically straightforward, cost-effective, and does not require microvascular anastomosis. Preservation of vascularity at one end facilitates union and promotes graft hypertrophy. Operative time is shorter, morbidity is confined to a single limb, and the reduced bulk facilitates wound closure after fibular medialization. The reduced implant burden may also decrease the risk of deep infection, a significant consideration in patients receiving chemotherapy.

However, the fibula's relatively small cross-section predisposes it to early fractures before hypertrophy occurs. Prolonged protected weight-bearing is usually required, and there is a risk of graft resorption or nonunion, necessitating secondary procedures. Ankle arthrodesis, often required with this technique, eliminates ankle motion, and in skeletally immature patients there is a risk of leg length discrepancy.

Puri et al. [9] achieved union in 12 of 13 patients treated with this technique, although 10 of the 26 junctions required further surgery. The mean MSTS score was 24.7/30, with superior function in intercalary reconstructions compared to ankle fusions. Kundu et al. [10] reported nine patients with distal tibial tumors managed with fibular centralization and ankle arthrodesis. Weight-bearing was restricted for eight weeks and full loading delayed until radiological union, which occurred at a mean of 12.4 months. All patients demonstrated radiological hypertrophy of the fibula, with a mean MSTS score of 22.75/30. Complications included two nonunions, one local recurrence, and one leg length discrepancy, but notably no deep infections or implant-related failures.

Finite element analysis by Zhao et al. [11] compared ipsilateral fibular centralization with double-strut fibula

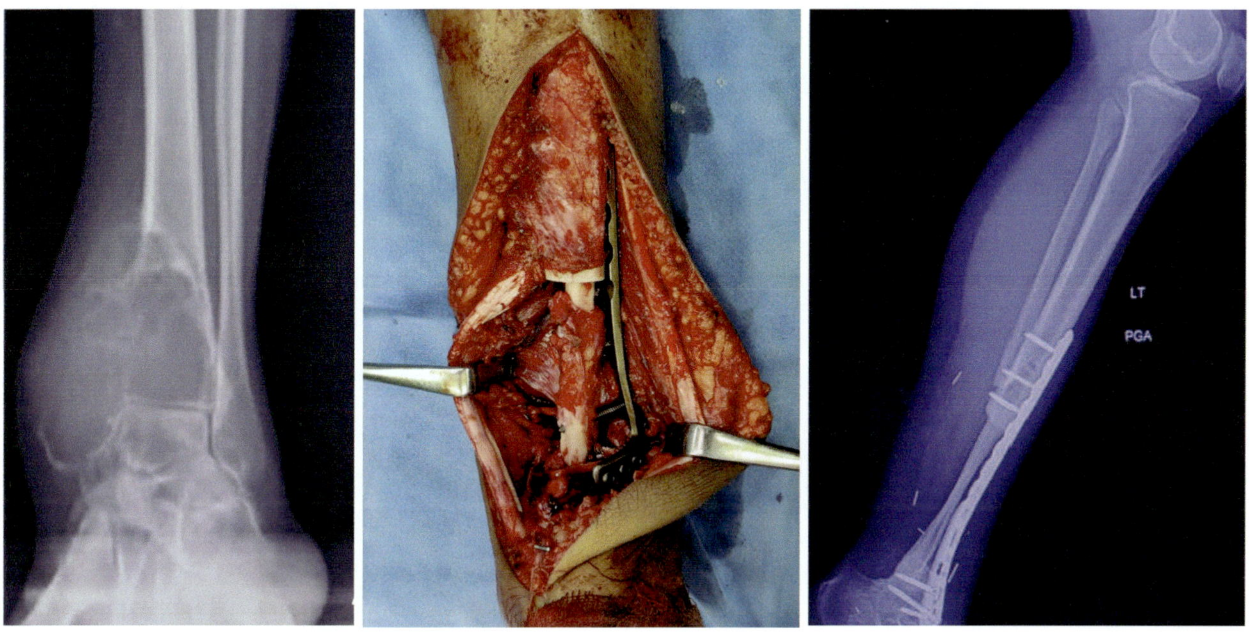

FIGURE 12.2 A 24-year-old female with a Giant Cell Tumor of the distal tibia. Patient underwent en bloc resection and fibular translocation. Follow-up radiographs at 24 months showed radiological union at the proximal and distal junctions.

reconstruction, revealing similar stress distribution but higher displacement and lower stiffness in fibular centralization. Implant stress was significantly greater, suggesting a higher risk of fixation failure and indicating that this method requires prolonged protection before weight-bearing.

Vascularized Fibular Autograft

In younger patients with long diaphyseal defects or compromised healing potential, vascularized fibular grafts provide superior biological potential. Harvested with their peroneal vascular pedicle from the contralateral leg, they are microvascularly anastomosed to recipient vessels and fixed between host bone ends. The fibular head may be preserved in pediatric patients to reconstruct the ankle joint.

The intrinsic vascularity of these grafts allows earlier union, better resistance to infection (particularly in irradiated fields), and marked hypertrophy under mechanical stress. However, the procedure is technically demanding, time-consuming, and dependent on microsurgical expertise and suitable recipient vessels. There is a risk of vascular thrombosis and donor site morbidity, including peroneal nerve injury or ankle instability.

Zhang et al. [12] described a trapezoidal double-barrel vascularized fibula configuration for ankle arthrodesis while preserving the subtalar joint. The mean union time was 10.1 ± 2.9 months, with hypertrophy in most grafts. MSTS scores averaged 81.5%, and graft survival was 100% at a mean follow-up of 46 months.

Recycled Autograft Reconstructions

Recycled autografts use the patient's own tumor-bearing bone, treated ex vivo to eradicate tumor cells before reimplantation. This preserves anatomical match and avoids graft procurement or immune compatibility issues. The two most common methods are extracorporeal irradiation (ECRT) and liquid nitrogen freezing.

Extracorporeal Irradiation and Reimplantation (ECRT)

The tumor-bearing bone is excised en bloc and irradiated outside the body with a single fraction of 50 Gy. Soft tissue is removed and the devitalized bone is reimplanted, often with a supplementary fibular graft. For distal tibial cases, ECRT segments are frequently combined with an ipsilateral nonvascularized fibula and ankle arthrodesis, which is fixed using locking plates (Figure 12.3).

ECRT ensures precise anatomical restoration without the risks of disease transmission or immune reaction, and is feasible in institutions lacking allograft facilities. However, it does not restore cartilage if the articular surface is involved, and the irradiated bone is avascular, requiring biological augmentation for integration.

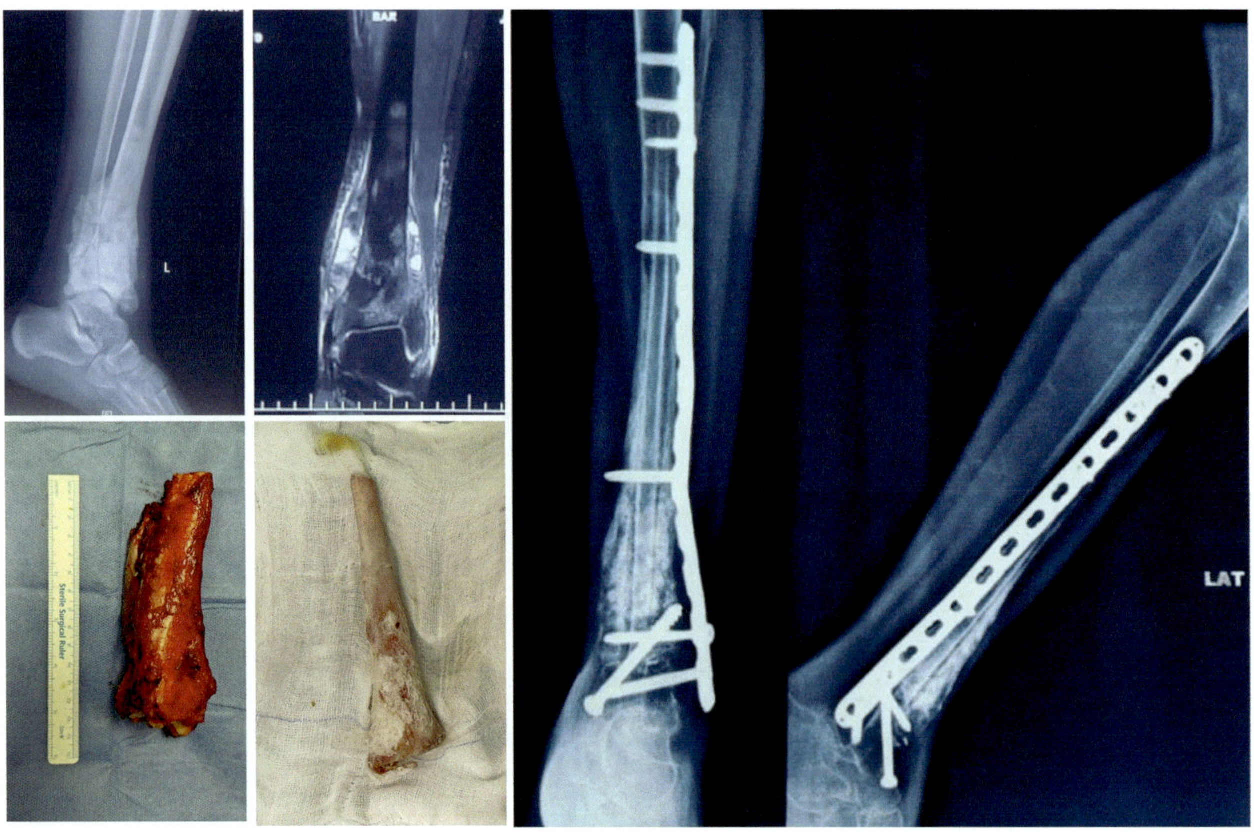

FIGURE 12.3 A 19-year-old male with Osteosarcoma distal tibia. Wide resection was performed, followed by tumor sterilization with irradiation and re-implantation of the irradiated bone and stabilization with a plate.

Gundavda et al. [13] compared ECRT with fibular centralization alone and found significantly better results for ECRT plus fibula: MSTS scores were 28.25 versus 23.67 ($p = 0.0003$), AOFAS scores were 83 versus 63 ($p < 0.0001$), and weight-bearing commenced earlier (26.75 vs 80.75 weeks). All patients in the ECRT group achieved union, with no implant failures or infections.

Liquid Nitrogen–Treated Autograft

This technique involves deep-freezing the resected bone segment in liquid nitrogen for 20 minutes, then thawing at room temperature and in warm saline before reimplantation. Fixation is achieved with plates or nails, frequently augmented with fibular grafts.

Liquid nitrogen treatment effectively kills tumor cells while preserving the bone matrix and precise anatomical contour. It is cost-effective and straightforward, but risks include fracture, infection, and delayed union due to bone devitalization. The requirement for cryogenic equipment and meticulous handling can limit its use.

Gede et al. [14] reported union in the majority of 17 patients reconstructed with frozen autografts, with a mean union time of 7.8 months. Complications occurred in two cases (fracture and infection). The mean MSTS score was 26.7, reflecting satisfactory function. Zhao et al.'s meta-analysis concluded that recycled autografts, whether irradiated or frozen, yield acceptable union rates and functional outcomes, particularly when augmented biologically with fibular grafts.

In summary, reconstruction after distal tibial tumor resection requires a balance between oncologic safety, biological potential, mechanical stability, and available resources. Allografts offer precise anatomical restoration but carry a high complication rate and delayed healing. Fibular autografts—whether centralized or vascularized—are biologically reliable, with vascularized grafts providing faster union and greater infection resistance at the cost of surgical complexity. Recycled autografts preserve native bone architecture and avoid donor morbidity, with ECRT combined with fibula showing particularly favorable outcomes. The optimal choice depends on patient factors, tumor extent, available expertise, and institutional resources, with long-term surveillance essential to detect complications and ensure functional preservation.

ENDOPROSTHETIC RECONSTRUCTION

Endoprosthetic replacement represents a nonbiological limb salvage solution for distal tibial defects following tumor resection. Although less frequently performed than in proximal limb segments due to anatomical constraints and biomechanical challenges, it remains a valuable option in selected cases where immediate stability, early ambulation, and shortened rehabilitation are priorities (Figure 12.4).

Most distal tibial endoprostheses are custom-made to accommodate individual anatomical variations, as commercially available modular options are scarce. Typically fabricated from titanium alloys with cobalt–chromium articulation surfaces, these implants incorporate a proximally fixed intramedullary stem, usually cemented, and often feature a hydroxyapatite (HA) collar to enhance osseointegration at the bone–implant interface. The talar component poses unique challenges due to its small surface area and limited bone stock, necessitating designs with dome-shaped contours and dual flanges or fins for secure anchorage.

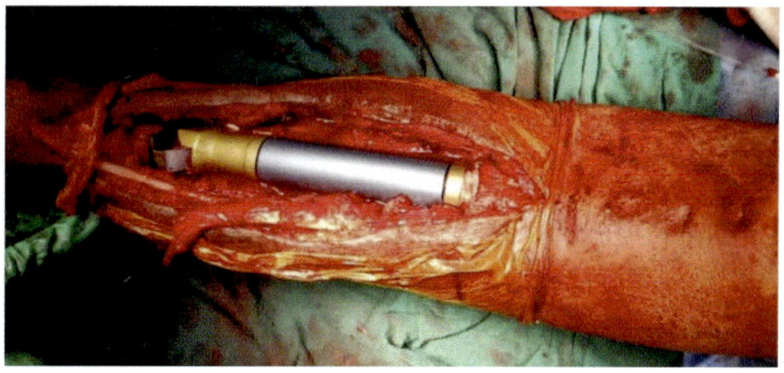

FIGURE 12.4 Intraoperative images of distal tibia endoprosthetic reconstruction. The endoprosthesis restores limb length and alignment while providing stable fixation and functional joint replacement, with the benefit of modularity.

Indications for endoprosthetic reconstruction include high-grade sarcomas with minimal extraosseous spread, preserved neurovascular integrity of the foot, and patients either with limited life expectancy or those in whom lengthy rehabilitation is undesirable. Contraindications include prior radiotherapy, severe soft tissue compromise, and systemic comorbidities such as diabetes or obesity, which elevate infection risk.

Advantages of this method include immediate structural stability, the ability to commence early full weight-bearing, avoidance of donor site morbidity, and a single-stage surgical protocol. It also offers a reproducible technique that can be standardized with modular systems. However, drawbacks are significant: reported deep infection rates reach 16%, aseptic loosening occurs in 13.5% of cases [1], and unique to distal tibia reconstruction is the risk of talar component failure due to collapse or inadequate fixation. Functional deterioration over time has been observed; Abudu et al. reported MSTS scores declining from 81% at one year to 65% at final review, largely due to mechanical failures [15]. Revision surgery options are limited, with salvage often requiring amputation—sometimes at a higher level than if performed initially. Additionally, custom manufacture increases cost and logistical complexity.

Outcomes vary across series. Yang et al. [16], in the largest single-center report of eight patients with custom megaprostheses, observed a median follow-up of 77 months, MSTS scores averaging 66%, and 5- and 10-year implant survival rates of 63% and 42%, respectively. Complications occurred in 37% of patients, including one deep infection, one superficial wound infection, and one asymptomatic talar loosening, though no revisions were necessary. Shekkeris et al. [17] reported on six patients with a mean follow-up of 9.6 years; two required below-knee amputation for persistent infection, while the remaining four achieved mean MSTS and TESS scores of 70% and 71%, respectively. In the meta-analysis by Zhao et al., endoprostheses demonstrated statistically lower MSTS scores compared to biological reconstructions (72.2% vs. 78.4%, p = 0.017) and slightly higher complication rates (32.4% vs. 20.2%) [1].

Despite these limitations, distal tibial endoprostheses remain appropriate for selected patients—particularly those where rapid recovery and avoidance of prolonged protective weight-bearing are key goals, and in whom biological options are unsuitable.

DISTRACTION OSTEOGENESIS

Distraction osteogenesis offers a purely biological reconstruction method, harnessing the body's innate regenerative capacity by gradually separating osteotomized bone under controlled mechanical tension. Its use in distal tibial tumor reconstruction enables restoration of bone stock without allografts or implants, thereby avoiding immunogenicity, donor site morbidity, and the long-term risks of prosthetic failure.

A notable hybrid method described by Lou et al. [18] combines initial bone transport via circular external fixation with later conversion to internal fixation using locking plates. This approach facilitates definitive ankle arthrodesis while reducing external fixator duration. In their series of five patients (mean age 18.6 years, mean defect length 11.8 cm), the external fixation index (EFI) averaged 29.3 days/cm. All achieved ankle fusion and solid union, with a mean MSTS score of 88%, reflecting favorable function.

Despite such encouraging reports, the wider application of distraction osteogenesis in this context remains limited. Zhao et al.'s meta-analysis identified only four published studies, totaling ten cases, with a pooled mean MSTS score of 91% (range 83%–100%) [1]. These high scores must be weighed against the demanding treatment course: prolonged use of external fixators, risk of pin or wire tract infection, and a 20% incidence of docking-site nonunion. In addition, reported bone transport distances did not exceed 15 cm, raising concerns about feasibility in extensive segmental defects.

The main advantages are the biological nature of the reconstruction, absence of foreign body implants, and the ability to create living bone capable of remodeling and hypertrophy. However, limitations include the extended rehabilitation period, risk of joint stiffness, soft tissue tethering, patient discomfort, and a steep learning curve for surgeons.

In practice, distraction osteogenesis is best suited for younger, compliant patients with moderate bone loss, preserved soft tissue envelopes, and no major comorbidities. For such cases, it can yield high functional scores and durable reconstruction, provided the patient is willing to accept the prolonged treatment timeline and potential complications.

SUMMARY

- **Distal tibia tumor resection** poses unique surgical and reconstructive challenges due to limited soft tissue coverage, weight-bearing demands, and proximity to the ankle joint.
- **Biological reconstructions** (allografts, fibular autografts, recycled autografts) provide long-term durability with good functional outcomes but are limited by delayed union and complications like nonunion or fracture.
- **Endoprosthetic reconstruction** allows early weight-bearing and functional recovery but has higher rates of infection, mechanical failure, and long-term decline in function.
- **Distraction osteogenesis** offers a graft-free, biologically sound option for selected patients but is constrained by long treatment duration, docking-site complications, and limited applicability for large defects.
- **Fibular centralization and vascularized fibular grafts** are effective, particularly in younger patients, providing hypertrophy and incorporation with acceptable MSTS scores.
- **Recycled autografts** (irradiated or frozen) maintain joint anatomy and avoid allograft risks but require meticulous technique and careful monitoring for graft-related complications.
- **Reconstruction strategy should be individualized**, integrating oncological safety, biomechanics, patient factors, and available expertise to optimize both functional and oncological outcomes.

REFERENCES

1. Zhao Z, Yan T, Guo W, Yang R, Tang X, Wang W. Surgical options and reconstruction strategies for primary bone tumors of distal tibia: A systematic review of complications and functional outcome. *J Bone Oncol.* 2019;14:100209.
2. Mavrogenis AF, Abati CN, Romagnoli C, Ruggieri P. Similar survival but better function for patients after limb salvage versus amputation for distal tibia osteosarcoma. *Clin Orthop Relat Res.* 2012;470(6):1735–1748.
3. Abudu A, Grimer RJ, Tillman RM, Carter SR. Endoprosthetic replacement of the distal tibia and ankle joint for aggressive bone tumours. *Int Orthop.* 1999;23(5):291–294.
4. Ebeid W, Amin S, Abdelmegid A, Refaat Y, Ghoneimy A. Reconstruction of distal tibial defects following resection of malignant tumours by pedicled vascularised fibular grafts. *Acta Orthop Belg.* 2007;73(3):354–359.
5. Natarajan MV, Annamalai K, Williams S, Selvaraj R, Rajagopal TS. Limb salvage in distal tibial osteosarcoma using a custom mega prosthesis. *Int Orthop.* 2000;24(5):282–284.
6. Lee SH, Kim HS, Park YB, Rhie TY, Lee HK. Prosthetic reconstruction for tumours of the distal tibia and fibula. *J Bone Joint Surg Br.* 1999;81(5):803–807.
7. Shalaby S, Bassiony AA, Shalaby H. Reconstruction of large bone defect after resection of osteosarcoma of the distal tibia. *J Bone Joint Surg Br.* 2006;88(7):995–1000.

8. Xu L, Zhou J, Wang Z, Xiong J, Qiu Y, Wang S. Reconstruction of bone defect with allograft and retrograde intramedullary nail for distal tibia osteosarcoma. *Foot Ankle Surg.* 2017;23(4):302–307. doi:10.1016/j.fas.2017.01.006
9. Puri A, Subin BS, Agarwal MG. Fibular centralisation for the reconstruction of defects of the tibial diaphysis and distal metaphysis after excision of bone tumours. *J Bone Joint Surg Br.* 2009;91(2):234–239. doi:10.1302/0301-620X.91B2.21272
10. Kundu ZS, Gogna P, Gupta V, et al. Ankle fusion with centralisation of the fibula after distal tibia bone tumour resection. *J Orthop Traumatol.* 2014;15(2):95–101. doi:10.1007/s10195-013-0279-2
11. Zhao Z, Yan T, Guo W, Yang R, Tang X. Is double-strut fibula ankle arthrodesis a reliable reconstruction for bone defect after distal tibia tumor resection? A finite element study based on promising clinical outcomes. *J Orthop Surg Res.* 2021;16(1):230. doi:10.1186/s13018-021-02362-0
12. Zhang C, Zeng B, Zhu K, Zhang L, Hu J. Limb salvage for malignant bone tumours of distal tibia with dual ipsilateral vascularized autogenous fibular graft in a trapezoid-shaped array with ankle arthrodesis and preserving subtalar joint. *Foot Ankle Surg.* 2019;25(3):278–285. doi:10.1016/j.fas.2017.11.006
13. Gundavda MK, Agarwal MG, Reddy R, Bary A. Reconstructive challenges of distal tibia bone tumors: Extracorporeally irradiated autograft combined with a nonvascularized autograft fibula for superior reconstruction and functional outcomes when compared to ipsilateral pedicled fibula transfer alone. *Sarcoma.* 2021;2021:6624550. doi:10.1155/2021/6624550
14. Gede IK, Erawati DA, Junaidi A, Reksoprodjo S, Asikin MZ. Frozen autograft for biological reconstruction following bone tumor resection: A single-center experience. *Orthop Rev (Pavia).* 2017;9(2):7257.
15. Abudu A, Grimer RJ, Tillman RM, Carter SR. Endoprosthetic replacement of the distal tibia and ankle joint for aggressive bone tumours. *Int Orthop.* 1999;23(5):291–294.
16. Yang P, Evans S, Khan Z, Abudu A, Jeys L, Grimer R. Reconstruction of the distal tibia following resection of aggressive bone tumours using a custom-made megaprosthesis. *J Orthop.* 2017;14(3):406–409.
17. Shekkeris AS, Hanna SA, Sewell MD, et al. Endoprosthetic reconstruction of the distal tibia and ankle joint after resection of primary bone tumours. *J Bone Joint Surg Br.* 2009;91(10):1378–1382. doi:10.1302/0301-620X.91B10.22643
18. Lou TF, Li H, Chai YM, et al. Resection arthrodesis using distraction osteogenesis then plating as a hybrid surgical technique for the management of bone sarcomas of the distal tibia. *Int Orthop.* 2018;42(3):705–711. doi:10.1007/s00264-018-3811-4

13 Fibular Resections

INTRODUCTION

Tumors of the fibula are uncommon, accounting for a small fraction of both primary and metastatic bone tumors. Among the different segments, the proximal fibula is most frequently affected, followed by the diaphysis and the distal fibula [1–3]. Historically, above-knee amputation was the standard approach for managing primary sarcomas of the fibula, primarily due to concerns about local control and the proximity of critical neurovascular structures. However, advancements in cross-sectional imaging, surgical techniques, and adjuvant therapies have led to a paradigm shift in favor of limb-sparing resections. These approaches have demonstrated that, with careful preoperative planning and meticulous surgical execution, tumors of the fibula can be resected safely without compromising oncological outcomes or limb function [4–6].

ANATOMIC CONSIDERATIONS

The fibula can be anatomically divided into three distinct regions, each with specific surgical implications.

PROXIMAL FIBULA

The proximal fibula serves as the attachment site for the lateral collateral ligament (LCL) and the biceps femoris tendon, playing a critical role in maintaining lateral stability of the knee joint. Importantly, the common peroneal nerve winds around the neck of the fibula and enters the peroneus longus tunnel, making it highly vulnerable during surgical dissection.

FIBULAR DIAPHYSIS

The diaphyseal segment of the fibula is circumferentially enveloped by muscle origins across all aspects and levels. Its resection, in general, does not compromise the stability of adjacent joints or the overall biomechanics of the lower extremity.

DISTAL FIBULA

The distal fibula is a subcutaneous structure with minimal soft tissue coverage. It forms an integral part of the lateral ankle complex, providing attachment to the tibiofibular and calcaneofibular ligaments, thereby contributing significantly to lateral ankle stability.

Preoperative Considerations

A thorough preoperative evaluation is critical to optimize surgical planning for fibular tumors. Key factors assessed with radiological imaging include the extent of bone destruction, intramedullary involvement, and soft tissuc extension. Particular attention is directed toward evaluating the relationship of the tumor to adjacent critical structures, notably the common peroneal nerve, major blood vessels, and the tibia.

Plain radiographs are essential for delineating the degree of cortical destruction and the anatomical boundaries of the lesion (Figure 13.1). Magnetic resonance imaging (MRI) further complements this evaluation by accurately assessing medullary canal involvement and extraosseous soft tissue extension, thereby guiding decisions regarding the need for nerve preservation or sacrifice (Figure 13.2). CT angiography may be employed to assess the relationship between the tumor and adjacent vessels.

Surgical Management

Positioning

Patients are positioned in a semi-supine posture with approximately 45-degree elevation of the operative side. This orientation facilitates easy access to the anterior and lateral compartments of the leg and enables dissection within the popliteal space if needed. Importantly, the entire lower extremity—from the inguinal ligament to the foot—is prepared within the sterile field. This preparation ensures the ability to monitor distal pulses intraoperatively and allows for swift conversion to an above-knee amputation should oncological or vascular considerations arise.

Incision

A utilitarian fibular incision is employed, offering versatile exposure across all segments of the fibula. The incision begins proximal to the biceps femoris tendon above the knee joint, extends over the midportion of the fibula, passes anteriorly toward the tibial crest, and then curves posteriorly and distally toward the ankle. This approach permits the creation of large anterior and posterior fasciocutaneous flaps, providing excellent visualization and maneuverability.

Through this incision, the anterior compartment (housing extensor musculature), the lateral compartment (peroneal musculature), and the superficial posterior compartment (lateral gastrocnemius and soleus muscles) are systematically exposed. In cases of prior biopsy, the biopsy tract is excised en bloc with the tumor specimen to ensure oncologic safety.

PROXIMAL FIBULA RESECTIONS

Proximal fibular tumors requiring surgical excision are managed through two main types of resections, depending on the tumor grade, cortical destruction, and extent of soft tissue involvement. Malawer [7] first described the classification of resections (Table 13.1).

DOI: 10.1201/9780367822002-16

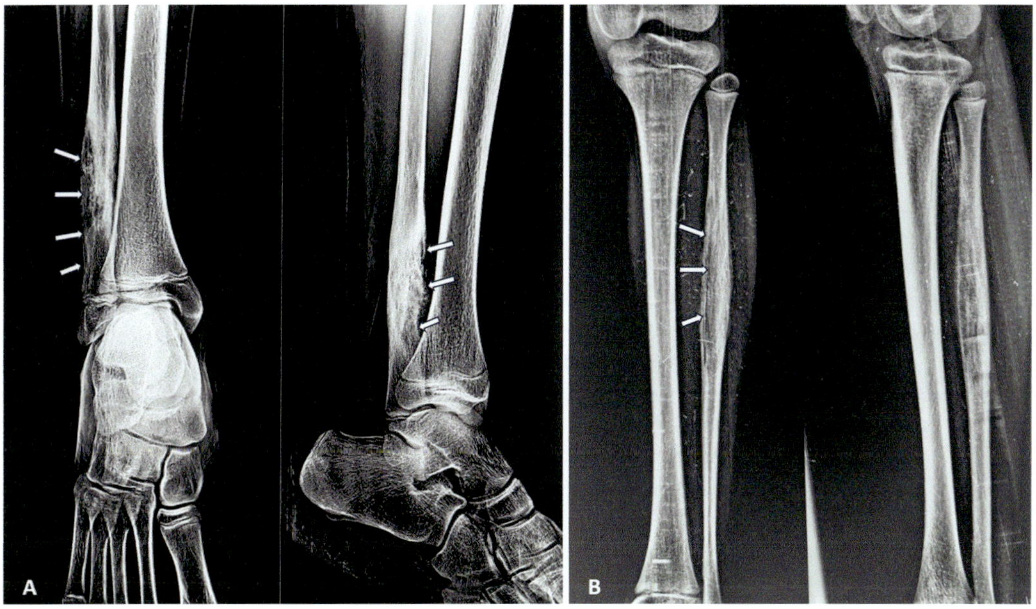

FIGURE 13.1 Plain radiographs of fibular lesions. (A) Anteroposterior and lateral views demonstrating an ill-defined, permeative, destructive lesion involving the meta-diaphyseal region of the distal fibula, associated with cortical thinning and subtle periosteal reaction. (B) Anteroposterior view showing an ill-defined diaphyseal lesion of the fibula characterized by cortical destruction and intramedullary expansion. Both patterns are suggestive of aggressive pathology, warranting further evaluation with MRI and histopathological correlation.

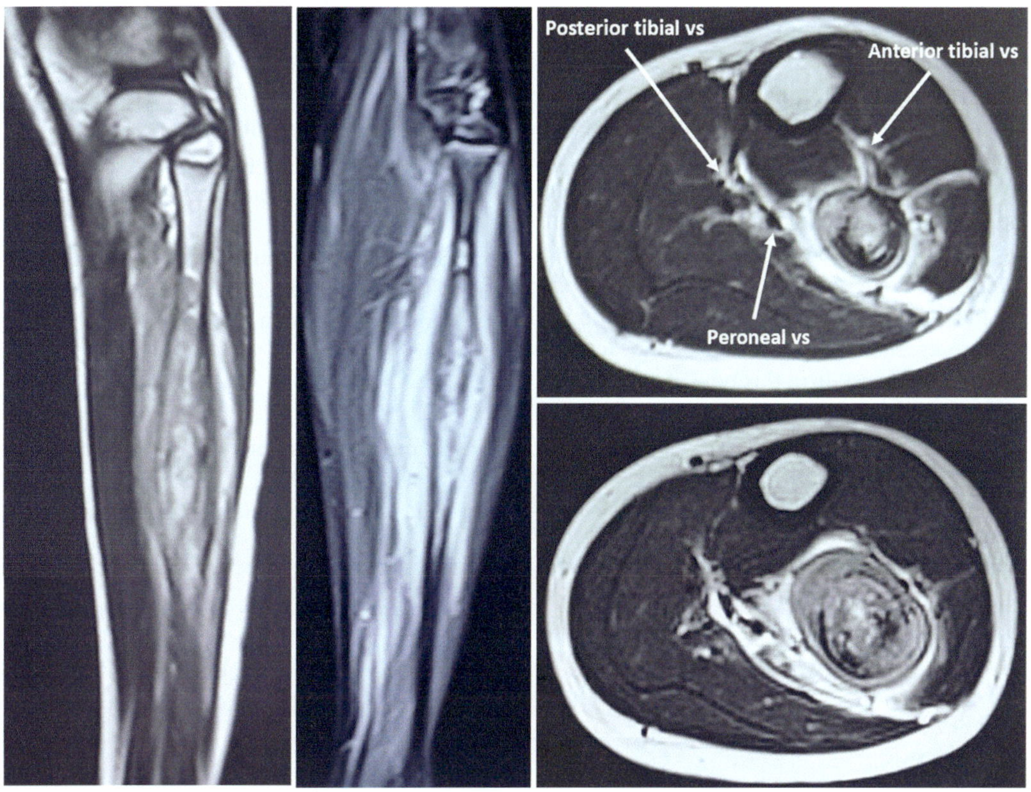

FIGURE 13.2 MRI of Ewing sarcoma involving the fibula in a 9-year-old male. Sagittal (left) and coronal (middle) images reveal an expansile lesion with cortical destruction and intramedullary involvement of the fibula, associated with soft tissue extension. Axial T2-weighted sections (right, upper, and lower) demonstrate a large heterogeneous soft tissue mass encasing the fibula, with close proximity to the anterior tibial, posterior tibial, and peroneal vascular structures, as marked. The lesion shows a hyperintense signal with areas of necrosis, highlighting both osseous and extraosseous disease extent.

TABLE 13.1
Comparison of Type I and Type II Proximal Fibula Resections

Feature	Type I Resection	Type II Resection
Tumor Type	Benign-Aggressive or Low-Grade	High-Grade Sarcomas
Peroneal Nerve	Preserved	Sacrificed
Anterior Tibial Artery	Preserved	Ligated
Muscle Compartment Involvement	Minimal	Anterior and lateral Compartments excised
Tibiofibular Joint Management	Intra-articular excision	Extra-articular disarticulation
Functional Morbidity	Minimal	Foot drop requiring AFO
Additional Vascular Steps	Not required	Possible ligation of peroneal vessels
Postoperative Concerns	LCL reconstruction critical	LCL reconstruction and foot-drop management necessary

Type I Resection

Type I resection involves en bloc excision of the proximal fibula, a thin muscle cuff circumferentially, and the LCL attachment site. The common peroneal nerve and its motor branches are preserved, and the proximal tibiofibular joint is excised intra-articularly. This technique is typically indicated for benign-aggressive tumors and low-grade sarcomas that have significant cortical destruction without extensive soft tissue extension.

During the procedure, the LCL and the biceps femoris tendon are released from their insertions on the fibular head, muscle origins are divided by electrocautery, and a fibular osteotomy is performed approximately 2–3 cm distal to the lesion. Careful mobilization and protection of the common peroneal nerve are essential. Preservation of the anterior tibial artery is generally possible in this type of resection.

Type II Resection

Type II resection is indicated for high-grade sarcomas with considerable cortical destruction and extraosseous extension. It involves wider resection of the proximal fibula, proximal tibiofibular joint, anterior and lateral muscle compartments, and necessitates sacrifice of the common peroneal nerve and anterior tibial artery.

SURGICAL STEPS: PROXIMAL FIBULA RESECTIONS

Exposure of Neurovascular Structures

Large tumors of the proximal fibula often extend posteriorly, potentially displacing or compressing the popliteal vessels.

- Exposure begins by reflecting the lateral gastrocnemius muscle along its entire length. If necessary, the proximal origin of the gastrocnemius from the lateral femoral condyle is released.
- The underlying soleus muscle is then detached from its fibular origin, allowing full visualization of the posterior fibular region.
- Key neurovascular landmarks include the anterior tibial artery (coursing through the interosseous membrane approximately 2–3 cm distal to the inferior border of the popliteus) and the peroneal artery, which runs posteriorly along the tibia.
- The posterior tibial nerve lies most superficially, while the popliteal vein and posterior tibial artery course deeper. Early identification of these structures is crucial to assess tumor resectability and determine if vascular reconstruction may be required.
- A simple traction maneuver on the popliteal artery facilitates visualization of the anterior tibial artery's origin. If needed, the anterior tibial vessels are ligated to allow posterior mobilization of the vascular bundle.

Type I Resection (Figure 13.3)

- The LCL and biceps femoris tendon are divided at their insertions on the fibular head.
- The common peroneal nerve is preserved by careful mobilization, typically after unroofing the peroneus longus tunnel.
- Muscle origins are detached using electrocautery, preserving vital soft tissues as much as possible.
- The anterior tibiofibular capsule is exposed and incised intra-articularly.
- An osteotomy is performed approximately 2–3 cm distal to the lower margin of the tumor to complete the resection.
- If exposure or tumor excision leads to a breach in the knee capsule, it is repaired meticulously to avoid postoperative complications such as synovial fistula formation.

Type II Resection

- In cases with extensive tumor spread, a wider resection is undertaken.
- The anterior and lateral muscle compartments and the overlying deep fascia are excised en bloc.
- The peroneal nerve is sacrificed approximately 2.5 cm proximal to its entry into the peroneus longus muscle.
- The anterior tibial artery, and often the peroneal vessels, are ligated to achieve complete vascular control.
- The origin of the anterior musculature from the tibia is transected at the musculotendinous junction to facilitate en bloc resection.
- A semicircular transection of the popliteus muscle is performed toward the posterior tibial condyle.
- An extra-articular disarticulation of the proximal tibiofibular joint is performed using a curved osteotome or high-speed burr, including a small portion of the lateral tibial plateau en bloc, ensuring that the tibiofemoral articulation is not violated.

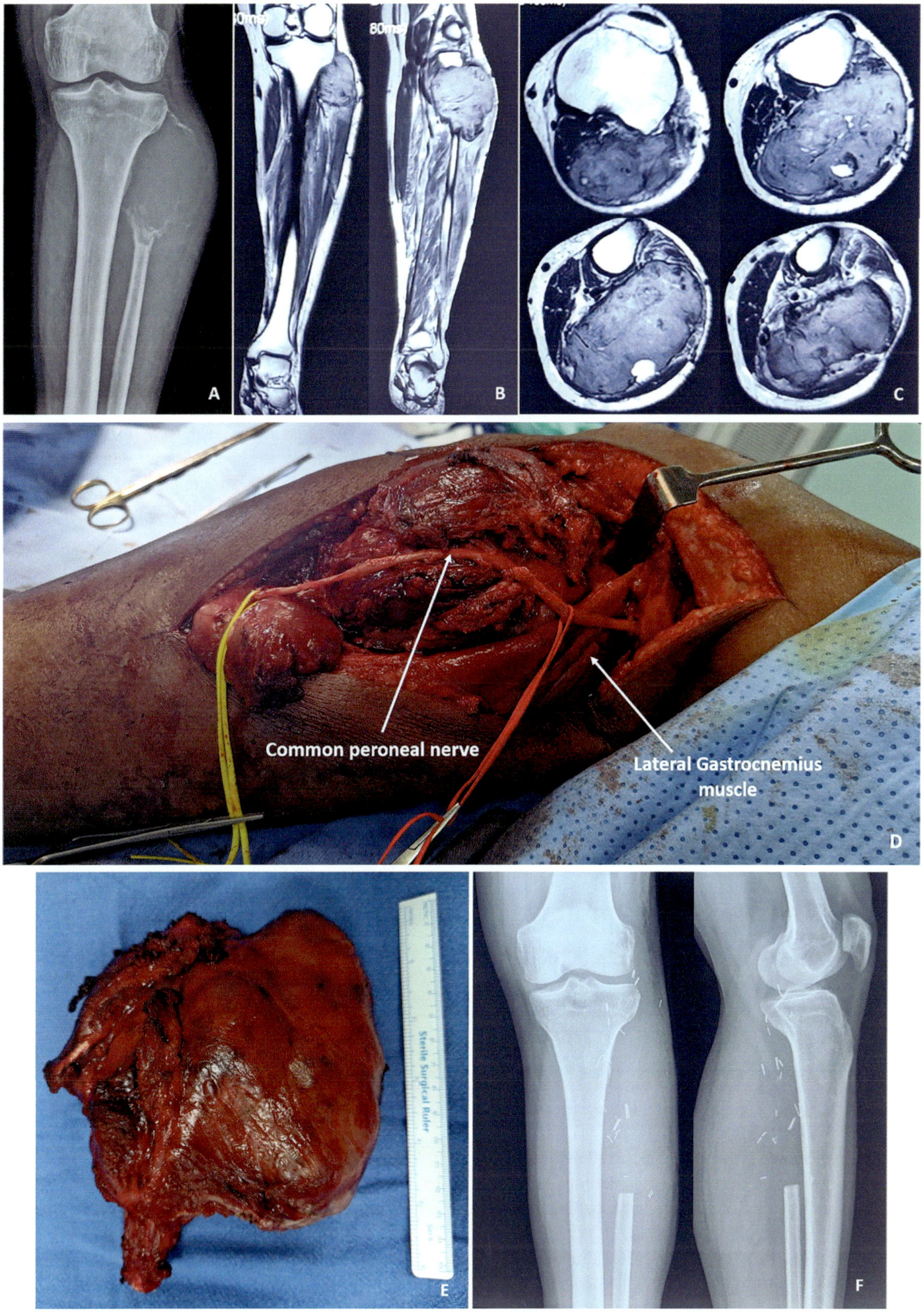

FIGURE 13.3 Plain radiographs (A) and MRI images (B & C) of Giant Cell Tumor involving the proximal fibula. Intra-operative images (D) showing the common peroneal nerve dissected and isolated from the tumor mass. En bloc resection (Type 1) was performed (E). (F) Post-operative radiographs following resection.

RECONSTRUCTION AND WOUND CLOSURE

Type I and Type II Resections

Following proximal fibula resection, meticulous soft tissue reconstruction is vital to restore stability and minimize functional morbidity.

- **LCL Reconstruction**: The LCL plays a pivotal role in maintaining knee stability, particularly by resisting varus stresses across all degrees of flexion. Together with the biceps femoris tendon, which provides posterior and rotational support, the LCL ensures lateral and anteroposterior stability of the knee [8]. Their loss can lead to varying degrees of knee instability, as demonstrated by biomechanical studies and clinical observations. In particular, the absence of the LCL constraint has been shown to significantly increase varus opening of the knee joint under stress, thereby predisposing to functional impairment and potential early degenerative changes [9].

  The necessity for LCL reconstruction after fibular resections remains an area of discussion. Evidence strongly suggests that patients who undergo reconstruction of the LCL and biceps femoris tendon exhibit better knee stability and functional outcomes. In a comparative study by Zhao et al, 83.3% of patients in the reconstruction group had a stable knee versus only 36.4% in the nonreconstruction group. Furthermore, functional outcomes, assessed by the Musculoskeletal Tumor Society (MSTS) score, were significantly superior in the reconstruction cohort (93% vs. 87%) [10]. Similarly, a more recent study found that reattachment of the LCL and biceps femoris tendon using suture anchors resulted in excellent lateral knee stability, with no knees classified as abnormal based on IKDC (International Knee Documentation Committee) criteria, and a significantly higher MSTS score in Type I resections compared to Type II resections (92.7% vs. 84.4%) [11].

  Several techniques for LCL reconstruction have been described in the literature:
  - **Suture anchor fixation**: Zhao et al. described reattachment of the LCL and biceps femoris tendon to the lateral tibial metaphysis using suture anchors, usually performed with the knee flexed at 20°, providing a straightforward and reliable technique [10].
  - **Staple fixation**: Abdel et al reported the use of metallic staples to reattach ligamentous structures to the tibia, offering a quick but less biologically favorable fixation [12].
  - **Drill holes with suture fixation**: Saini et al utilized nonabsorbable sutures passed through drill holes in the proximal tibia for ligament reconstruction.
  - **Reinforcement with iliotibial band**: Some authors have advocated for additional reinforcement by suturing the reconstructed structures to the iliotibial tract to enhance lateral knee stability [13].

  While some studies suggest that knee function can remain acceptable without formal reconstruction in selected cases [14, 15], the consensus emerging from most series supports active reconstruction to optimize mechanical integrity and minimize the risk of long-term complications such as instability and degenerative arthritis.
- In resections where the surgical field extends distally into the leg, the peroneal and extensor digitorum longus tendons are mobilized proximally to advance the foot into a neutral position. These tendons are then tenodesed to the tibial shaft to reduce foot-drop severity, potentially obviating the need for an ankle-foot orthosis.
- The lateral head of the gastrocnemius muscle is rotated anteriorly to cover the exposed tibial surface and defect. The gastrocnemius muscle is sutured to the deep fascia, soleus muscle, and the lateral capsule of the knee to achieve a robust soft tissue envelope.

  Additionally, the biceps femoris tendon is anchored to the transferred gastrocnemius muscle to enhance dynamic stability around the knee.

FIBULAR DIAPHYSIS RESECTION

Indications and Resection Principles

Tumors involving the fibular diaphysis, whether benign or malignant, are typically managed through intercalary resection of the involved segment. Due to the narrow diameter and limited soft tissue coverage in this region, curettage is neither practical nor oncologically safe. Resection of the fibular diaphysis generally does not compromise knee or ankle stability, nor does it adversely affect overall limb function, owing to the fibula's non-weight-bearing role.

In benign tumors, excision of the bone alone is often sufficient. However, for high-grade sarcomas, a wide resection including a cuff of surrounding musculature is mandatory to achieve clear oncologic margins.

Surgical Exposure

Surgical access is obtained using the middle portion of the utilitarian fibular incision, with proximal or distal extension based on the tumor's anatomical location. The exposure involves the following steps:

- The deep fascia is incised in line with the skin incision.
- The intermuscular septum between the peroneal muscles (laterally) and the soleus (medially) is identified.
- The soleus is carefully detached from its fibular origin and, along with the lateral gastrocnemius, is retracted medially and proximally to expose the posterior crest of the fibula.
- The flexor hallucis longus may be preserved or sacrificed depending on tumor involvement.
- The peroneal muscles are mobilized anteriorly, and retractors are placed under the fibula to deliver the bone.

This exposure allows safe dissection while preserving surrounding neurovascular structures.

Tumor resection is performed at predetermined osteotomy levels based on preoperative imaging. Care must be taken to protect the peroneal vessels, which course posterior and parallel to the fibula. In malignant cases, wide margins are ensured by including a cuff of adjacent soft tissue in the resection.

RECONSTRUCTION AND WOUND CLOSURE

In most cases, osseous reconstruction is not required following intercalary fibular resections due to the minimal mechanical role of the diaphysis. However:

- In low diaphyseal resections, where only a short segment of the distal fibula remains, reinforcement of the lateral malleolus may be necessary to prevent ankle instability.
- This reinforcement can be achieved through screw fixation or, in more extensive cases, structural grafting using ipsilateral or contralateral fibular segments.

Soft tissue closure is completed over a drain, with layered approximation of fascia and skin. When extensive soft tissue dissection is involved, local muscle flaps may be employed for coverage.

DISTAL FIBULA RESECTION AND RECONSTRUCTION

Malignant tumors involving the distal fibula are rare, comprising only 8–18% of all primary fibular sarcomas [16]. Despite the fibula being a non-weight-bearing bone, the distal fibula contributes critically to ankle stability, particularly by functioning as the lateral buttress of the ankle mortise. Resection of this segment, therefore, risks valgus ankle instability and deformity, especially when the lateral malleolus is compromised [17].

Surgical resection is indicated in high-grade sarcomas or locally aggressive lesions requiring negative margins. If the resection is >15–20 mm above the distal tibiofibular joint in adults, or 5 mm above the growth plate in children, lateral ankle stability may be preserved and reconstruction may not be needed [18, 19]. In most other cases, reconstruction is advocated to prevent long-term mechanical complications.

Several **reconstructive strategies** have been described:

- **Tibiotalar Arthrodesis**: This technique eliminates motion at the ankle joint but ensures maximum mechanical stability. Fixation is usually achieved with screws and may be reinforced with autologous or allogeneic fibular grafts. It is preferred when the entire distal fibula and part of the tibia are resected [16, 20]. Despite loss of range of motion, MSTS scores remain high, indicating good functional adaptation.
- **Rotational Vascularized Fibula Transposition**: The proximal fibula, including its vascular pedicle, is rotated 180° and fixed to the distal tibia to replicate the lateral malleolus. This biologic reconstruction provides dynamic stability and preserves joint motion. Although technically demanding, it is a viable option, especially in younger patients [18, 21].
- **Non-Vascularized Fibular Graft**: A segment of the ipsilateral fibular diaphysis is transposed distally to reconstruct the malleolus. This method is simpler and effective, with acceptable fusion rates and ankle stability when properly fixated [16, 17].
- **Intercalary Allograft**: Used when the lateral malleolus is preserved, this technique employs a frozen fibular strut to bridge the defect. Fixation is secured with screws. Bone integration is reliable, though risks of infection and mechanical failure exist if soft tissue coverage is inadequate [22].
- **No Reconstruction**: In selected cases where the peroneal malleolus is preserved, simple fixation of the remnant fibula to the tibia with screws may suffice. However, long-term risks of valgus drift or joint instability remain, particularly without syndesmotic stabilization [23] (Figure 13.4).

In the series reported by Khal et al., reconstruction techniques yielded stable ankles and high MSTS scores (mean 26.7), although complications such as peroneal nerve palsy, deep infections, and equinus deformity were noted. Tibiotalar arthrodesis was associated with the fewest mechanical complications, while biologic reconstructions carried the benefit of preserved motion but had higher technical demands [16].

In summary, the choice of reconstruction after distal fibula resection should be individualized. When the lateral malleolus is sacrificed, arthrodesis or fibular transposition is preferred. If the lateral malleolus is intact, screw fixation or intercalary grafting may suffice. Surgeon expertise, patient age, and adjuvant therapy requirements all influence the selection of the reconstructive method [16].

POSTOPERATIVE REHABILITATION PROTOCOL

Proximal Fibula Resection

Following resection, continuous suction drainage is maintained for three to five days, and intravenous antibiotics are continued until the drains are removed.

- Type I and Type II Resections: The limb is immobilized in a cast at 20° of knee flexion for 3 weeks to facilitate soft tissue healing. Thereafter, full weight-bearing and unrestricted knee motion are initiated.
- Type II resections often result in peroneal nerve dysfunction, necessitating the use of an ankle-foot orthosis (AFO) to manage foot drop.

Fibular Diaphysis Resection

Standard postoperative care includes drainage and IV antibiotics for three to five days. Early mobilization is encouraged with

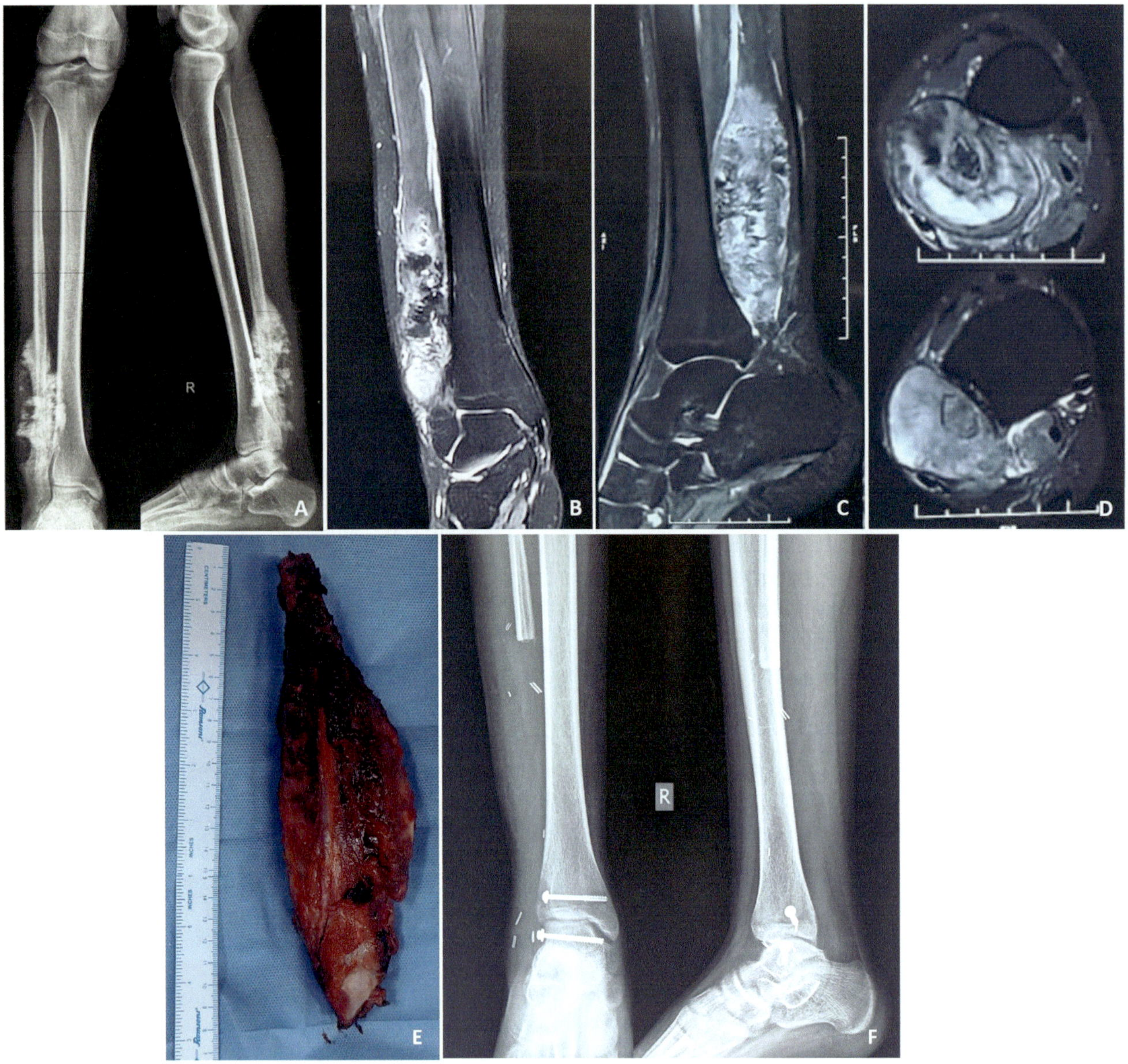

FIGURE 13.4 Plain radiographs (A) and coronal (B), sagittal (C), and axial (D) MRI images of Osteosarcoma involving the distal fibula. Wide resection was performed (E). Lateral ankle stability was restored using a Prolene mesh sleeve secured with screws into the distal tibia and talus to provide a lateral buttress to the ankle mortise and prevent valgus ankle instability. (F) Post-operative radiographs following resection and reconstruction.

- partial weight-bearing and active/passive knee range of motion exercises starting in the early postoperative phase and
- full weight-bearing is permitted following wound healing and satisfactory radiographic review.

Distal Fibula Resection

Rehabilitation after distal fibula reconstruction is tailored to the type of procedure performed.

- Initially placed in a cast or splint for 4 weeks with strict non-weight-bearing.
- Partial weight-bearing begins after the first month, progressing gradually over the next 8 weeks.
- Ankle mobilization exercises are initiated upon cast removal to prevent stiffness and muscular atrophy.
- In cases involving arthrodesis, permanent ankle immobility is expected, whereas in biological reconstructions (e.g., fibular transpositions or allografts), preservation of ankle motion is emphasized.

Complications

Surgical resections of the fibula—whether proximal, diaphyseal, or distal—are generally well-tolerated, but several complications may arise depending on the extent of resection, reconstruction technique, and adherence to rehabilitation protocols.

- **Peroneal Nerve Injury**: Commonly encountered during curettage or Type I proximal fibula resections, particularly if nerve dissection is inadequate. Injuries may be transient or, in rare cases, permanent, requiring supportive measures such as an AFO.
- **Lateral Knee Instability**: Occurs when the LCL is not adequately reconstructed or if rehabilitation is insufficient, particularly after Types I and II proximal fibula resections.
- **Lateral Ankle Instability**: May result from inadequate fixation or lack of malleolar reconstruction in low intercalary resections of the fibular diaphysis or after distal fibula resections without stabilization. This may lead to valgus deformity and progressive functional decline.
- **Deep Surgical Site Infections**: Can occur after extensive reconstructions, particularly with allograft usage or arthrodesis, and may require surgical debridement and prolonged antibiotic therapy.

SUMMARY

- Fibular resections are uncommon but essential in managing primary bone tumors, with limb-sparing techniques replacing traditional amputations.
- The proximal fibula contributes to knee stability, necessitating LCL reconstruction—especially in Type I resections—to prevent varus instability.
- The fibular diaphysis can be safely resected without reconstruction in most cases, owing to its minimal role in weight-bearing.
- Distal fibula resections compromise ankle stability and often require reconstruction (arthrodesis, fibular transposition, or allograft) if the lateral malleolus is sacrificed.
- Postoperative care includes staged mobilization, protection of soft tissue repairs, and orthotic support when indicated; complications are uncommon with proper technique.

REFERENCES

1. Guo C, Zhang X, Gao F, Wang L, Sun T. Surgical management of proximal fibular tumors: risk factors for recurrence and complications. *J Int Med Res.* 2018 May;46(5):1884–1892. doi: 10.1177/0300060518762677
2. Sun T, Wang L, Guo C, Zhang G, Hu W. Symptoms and signs associated with benign and malignant proximal fibular tumors: a clinicopathological analysis of 52 cases. *World J Surg Oncol.* 2017 May 2;15(1):92. doi: 10.1186/s12957-017-1162-z
3. Dorfman HD, Czerniak B. General considerations. In: Dorfman HD, Czerniak B, eds. *Bone Tumors*. St. Louis, MO: CV Mosby, 1998: 1–33.
4. Erler K, Dcmiralp B, Ozdcmir T, et al. Treatment of proximal fibular tumors with en bloc resection. *Knee.* 2004;11:489–496.
5. Faczypour H, Davis AM, Griffin AM, et al. Giant cell tumor of the proximal fibula: surgical management. *J Surg Oncol.* 1996;61:34–37.
6. Farooquc M, Biyani A, Adhikari A. Giant cell tumours of the proximal fibula. *J Bone Joint Surg Br.* 1990;72B:723–724.
7. Malawer MM. Surgical management of aggressive and malignant tumors of the proximal fibula. *Clin Orthop Relat Res.* 1984;186:172–181.
8. Grood ES, Noyes FR, Butler DL, Suntay WJ. Ligamentous and capsular restraints preventing straight medial and lateral laxity in intact human cadaver knees. *J Bone Joint Surg Am.* 1981;63:1257–1269.
9. Draganich LF, Nicholas RW, Shuster JK, Sathy MR, Chang AF, Simon MA. The effects of resection of the proximal part of thc fibula on stability of the knee and on gait. *J Bone Joint Surg Am.* 1991;73:575–583.
10. Zhao SC, Zhang CQ, Zhang CL. Reconstruction of lateral knee joint stability following resection of proximal fibula tumors. *Exp Ther Med.* 2014;7(2):405–410. doi:10.3892/etm.2013.1429
11. Buyukdogan K, Işık S, Ayık G, Tokgözoğlu M, Ayvaz M. Lateral collateral ligament and biceps femoris tendon fixation with a suture anchor to the tibial metaphysis after proximal fibula en bloc resections preserve lateral knee stability. *J Knee Surg.* 2023;36(8):878–885. doi:10.1055/s-0042-1744220
12. Abdel MP, Papagelopoulos PJ, Morrey ME, et al. Malignant proximal fibular tumors: surgical management of 112 cases. *J Bone Joint Surg Am.* 2012;94:e165.
13. Saini R, Bali K, Gill SS, Mootha AK, Dhillon MS. En bloc resection of osteosarcoma of the proximal fibula. An analysis of 8 cases. *Acta Orthop Belg.* 2010;76:806–810.
14. Einoder PA, Choong PF. Tumors of the head of the fibula: good function after resection without ligament reconstruction in 6 patients. *Acta Orthop Scand.* 2002;73:663–666.
15. Takahashi S, Ogose A, Tajino T, Osanai T, Okada K. Osteosarcoma of the proximal fibula. An analysis of 13 cases in the northern Japan. *Ups J Med Sci.* 2007;112:366–372.
16. Khal AA, Zucchini R, Giannini C, Sambri A, Donati DM, De Paolis M. Distal fibula reconstruction in primary malignant tumours. *Curr Oncol.* 2021;28(5):3463–3473. doi:10.3390/curroncol28050299
17. Leibner ED, Ad-El D, Liebergall M, Ofiram E, London E, Peyser A. Lateral malleolar reconstruction after distal fibular resection. A case report. *J Bone Joint Surg Am.* 2005;87:878–882.
18. Capanna R, van Horn JR, Biagini R, Ruggieri P, Bettelli G, Campanacci M. Reconstruction after resection of the distal fibula for bone tumor. *Acta Orthop Scand.* 1986;57:290–294.
19. Abuhassan FO, Shannak AO. Subperiosteal resection of aneurysmal bone cysts of the distal fibula. *J Bone Joint Surg Br.* 2009;91:1227–1231.
20. Dieckmann R, Ahrens H, Streitbürger A, Budny TB, Henrichs MP, Vieth V, Gebert C, Hardes J. Reconstruction after wide resection of the entire distal fibula in malignant bone tumours. *Int Orthop.* 2011;35:87–92.
21. de Gauzy JS, Kany J, Cahuzac JP. Distal fibular reconstruction with pedicled vascularized fibular head graft: a case report. *J Pediatr Orthop B.* 2002;11:176–180.
22. Jamshidi K, Mazhar FN, Masdari Z. Reconstruction of distal fibula with osteoarticular allograft after tumor resection. *Foot Ankle Surg.* 2013;19:31–35.
23. Ozaki T, Hillmann A, Lindner N, Winkelmann W. Surgical treatment of bone sarcomas of the fibula. Analysis of 19 cases. *Arch Orthop Trauma Surg.* 1997;116:475–479.

Section IV

Pelvic and Sacral Resections

14 Pelvic Resections and Reconstructions

INTRODUCTION

Pelvic bone tumors present complex challenges in orthopedic oncology due to the intricate anatomy of the pelvic ring, its critical role in weight transmission, and the close relationship to major neurovascular and visceral structures. Primary malignancies such as chondrosarcoma, Ewing sarcoma, and osteosarcoma are relatively common in this region and are often diagnosed late, as the capacious pelvic cavity allows tumors to grow substantially before producing specific symptoms.

Compared to appendicular tumors, pelvic lesions have a poorer prognosis, largely because of the difficulty in obtaining wide surgical margins, the higher incidence of local recurrence, and limitations in delivering adjuvant therapy after extensive resections. Achieving oncologic clearance requires meticulous preoperative planning, with detailed imaging to map tumor extent and its relationship to the sacral plexus, iliac vessels, bladder, bowel, and ureter. Modern strategies often employ advanced MRI, CT angiography, preoperative embolization, and computer-assisted navigation to optimize surgical accuracy and safety.

Reconstruction after pelvic resection is uniquely challenging. Techniques must restore skeletal continuity and stability while preserving function, ensuring adequate soft tissue coverage, and minimizing complications. Despite advances in biological grafting and prosthetic reconstruction, complication rates remain high and functional results are modest. This chapter reviews the anatomy, classification, surgical principles, and reconstruction options in pelvic tumor surgery, with emphasis on balancing oncologic control and functional preservation.

CLASSIFICATION AND TYPES OF RESECTIONS

Pelvic and sacral tumor resections vary considerably in their extent and complexity, depending on tumor size, location, and involvement of adjacent neurovascular or visceral structures. To standardize surgical planning and reporting, **Enneking and Dunham** proposed a classification in 1978 that remains the cornerstone in orthopedic oncology [1]. This system divides the pelvis into four anatomical zones, with later refinements introducing subtypes based on the extent of resection and associated soft tissue involvement (Figure 14.1). Combinations such as Types I–II or Types I–IV resections are frequent in advanced tumors, and suffixes (e.g., "A" for associated muscle resection, "S" for sacral extension) add precision to operative planning (Table 14.1).

Type I – Iliac Wing

This resection removes part or all of the ilium, sparing the acetabulum. The ilium connects the acetabulum to the spine via the sacroiliac joint and anchors important musculature, including the abdominal wall, gluteals, pelvic floor, and iliacus.

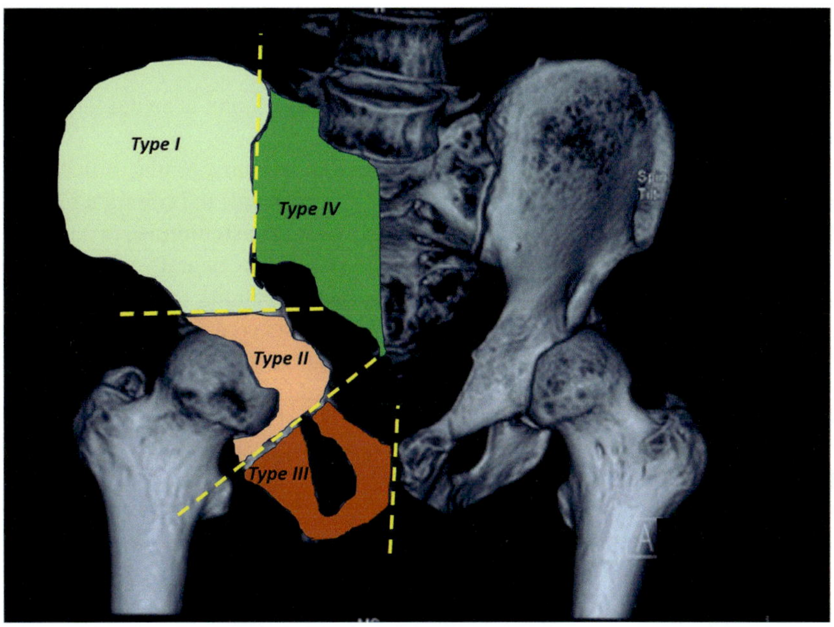

FIGURE 14.1 Schematic illustration of the Enneking and Dunham classification of pelvic resections, depicting the different types of resections based on anatomical location within the pelvis. This classification provides a systematic framework for planning surgical management of pelvic tumors.

DOI: 10.1201/9780367822002-18

TABLE 14.1
Enneking–Dunham Pelvic Resection Types

Type	Anatomic Zone	Structures Involved	Reconstruction Need
I	Iliac wing	Iliac bone, gluteal muscles, SI joint (variable)	Variable; often not required
II	Periacetabular region	Acetabulum, femoral head (Type II-A)	Hip reconstruction necessary
III	Ischiopubic region	Pubis, ischium	Not always; depends on stability
IV	Sacrum	Sacral ala, sacral nerve roots (S1–S4)	Requires spinopelvic fixation if >S1

- *Type I-A* includes removal of gluteal musculature, potentially compromising flap viability.
- *Type I-S* extends into the sacrum (extended hemipelvectomy).

  Complete ilium resection disrupts pelvic ring continuity and may cause acetabular rotation and instability, whereas partial resections preserving the sacroiliac joint often require no reconstruction.

Type II – Periacetabular Region

This resection involves the acetabulum, the main weight-bearing component of the hip. It is the most disabling type due to the need for hip joint reconstruction and limb-length preservation.

- *Type II-A* (extra-articular hip resection) includes femoral head removal with osteotomies through the ilium, ischium, and pubis.

Type III – Ischiopubic Region

This involves resection of the pubis and ischium medial to the acetabulum. While these bones are not weight-bearing, they maintain pelvic ring integrity and serve as muscle attachment points. Because the acetabulum and hip joint are preserved, reconstruction is rarely necessary.

Type IV – Sacrum

Sacral resections can be transverse, sagittal, or combined, and may occur in isolation or with pelvic resections (e.g., Types I–IV).

Kapoor et al. [2] have proposed "transacetabular resections" to preserve part of the acetabulum when feasible. In *Type I + II* patterns, the superior acetabulum may be resected while preserving the inferior portion (*Type I + half*). In *Types II + III* cases, the inferior acetabulum may be resected while sparing the superior dome (*Type III + half*). These modifications have shown functional benefits without compromising oncologic margins, emphasizing the value of acetabular preservation in select cases.

ANATOMICAL CONSIDERATIONS

Pelvic tumor resections demand a highly detailed knowledge of regional anatomy due to the dense concentration of osseous, neurovascular, and visceral structures within a confined space. Large tumors frequently distort normal landmarks, making the orientation and protection of vital structures more challenging.

OSSEOUS FRAMEWORK

The pelvis is formed by the ilium, ischium, and pubis, converging at the acetabulum, and articulates with the sacrum at the sacroiliac joint.

- **Iliac wing** resections are often possible without reconstruction due to their non-weight-bearing role and soft tissue coverage from the iliacus and gluteals.
- **Acetabular involvement** poses the greatest reconstructive challenge, as it is critical for hip articulation and load transmission.

HIP JOINT CONSIDERATIONS

Extra-articular hip resections are required when tumors involve the acetabulum or proximal femur.

- Fractures necessitate assuming intracapsular contamination and sacrificing the joint.
- Preserving abductors via trochanteric osteotomy can retain partial hip function.
- Surgeons must note that the anterior capsule extends more distally than the posterior, risking inadvertent breach in anterior approaches.

SACRUM AND SACROILIAC JOINT

The sacroiliac joint is a vital landmark.

- Major neurovascular structures, including the lumbosacral trunk and common iliac vessels, lie medial to it.
- **Lateral osteotomies** avoid sacral root injury; **medial cuts** risk neural compromise and require direct visualization.
- Tumors crossing midline foramina often require bilateral sacral nerve sacrifice, causing severe bowel and bladder dysfunction, making limb salvage less feasible.

SCIATIC NOTCH REGION

The greater sciatic notch transmits the **sciatic nerve** (inferior to piriformis) and the **superior gluteal bundle** (superior to piriformis).

- Large tumors blocking the notch may preclude safe dissection, leading to external hemipelvectomy.
- Dividing sacrotuberous and sacrospinous ligaments enlarges exposure for neurovascular protection.

NEUROVASCULAR ANATOMY

- Arterial Landmarks:
  - The aorta bifurcates at L4 into common iliac arteries, which split into external and internal branches at S1.
  - The **external iliac artery** becomes the femoral artery under the inguinal ligament; its **inferior epigastric branch** is at risk during anterior approaches.
  - The **internal iliac artery** supplies pelvic walls via obturator, gluteal, iliolumbar, and pudendal branches; these must be preserved to maintain flap viability.
  - **Corona mortis**, an obturator-external iliac anastomosis, can cause life-threatening bleeding if injured.
- **Venous Considerations**: Internal iliac veins are thin-walled and fragile; the iliolumbar vein may be damaged during exposure.
- Nerves:
  - The sciatic nerve must be preserved in most Types I and II resections.
  - Femoral nerve preservation is generally possible except in anterior pubic resections.
  - The obturator nerve is often sacrificed in Type III resections.
  - Internal pudendal structures lie near the sacrospinous ligament and are at risk during ligament division.
  - Superficial sensory nerves (iliohypogastric, ilioinguinal, genitofemoral) are often sacrificed with minimal functional deficit.

INGUINAL AND ANTERIOR PELVIC REGION

The inguinal canal runs between the ASIS and pubic tubercle, containing the spermatic cord or round ligament. These structures can be disrupted during anterior dissection.

VISCERAL RELATIONSHIPS

- **Bladder and urethra**: At risk in pubic symphyseal division; tumors near bladder base may require partial cystectomy.
- **Ureter**: Crosses the pelvic brim near the common iliac bifurcation; it is at risk in medial ilium or sacral ala resections. Preoperative stenting aids identification.

MUSCULAR CONSIDERATIONS

The **iliacus** often acts as a barrier in primary tumors but may be breached in aggressive lesions.

- **Gluteal muscles** are essential for flap closure and ambulation; preservation, particularly of gluteus maximus, is critical.
- Disruption of muscle origins and insertions impacts postoperative gait and stability, influencing reconstructive planning.

PREOPERATIVE CONSIDERATIONS AND EVALUATION

Pelvic tumor resections require meticulous preoperative assessment to ensure oncologic clearance and functional preservation, and to minimize complications.

CLINICAL ASSESSMENT

A comprehensive history should address pain characteristics, neurological symptoms (sciatica, bowel/bladder disturbance), gait changes, and signs of pelvic instability. Examination must evaluate limb-length discrepancy, pelvic stability, and neurovascular status. General health, comorbidities, and patient expectations are integral to surgical decision-making.

IMAGING EVALUATION (FIGURE 14.2)

- **Plain radiographs**: Identify cortical destruction, acetabular involvement, or pelvic ring disruption.
- **CT scan**: Define cortical destruction and sacroiliac proximity, and facilitate osteotomy planning.
- **MRI**: Serve as gold standard for soft tissue extension, marrow infiltration, neurovascular encasement, and joint involvement; contrast may highlight tumor viability and vascularity.
- **PET-CT/Bone scan**: Use for staging, detecting metastases, and assessing treatment response.
- **Angiography/CT angiography**: Map vessel anatomy, displacement, or encasement; guide vascular control or reconstruction needs.
- **MR urography/CT urogram**: Recommended for lesions near the bladder, ureter, or pelvic floor.

BIOPSY PLANNING

Biopsy must be coordinated with the definitive surgical plan, placing the tract within a resectable zone. **Image-guided core biopsy** is preferred to reduce contamination and diagnostic errors. Poorly planned biopsies risk compromising limb salvage.

MULTIDISCIPLINARY COORDINATION

Orthopedic oncologists, radiologists, vascular surgeons, urologists, and plastic surgeons should jointly plan resection extent, reconstruction type, adjuvant therapy timing, and need for preoperative embolization or flap coverage.

For anatomically complex or high-risk cases, 3D reconstructions or patient-specific, 3D-printed models can significantly enhance precision in planning osteotomies and

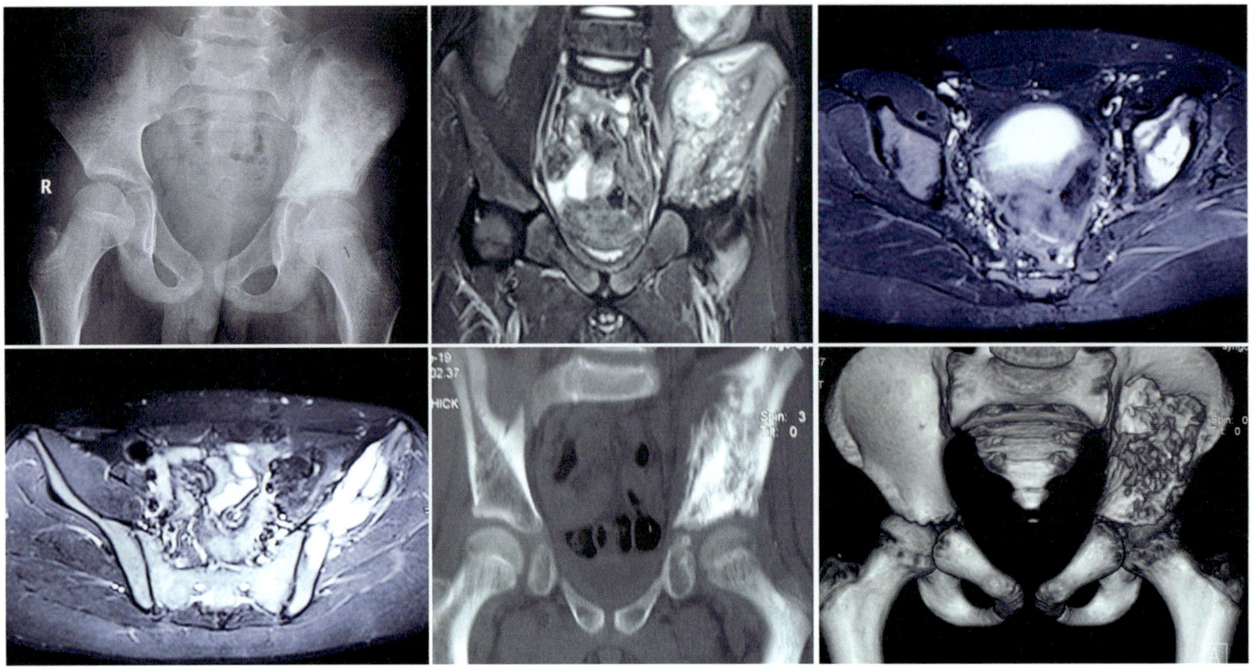

FIGURE 14.2 Imaging evaluation of Ewing sarcoma of the hemipelvis. Radiological workup includes plain radiographs, MRI, and CT scans to assess cortical destruction, marrow infiltration, soft tissue extension, neurovascular involvement, and sacroiliac proximity. These modalities also delineate acetabular and joint involvement, thereby facilitating precise surgical planning and osteotomy execution.

reconstructions. Additionally, vascular road-mapping and ureteric stenting may be employed preoperatively to avoid intraoperative injury. For tumors involving the left hemipelvis or adjacent colon, preoperative imaging and colonoscopy help assess the need for a diverting colostomy. In such scenarios, collaboration with colorectal surgery and preoperative stoma site marking and patient training are critical steps to reduce morbidity and facilitate recovery.

SURGICAL TECHNIQUES AND RESECTION PLANNING

Surgical management of pelvic tumors demands individualized, meticulously executed approaches based on tumor location, size, extent, and involvement of adjacent structures. The dual objectives are to achieve negative margins for oncologic clearance and to preserve functional capacity by safeguarding neurovascular structures and optimizing reconstructive possibilities. The intricate pelvic anatomy, vital structure proximity, and high risk of massive hemorrhage necessitate advanced preoperative planning, frequently aided by high-resolution imaging, three-dimensional modeling, and multidisciplinary team coordination.

GENERAL SURGICAL PRINCIPLES

Wide surgical excision remains the standard for curative treatment of malignant pelvic tumors. Resection type is determined by tumor site using the Enneking–Dunham classification, with modern refinements—such as transacetabular and partial resections—allowing preservation of critical elements like the acetabulum when oncologically safe. Surgical approaches are customized to anticipated osteotomy planes, tumor bulk, neurovascular relationships, and the chosen reconstruction strategy.

Positioning is often **lateral decubitus with posterior tilt**, providing simultaneous anterior and posterior access. For specific cases, supine or prone positioning may be used. **Combined anterior-posterior or extensile utilitarian pelvic incisions** are preferred for extensive tumors to ensure optimal exposure for resection and reconstruction.

SURGICAL EXPOSURE AND INCISION PLANNING

Utilitarian Pelvic Incision

The most versatile approach, the utilitarian pelvic incision, provides access to all pelvic zones. Starting at the posterior inferior iliac spine, it runs along the iliac crest to the anterior superior iliac spine, then bifurcates:

- **Anterior limb**: follows the inguinal ligament to the symphysis pubis.
- **Posterior limb**: extends over the proximal anterior thigh, curving laterally behind the femur below the greater trochanter, ending at the gluteus maximus insertion (Figure 14.3).

A posterior fascio-cutaneous flap exposes the retro-gluteal space, sciatic notch, gluteal musculature, and sacrum. Large skin and muscle flaps are elevated to facilitate safe

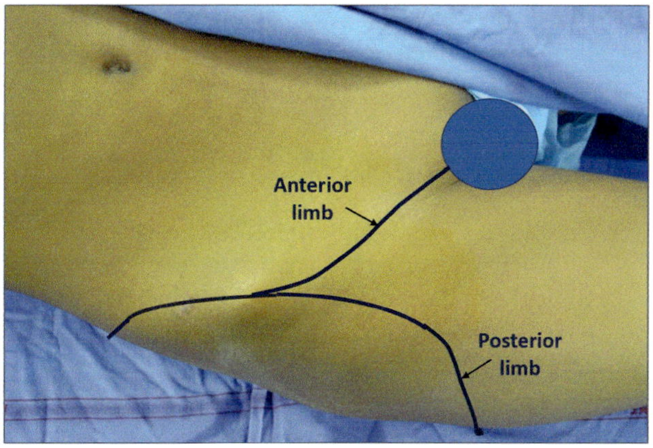

FIGURE 14.3 The utilitarian pelvic incision starts at the posterior inferior iliac spine, runs along the iliac crest to the anterior superior iliac spine, then bifurcates into an anterior limb that follows the inguinal ligament to the symphysis pubis, and a posterior limb that extends over the proximal anterior thigh, curving laterally behind the femur below the greater trochanter.

resection and reconstruction. Previous biopsy tracts should be incorporated into the incision to prevent tumor contamination of uninvolved compartments.

Type I – Iliac Resections

For tumors confined to the ilium, the **ilioinguinal extension** reaches the symphysis pubis, with the posterior arm terminating at the sacroiliac joint. The abdominal wall, sartorius, and tensor fasciae lata are detached from the iliac crest and reflected. The iliacus, gluteus minimus, and portions of gluteus medius are excised en bloc with the tumor.

The femoral nerve, lying between the iliacus and psoas, is mobilized medially for protection. Osteotomy is performed with a malleable retractor via the sciatic notch to shield viscera, followed by sacroiliac joint disarticulation. Preservation of the rectus femoris origin and acetabular roof is prioritized when feasible.

Soft tissue reconstruction involves reattaching the gluteus medius to abdominal musculature, with sartorius and tensor fasciae lata support, preferably with the limb abducted to reduce tension.

Type II – Periacetabular Resections

These are the most technically challenging resections due to acetabular involvement. Exposure combines anterior retroperitoneal and posterior gluteal approaches. External and internal iliac vessels are mobilized with hypogastric artery ligation to reduce blood loss. The sciatic and femoral nerves are identified and protected.

A gluteus maximus–based posterior flap exposes the ischium, sciatic notch, hip joint, and acetabulum. Standard osteotomies include the following:

- **Supra-acetabular cut** through the ilium
- **Superior pubic ramus cut** after vessel mobilization
- **Ischial osteotomy** above the biceps femoris insertion

In cases requiring hip replacement, total hip exposure is achieved, the femoral neck is osteotomized proximal to the lesser trochanter, and capsulotomy is performed. Posterior column osteotomy is undertaken with care to avoid sciatic nerve injury.

Type III – Ischiopubic and Pelvic Floor Resections

Access involves a three-incision strategy: **ilioinguinal**, **lateral thigh**, and **perineal** extensions, enabling visualization of the obturator foramen, adductor compartment, and ischiopubic rami.

The spermatic cord or round ligament is retracted medially; the inguinal ligament is released for better exposure. Resection begins with detachment of the adductor magnus, gracilis, and pectineus from the pubis, followed by hamstring detachment from the ischium. The symphysis pubis and rami are osteotomized with retractors protecting pelvic viscera, and sharp edges are smoothed to avoid bladder injury.

Precise incision planning, mastery of pelvic anatomy, and preservation of key neurovascular structures are crucial to the success of pelvic tumor resections. Each resection type presents unique exposure challenges and reconstructive demands, making preoperative planning and intraoperative adaptability essential for optimal oncologic and functional outcomes.

RECONSTRUCTION CONSIDERATIONS

Pelvic reconstruction after oncologic resection is a highly individualized process, requiring careful assessment of the anticipated biomechanical and functional benefits against the potential risks of added operative complexity. The pelvis not only provides structural continuity for load transfer between the spine and lower limbs but also houses essential viscera and supports numerous muscular attachments. Disruption of this anatomy can significantly affect gait, stability, and visceral function, making reconstruction crucial in selected cases.

Reconstruction after pelvic tumor surgery should aim for optimal stability and function without disproportionately increasing perioperative risk. The decision requires a holistic view of tumor characteristics, patient factors, available expertise, and long-term goals, ensuring that chosen techniques offer durable, safe, and functional outcomes.

INDICATIONS FOR RECONSTRUCTION

Reconstruction is typically indicated in two primary scenarios:

1. **Loss of Pelvic Continuity** – Seen in complete Type I, I-A, or I-S resections, where the mechanical link between the sacrum and acetabulum is interrupted, impairing load transfer. Reconstruction restores skeletal stability and allows functional rehabilitation.
2. **Acetabular Resection** – Following Type II or II-A resections, the hip's primary articulation is lost, leading to profound mobility and weight-bearing limitations. Here, structural hip joint reconstruction is essential for ambulation and daily activities [3].

In contrast, **reconstruction is often not necessary** in:

- **Partial Type I resections**, which preserve pelvic ring integrity (Figure 14.4).
- **Complete Type III resections**, involving the ischiopubic region without significantly affecting load-bearing biomechanics [3] (Figure 14.5).

KEY DECISION FACTORS

- **Patient profile** – Younger, active individuals benefit from durable biologic solutions; elderly or low-demand patients may be better served with simpler prosthetic options.
- **Oncological prognosis** – In patients with limited survival, low-morbidity options enabling rapid mobilization are prioritized.
- **Soft tissue coverage** – Adequate viable tissue is essential; prior radiotherapy or infection history increases complication risk.
- **Neurological status** – Nerve deficits may require constrained implants to prevent instability.
- **Healing capacity** – Compromised nutrition, diabetes, or immunosuppression warrant biologic preference over complex prosthetics.
- **Follow-up feasibility** – Prosthetic reconstructions demand ongoing surveillance; biologic techniques are favored where follow-up may be inconsistent.
- **Surgical expertise and available resources** – Institutional capability influences reconstruction selection.

RECONSTRUCTIVE OPTIONS

1. **Prosthetic** – Total hip arthroplasty, saddle prostheses, custom or modular hemipelvic endoprostheses.
2. **Biological** – Arthrodesis, massive allografts, vascularized or non-vascularized autografts, or acceptance of a functional pseudoarthrosis.
3. **Composite** – Allograft-prosthetic composites combining structural support with articulating capability.

RECONSTRUCTION OF TYPE I PELVIC RESECTIONS

Reconstruction following Type I pelvic resections—which involve complete or near-complete removal of the ilium (including variants such as Type I-A and Type I-S)—is essential to restore mechanical continuity between the axial skeleton and the acetabulum. Although the hip joint remains intact in these resections, the structural integrity of the pelvic ring is compromised, necessitating bony reconstruction to facilitate effective force transmission from the lower limb to the spine.

When the residual gap between the sacrum and remaining ilium is minimal, a direct iliosacral arthrodesis can be achieved. This involves cartilage denudation of the sacroiliac joint surfaces followed by stabilization using wire or heavy suture constructs to bring the hemipelvis into apposition, typically hinging anteriorly through the symphysis pubis. Despite minor alterations to hip biomechanics, this method promotes reliable union due to the broad cancellous surfaces involved. During this process, care must be taken to avoid sciatic nerve impingement; contouring the sciatic notch may be necessary to ensure an unobstructed exit for the nerve.

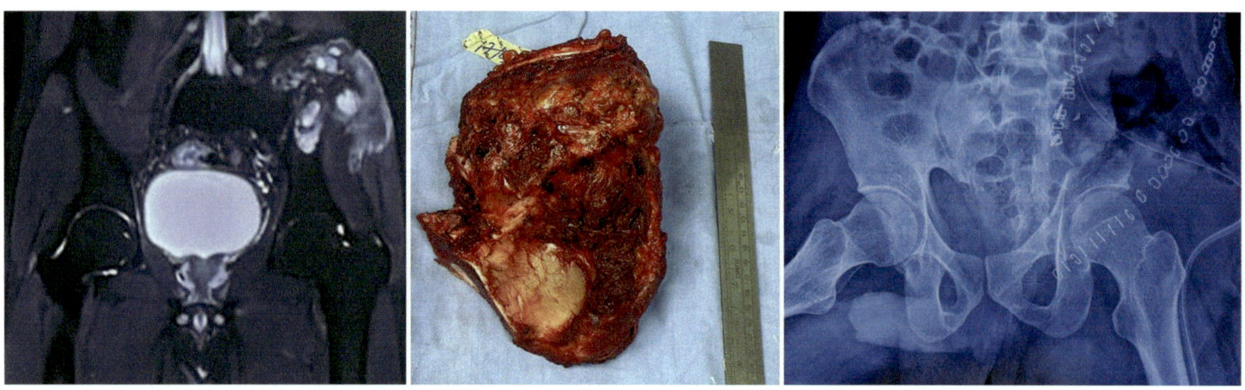

FIGURE 14.4 Ewing sarcoma of the ilium with involvement of the sacro-iliac joint. A Type I resection with extra-articular resection of the SI joint was performed, with preservation of pelvic ring integrity and the hip joint, obviating the need for reconstruction.

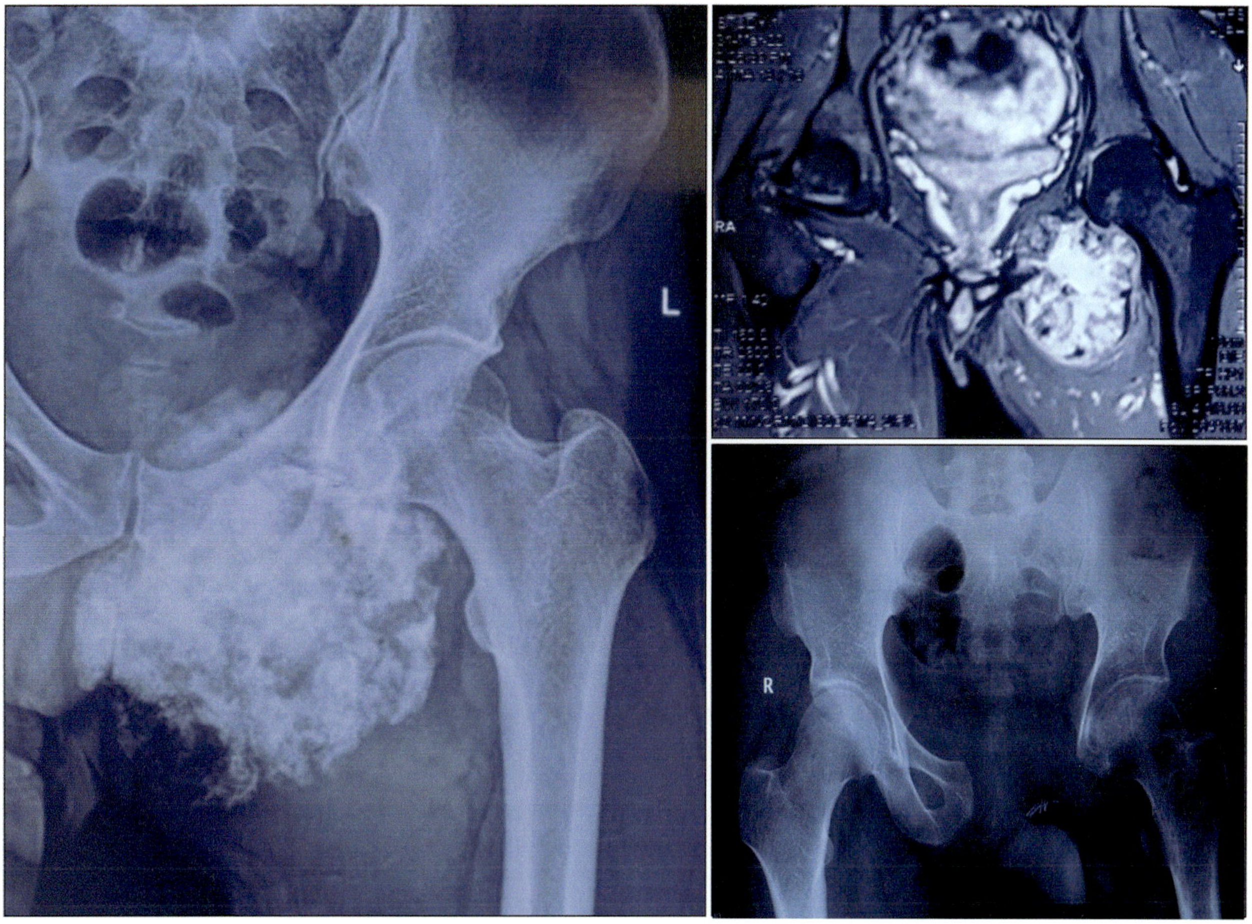

FIGURE 14.5 Type III pelvic resection in a case of chondrosarcoma involving the pubic bone.

In cases where the intersegmental gap is too wide for direct closure, structural grafting is required. Strut grafts using fibular autograft—vascularized or nonvascularized—are favored in biologically compromised environments, such as those involving prior infection, radiation exposure, smoking, or diabetes. These grafts enhance the osteogenic potential in challenging healing conditions. In young patients with robust soft tissue coverage, a nonvascularized allograft fibula is an effective alternative, offering good incorporation rates while eliminating donor site morbidity. Other described options include vascularized iliac crest autografts and autoclaved autografts, though these are less commonly employed [4].

RECONSTRUCTION OF TYPE II PELVIC RESECTIONS

Type II pelvic resections, involving the periacetabular region, pose some of the most complex reconstructive challenges due to loss of the hip joint. A wide spectrum of techniques has been developed to address these defects, with the choice of reconstruction tailored to the individual patient's anatomy, functional requirements, and biological factors.

Iliofemoral arthrodesis is a durable and time-tested method following acetabular resection. The technique involves osteotomy of the femoral head at or below the femoral neck to create a cancellous surface conducive to fusion. The femur is then apposed to the iliac osteotomy and stabilized, often using a contoured compression plate such as a cobra plate. The joint is positioned in a functional alignment—typically with 0° adduction, 0°–5° flexion, and 5° external rotation—to facilitate ambulation post-fusion. Postoperative immobilization in a hip spica cast for three to four months is critical to achieving union. While femoral intercalary allografts can reduce limb-length discrepancy, they may increase the risk of nonunion and infection [5].

Ischiofemoral arthrodesis is another fusion-based technique, particularly suitable when the ilium is insufficient for iliofemoral fixation. It offers the advantage of maintaining greater limb length but suffers from biomechanical instability due to increased shear forces across the arthrodesis site. Fusion rates are lower, and persistent motion at the symphysis pubis can lead to discomfort. A prolonged period of cast and brace immobilization is usually required [3].

Saddle prosthesis provides another reconstructive alternative when traditional fixation is not feasible. It was originally developed as a solution for extensive periacetabular defects following Type II pelvic resections, where conventional arthroplasty or biological reconstructions were not feasible. The implant consists of a curved, saddle-like component that straddles the remaining ilium, with a femoral stem articulating within this structure. Its design aims to maintain limb length and provide a degree of mobility by allowing the femoral component to "ride" within the iliac notch [6].

Surgical implantation involves fashioning a notch or groove within the residual ilium to accommodate the saddle component. This notch is ideally medialized to minimize torque forces on the pelvis. The femoral stem is then inserted, often via a standard femoral osteotomy and canal preparation. Fixation of the prosthesis relies on mechanical seating within the iliac notch rather than biologic integration, and soft tissue tensioning—particularly with preserved abductor mechanisms—is critical to ensure initial stability. Sutures or cerclage wires may be used to reinforce the construct during the early postoperative phase.

The saddle prosthesis offers a distinct set of advantages in managing large periacetabular defects following pelvic resections. It provides immediate structural stability without necessitating complex osteosynthesis or biologic grafting techniques, making it particularly suitable for elderly or low-demand patients who may not tolerate more extensive reconstruction. Additionally, it preserves lower limb length, which is beneficial for gait rehabilitation and maintaining overall limb alignment. However, the saddle prosthesis is not without significant drawbacks. Its design lacks a true articulation, resulting in abnormal load transmission across the pelvis. The absence of biologic fixation further predisposes the construct to loosening, and precise intraoperative positioning is technically demanding. These limitations contribute to its high failure rates.

Complications are frequent and well-documented, with studies highlighting a high incidence of mechanical failure, including prosthetic migration and erosion of the iliac bone. Dislocation and instability are also common, particularly in patients with compromised abductor function. Infection remains a major concern due to the large implant volume and surgical exposure, while persistent pain and limited functional outcomes often necessitate walking aids or lead to substantial mobility restrictions. As such, the use of a saddle prosthesis should be carefully considered and reserved for select cases where alternative reconstructive strategies are not feasible. Jansen et al. [6] reported poor functional scores, with limited ability to walk unassisted and high dependence on support devices. Many required revision surgery or prosthesis removal due to mechanical failure or persistent pain. While the saddle prosthesis represents a reconstructive option in selected cases of pelvic discontinuity, its high complication rates and suboptimal functional outcomes have limited its broader adoption. It is best considered as a salvage or temporizing measure when more biologically integrated or prosthetic composite options are not feasible.

The **ice-cream cone** and **pedestal cup prostheses** are modular, readily available implant systems developed to address complex periacetabular defects following pelvic tumor resections. The ice-cream cone prosthesis, initially derived from the McMinn acetabular component, features a conical iliac stem that is inserted into the remaining ilium and supports a modular acetabular component to reestablish hip articulation [7]. Similarly, the pedestal cup prosthesis consists of a titanium stem with a ribbed, conical design that is anchored into the dorsocranial ilium, serving as a stable base for a modular hip joint reconstruction [8].

Implantation of both systems typically involves iliofemoral exposure with reaming of the iliac bone, followed by the press-fit or cemented insertion of the implant, directed toward the posterior superior iliac spine while avoiding the sacroiliac joint. These prostheses offer the advantage of standardized manufacturing, eliminating delays associated with custom designs. Their modularity and ease of implantation reduce operative time and allow relatively quicker rehabilitation. Furthermore, these systems are particularly useful in patients where extensive biologic reconstructions are contraindicated due to factors such as advanced age, comorbidities, or limited life expectancy.

However, these designs have inherent limitations. Their effectiveness is constrained by the availability of sufficient healthy ilium for fixation, and they do not reconstitute pelvic ring continuity, which can lead to biomechanical alterations. In cases with massive bone loss or pelvic discontinuity, these implants may not offer adequate long-term stability.

The complication rates associated with both systems remain substantial. For the pedestal cup prosthesis, reported complications include infection (17%), dislocation (15%), and aseptic loosening (6%), with approximately 38% of patients requiring revision surgery at a median follow-up of 6.6 years [8]. The ice-cream cone prosthesis shows similarly high complication rates in the literature, ranging from 45% to 53%, primarily due to infection and instability [7]. Functional outcomes are modest; patients reconstructed with the pedestal prosthesis report a mean Musculoskeletal Tumor Society (MSTS) score of approximately 71%, indicating moderate restoration of limb function [8]. While they offer technical ease and timely availability, their application is tempered by a relatively high complication burden and limited durability, particularly in younger, high-demand patients.

The **PAR (periacetabular replacement) Endoprosthesis** is a viable reconstructive option following Type II and combined Types II–III pelvic resections. This system employs a prosthetic component featuring iliac flanges designed to sit bilaterally on the resected iliac wing, which is secured with bolts and further stabilized using bone cement. Unlike the saddle prosthesis, in which articulation occurs at the bone-prosthesis interface, the PAR Endo design incorporates a constrained liner that interfaces with the femoral component, effectively relocating the mobile articulation within the prosthetic system itself. This design mitigates the risk of iliac erosion often encountered with saddle prostheses.

Despite its mechanical advantages, the PAR Endo prosthesis is associated with a considerable complication profile. Menendez et al. [9] experienced deep infection in one-third of their patients, while prosthetic instability was reported in around 15% of cases. The cumulative rate of major complications underscores the technical and biological challenges of this reconstruction. Functional outcomes, as measured by the MSTS score, average around 67% of normal, reflecting moderate functional restoration following extensive pelvic resections.

Modular hemipelvic endoprosthesis is a reconstructive option designed to address large pelvic defects following tumor resection. The implant consists of multiple components—namely, an iliac fixation part, artificial acetabulum, and a pubic connection plate—allowing flexibility to accommodate various combinations of pelvic resections, including complex defects involving the iliosacral joint. The key advantages of the modular design include adaptability to diverse anatomical scenarios, relative ease of intraoperative assembly, early postoperative mobilization, and restoration of hip articulation. However, the technique is associated with a substantial complication profile.

In a cohort of 100 patients, wound healing disturbances (18%) and deep infections (15%) were the most common complications, with others including dislocation, aseptic loosening, and mechanical failure, such as breakage of the pubic connection plate. Implant survival at three years was 81.8%, and approximately 16% of patients required revision surgery. Functionally, the mean MSTS score was 57.2%, and the average Karnofsky Performance Score was 64.4, with better outcomes in resections sparing the iliosacral joint [10]. Despite the risks, this approach offers limb salvage with acceptable midterm oncological and functional results.

Custom-made prostheses, particularly those fabricated through advanced 3D printing technologies, have emerged as a highly individualized solution for pelvic reconstruction following oncologic resection. These implants are tailored to fit the patient's specific anatomic defect using high-resolution CT-based modeling, ensuring precise conformity to the residual pelvic anatomy. Typically constructed from porous titanium alloys, these prostheses enable biological fixation through bone ingrowth at the bone–implant interface, offering the potential for long-term stability [11].

The implantation technique involves extensive preoperative planning using computer-assisted design, followed by intraoperative placement that may incorporate screw fixation and cement augmentation depending on the defect's location and residual bone quality. This high degree of customization allows for optimal distribution of mechanical stress and better restoration of pelvic biomechanics, particularly in complex or large defects that are not amenable to standard modular systems [11, 12].

The principal advantage of custom-made prostheses lies in their anatomical fit, the ability to address unique defects involving complex zones such as the sacroiliac joint or pubic rami, and potential for osseointegration, which reduces the risks of mechanical failure, impingement, and improper load transmission. Additionally, these prostheses may accommodate constrained liners or integrate modular components to improve hip stability. However, the fabrication process is time-intensive and costly, which can delay surgery and limit accessibility in certain settings. Furthermore, despite their biomechanical advantages, complications such as infection and wound healing issues remain a concern. A recent study by Wang et al. [12] demonstrated encouraging midterm outcomes with 3D-printed custom-made pelvic prostheses. At a median follow-up of 27 months, patients showed significant improvement in pain and function, with the median VAS score improving from 5 to 2, MSTS-93 score from 14 to 23, and Harris Hip Score from 64 to 82. Importantly, no instances of deep infection, dislocation, implant breakage, aseptic loosening, or local recurrence were observed. Although two patients experienced delayed wound healing. Digital tomosynthesis confirmed successful osseointegration in all cases, supporting the reliability of porous implant surfaces in promoting biological fixation. These findings reinforce the clinical utility of custom-made prostheses in achieving durable functional outcomes with a favorable complication profile. However, long-term data are still evolving, and multicentric studies are needed to fully establish durability and complication profiles compared to other reconstructive modalities. Overall, custom-made 3D printed prostheses offer a cutting-edge approach for anatomically complex pelvic reconstructions, balancing mechanical precision with biological potential.

ALLOGRAFTS AND AUTOGRAFTS IN PELVIC RECONSTRUCTION

Biological reconstruction using allografts and autografts represents an important, albeit challenging, option for pelvic defect restoration following tumor resection. Hemipelvic allografts aim to anatomically restore the resected pelvic segment, particularly after Type II or Type II–III resections. Allografts are typically combined with cemented total hip arthroplasty or, in some cases, osteoarticular allografts of the acetabulum are used alone. These constructs allow for restoration of bony continuity and, when union is achieved, provide structural bone stock for potential future revisions. However, they are constrained by limited donor availability, potential host-donor anatomical mismatch, and a substantial risk of complications.

Allograft preparation involves shaping the donor bone to match the resected pelvic segment. It is then secured with internal fixation to achieve rigid stabilization. Optimal outcomes are more frequently observed in Type II resections, where compressive forces enhance graft-host union, as opposed to Types I–II or I–II–III resections, where shearing forces across the sacroiliac junction may predispose to nonunion. Reported rates of nonunion reach 10%–15%, often requiring secondary procedures such as morcellized bone grafting [13]. Infection remains a predominant complication, affecting up to 40% of patients in some series [14], while prosthetic dislocation is also prevalent, possibly due to proprioceptive loss or subtle anatomical mismatches. A study reported allograft resorption in three of nine patients, with five-year allograft survival of only 26.7% [15]. Despite these concerns, patients with intact reconstructions demonstrate moderate functional recovery, with MSTS scores ranging from 60% to 75% [13, 14].

Recycled autografts, another form of biological reconstruction, involve reimplantation of the patient's own resected bone following sterilization through irradiation, thermal treatment, or cryotherapy (Figure 14.6). This approach allows precise anatomical matching without dependence on donor tissue. However, it carries theoretical risks such as tumor cell persistence and precludes histopathologic assessment of surgical margins and chemotherapeutic response. The technique is also associated with a high failure rate, with graft fracture, infection, and prosthetic loosening being common.

In one report, only 4 of 14 reimplanted autografts remained intact at follow-up [16]. In a cohort of 18 patients undergoing pelvic reconstruction with extracorporeally irradiated autografts after Type II internal hemipelvectomy, the mean MSTS score among 16 evaluable patients was 77%, and the mean TESS score among 15 patients was 71%, indicating favorable functional outcomes. Despite a 17% rate of deep infection and three cases of local recurrence, the technique demonstrated acceptable morbidity and oncologic safety, supporting its validity as a reconstructive option [17]. Allograft-/autograft-endoprosthesis composites provide a prudent reconstruction option in cases with hip joint involvement by the tumor, necessitating extra-articular resections (Figure 14.7).

A systematic review analyzing surgical outcomes of limb-sparing pelvic resections and reconstruction revealed a consistently high complication burden. Despite varied reconstructive strategies—including allografts, allograft-prosthesis composites, saddle prostheses, custom endoprostheses, and irradiated autografts—the pooled nononcologic complication rate reached 49%, and the reoperation rate was 37%, underscoring the technical complexity and risk profile associated with these procedures [18].

The high complication and revision surgery rate, along with. the generally poor or modest functional outcome scores in all methods noted previously have led some orthopedic oncologists to advocate less extensive and nonanatomic reconstruction for large pelvic defects after sarcoma resection.

Hip transposition has emerged as a viable reconstructive alternative for large pelvic defects following periacetabular resections, particularly in the setting of Types I–II or Types I–II–III resections where traditional prosthetic or anatomical reconstruction methods may be associated with high complication and revision rates. This technique involves repositioning the femoral head to articulate with the sacral ala or a residual segment of ilium, creating a new articulation at a high hip center (Figure 14.8). When some inferior pelvic bone remains after resection, it can serve as a structural shelf to support the femoral head. In cases with intra-articular tumor extension, hemiarthroplasty may be used, attaching a prosthetic femoral head to the sacrum.

This technique involves creating a pseudo-capsule using synthetic mesh, typically polypropylene mesh, which is anchored to the remaining pelvic bone using sutures or anchors (Figure 14.9). Patients are often maintained on prolonged bed rest postoperatively to allow fibrosis to stabilize the construct before mobilization. Despite resulting in a

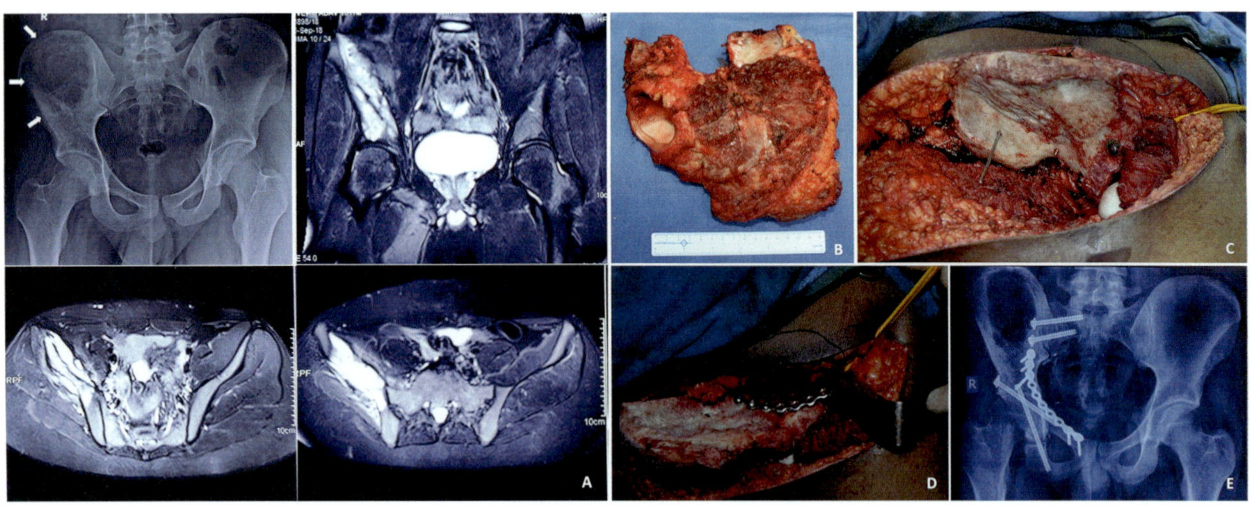

FIGURE 14.6 (A) Radiological images of an 18-year-old male with Ewing sarcoma involving the right ilium. (B) Type I + II resection was performed, followed by sterilization through irradiation, and re-implantation and fixation with screws and plates (C & D). (E) Postoperative radiographs at 24 months follow-up.

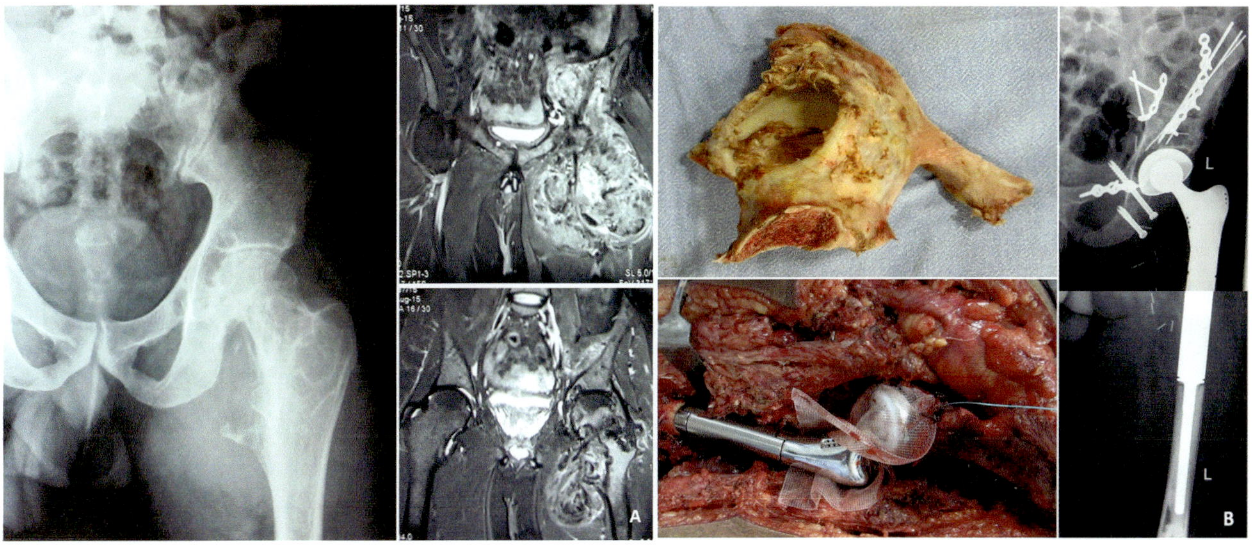

FIGURE 14.7 (A) Radiological images of a patient with chondrosarcoma involving the peri-acetabular region and the proximal femur. (B) A wide peri-acetabular, extra-articular resection was performed. Reconstruction was performed with an autograft-prosthesis composite, with the re-implantation of irradiated peri-acetabular bone and proximal femur endoprosthesis.

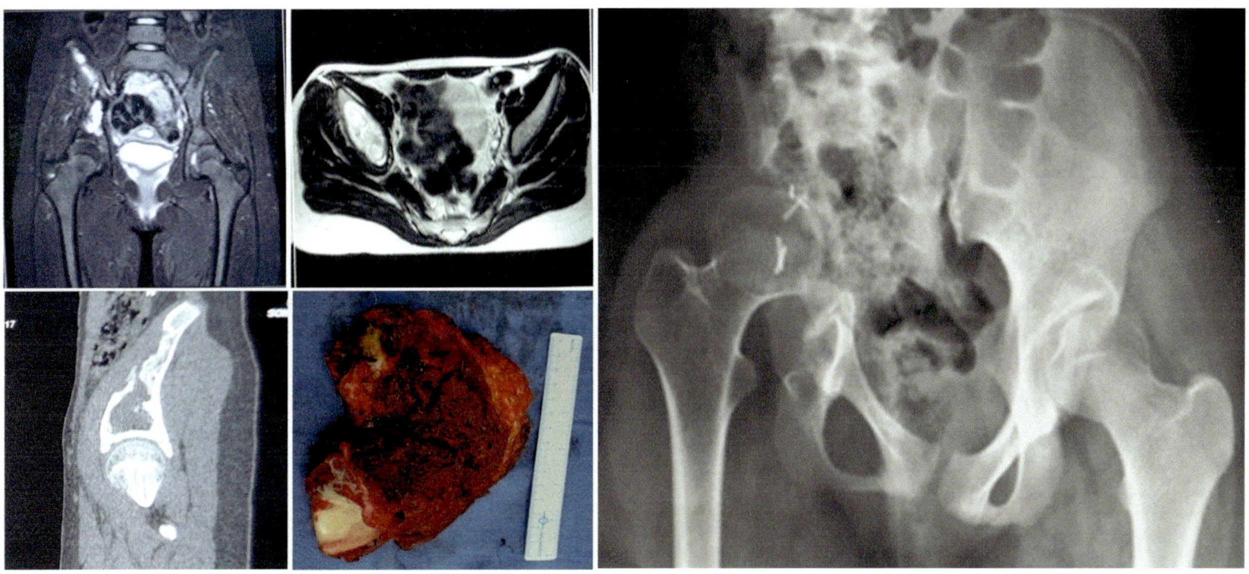

FIGURE 14.8 A case of Ewing sarcoma in a 15-year-old female, with involvement of the ilium and extension into the supra-acetabular region. A trans-acetabular resection was performed, including the ilium and superior half of the acetabulum, followed by repositioning the femoral head to articulate with the sacrum.

limb-length discrepancy, hip transposition avoids the use of large implants and enables tension-free soft tissue closure, which significantly reduces the risk of wound complications and deep infections commonly seen with prosthetic reconstruction.

Several clinical series have reported favorable functional outcomes with this method. Hoffman et al. [19] demonstrated that patients who underwent hip transposition after acetabular resections experienced notably improved functional outcomes and quality of life compared to those treated with prosthetic reconstruction or hindquarter amputation. Furthermore, in an analysis of complications following 110 pelvic resections, the highest functional outcomes were observed in patients who either underwent no reconstruction or had hip transposition, whereas the poorest results were associated with prosthetic reconstruction and amputation [20]. The absence of metallic implants and the ability to achieve tension-free wound closure likely

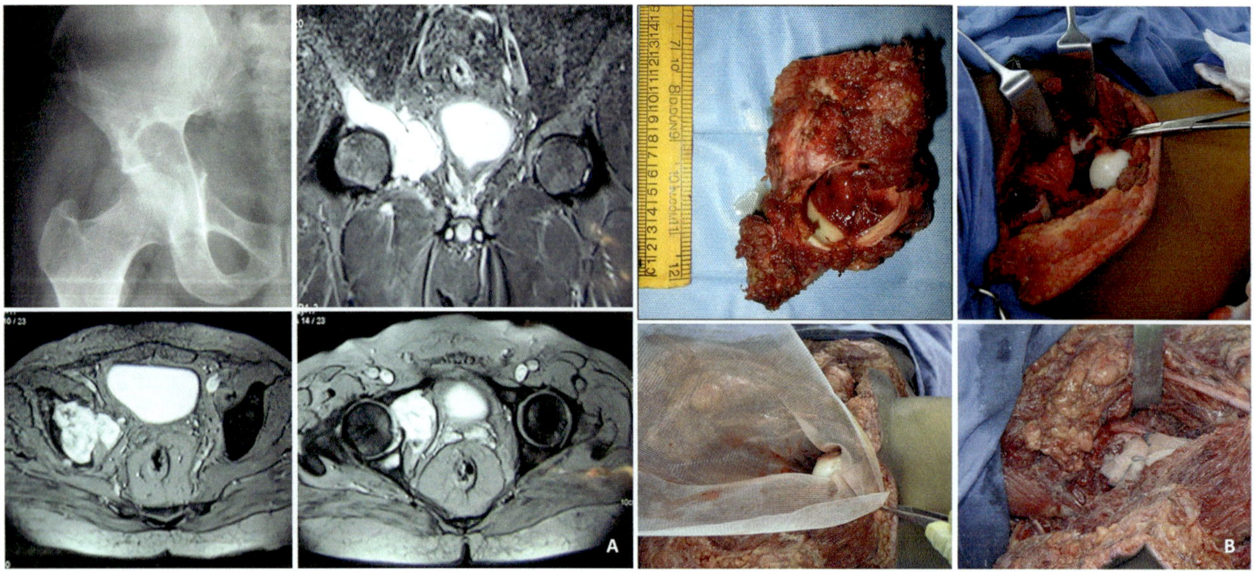

FIGURE 14.9 (A) Radiological images of a chondrosarcoma involving the peri-acetabular region. (B) Type II peri-acetabular resection was performed, followed by balanced suspension of the extremity by anchoring the femoral head to the residual pelvic bone using a Prolene mesh wrapped around the femoral head.

contribute to the reduced incidence of wound-related complications. Gebert et al. [21] documented a mean MSTS score of 62% following hip transposition. Another recent experience reported a mean MSTS-93 score of 21.25 (approximately 71%) and a Harris Hip Score of 87.2, with most patients regaining unassisted ambulation, squatting ability, and returning to work [2]. Notably, proximal migration of the transposed femoral head was prevented by the presence of residual bone, and over time, some cases demonstrated appositional bone formation that further stabilized the construct. Given its relative simplicity, lower complication profile, and acceptable functional outcomes, hip transposition represents a valuable and pragmatic reconstructive strategy following pelvic tumor resections.

RECONSTRUCTION OF TYPE III RESECTIONS

Type III pelvic resections, involving the pubis and ischium, typically do not necessitate bony reconstruction if acetabular stability is preserved (Figure 14.10). Functional outcomes in such cases are generally favorable, although patients may experience diminished adduction strength and are at risk for stress-related changes or fractures near the iliosacral region. Pring et al. reported that patients who underwent Type I or Type III resections had better functional outcomes than those after Type II resections [22].

A notable postoperative concern is the potential for visceral or bladder herniation due to anterior pelvic wall defects. Therefore, meticulous soft tissue reconstruction is essential, often employing synthetic sheet grafts or autologous flaps such as vertical rectus abdominis myocutaneous (VRAM) flaps to restore the pelvic floor and prevent herniation. Prolonged suction drainage (three to five days) and intravenous antibiotics until drain removal help reduce postoperative complications. In large defects, reinforcement of the pelvic floor with synthetic mesh may be required.

POSTOPERATIVE CARE AND REHABILITATION

Postoperative management following pelvic resections is critical to optimize functional recovery, minimize complications, and facilitate long-term rehabilitation. Immediate postoperative care focuses on pain control, wound care, infection prevention, and monitoring for neurovascular compromise. Given the extensive nature of pelvic surgeries, patients are at high risk for wound-related issues, especially in the presence of large dead spaces and compromised soft tissue envelopes; therefore, meticulous attention to drain management, tension-free closure, and, when necessary, the use of vacuum-assisted dressings is essential.

Immobilization protocols vary depending on the type and extent of resection and reconstruction. For example, patients undergoing iliosacral arthrodesis (following Type I resections) or hip arthrodesis (after Type II resections) are often immobilized in a spica cast or brace for 6–12 weeks to ensure bony fusion. In contrast, those with prosthetic reconstructions may begin mobilization earlier but require partial weight-bearing for six to eight weeks to allow for soft tissue healing and implant integration. Hip transposition patients typically undergo prolonged bed rest to allow fibrosis and soft tissue stabilization of the neo-articulation.

A structured physiotherapy program is essential and should be initiated as soon as feasible, beginning with passive range-of-motion exercises and progressing to active strengthening, gait training, and functional mobility. Rehabilitation goals include achieving independent ambulation, maximizing joint range, and restoring balance and coordination.

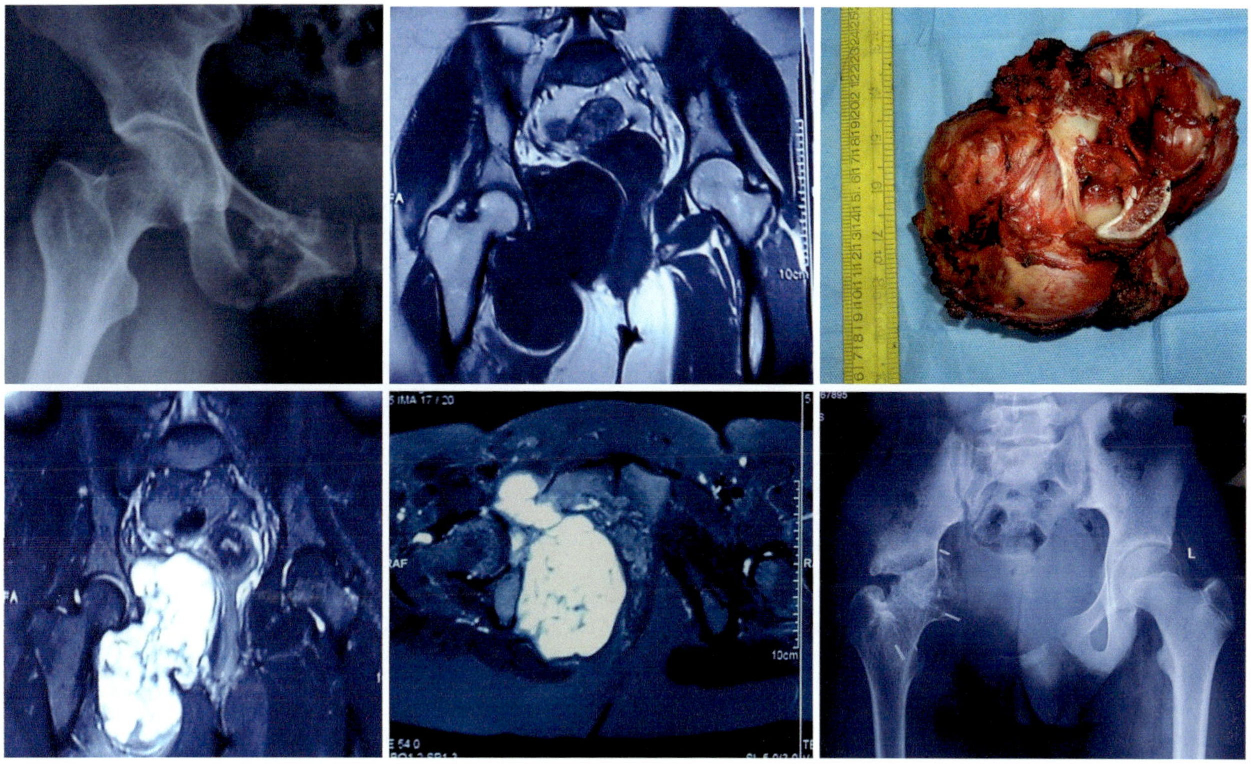

FIGURE 14.10 A case of chondrosarcoma of the pubis, with extension into the inferior part of the acetabulum. A Type III resection was performed, including the inferior half of the acetabulum. The preserved superior part of the acetabulum prevents superior migration of the femoral head. Type III resections do not require reconstruction as load-bearing biomechanics is not affected.

ROLE OF NAVIGATION IN PELVIC RESECTIONS

The application of computer-assisted navigation has significantly enhanced precision in pelvic tumor resections, addressing the unique challenges posed by complex three-dimensional pelvic anatomy and the proximity to vital neurovascular structures. In the prospective multicenter study by Gouin et al. [23], the use of navigation technology was shown to improve the accuracy of osteotomies, particularly in Types I and II pelvic resections, which often require intricate resection planes around the ilium and acetabulum.

The study demonstrated that navigated resections resulted in improved surgical margins, with a higher proportion of wide resections and reduced instances of intralesional cuts, compared to conventional techniques. Moreover, the authors reported a lower rate of local recurrence in the navigation-assisted group, suggesting an oncologic benefit. Importantly, this technique facilitated the preservation of uninvolved bone, thereby increasing the feasibility and durability of subsequent reconstruction, particularly with custom-made implants or allografts.

Despite these advantages, the study acknowledged certain limitations, including prolonged operative time, technical demand, and the need for preoperative planning with CT/MRI-based navigation protocols. Nevertheless, computer-assisted navigation represents a valuable adjunct in the surgical management of pelvic bone tumors, particularly when aiming to balance oncologic control with functional preservation.

SUMMARY

- **Pelvic resections for bone tumors require careful preoperative planning**, incorporating anatomical complexity, tumor location, and functional demands to determine the appropriate type of resection and reconstruction.
- **The Enneking–Dunham classification system remains the foundation for categorizing pelvic resections**, with evolving modifications such as trans-acetabular resections to preserve acetabular function and optimize outcomes.
- **Reconstruction strategies are highly individualized**, ranging from biological options (autografts/allografts), prosthetic solutions (saddle, pedestal, modular, or custom-made implants), to nonanatomic methods like hip transposition, each with distinct merits and complication profiles.
- **Outcomes vary significantly with the type of resection and reconstruction**, with Types I and III resections typically yielding good function without the need for bony reconstruction, while Type II reconstructions pose the greatest technical and functional challenges.
- **Hip transposition offers a promising alternative** to complex prosthetic reconstructions, particularly in low-resource settings or patients with high infection risk, showing comparable or superior functional results with fewer complications.

- **All reconstruction techniques are associated with significant complication risks**, necessitating careful patient selection, surgical expertise, and comprehensive postoperative care and rehabilitation to optimize functional recovery and long-term outcomes.

REFERENCES

1. Enneking WF, Dunham WK. Resection and reconstruction for primary neoplasms involving the innominate bone. *J Bone Joint Surg Am.* 1978;60(6):731–746.
2. Kapoor L, Sahoo B, Majeed A, et al. Leaving half the acetabulum in pelvic resections improves hip function. Is there a need to revisit conventional pelvic resections?. *J Surg Oncol.* 2022;125(6):1032–1041. doi:10.1002/jso.26806
3. Hugate R Jr, Sim FH. Pelvic reconstruction techniques. *Orthop Clin North Am.* 2006;37(1):85–97. doi:10.1016/j.ocl.2005.08.006
4. Cannon SR, Tillman RM, Grimer RJ, et al. Treatment of primary bone tumors of the ilium by local resection and fibular strut graft (non-vascularized) [abstract]. In: Companacci M, Capanna R, editors. *Proceedings of the Eighth International Symposium on Limb Salvage*. May 10–12, 1995, Vol. 77. Florence (Italy); 1995.
5. Fuchs B, O'Connor MI, Kaufman KR, Padgett DJ, Sim FH. Iliofemoral arthrodesis and pseudarthrosis: a long-term functional outcome evaluation. *Clin Orthop Relat Res.* 2002;(397):29–35.doi:10.1097/00003086-200204000-00005
6. Jansen JA, van de Sande MA, Dijkstra PD. Poor long-term clinical results of saddle prosthesis after resection of periacetabular tumors. *Clin Orthop Relat Res.* 2013;471(1):324–331. doi:10.1007/s11999-012-2631-x
7. Fisher NE, Patton JT, Grimer RJ, et al. Ice-cream cone reconstruction of the pelvis: a new type of pelvic replacement: early results. *J Bone Joint Surg Br.* 2011;93(5):684–688. doi:10.1302/0301-620X.93B5.25608
8. Hipfl C, Stihsen C, Puchner SE, et al. Pelvic reconstruction following resection of malignant bone tumours using a stemmed acetabular pedestal cup. *Bone Joint J.* 2017;99-B(6):841–848. doi:10.1302/0301-620X.99B6.BJJ-2016-0944.R1
9. Menendez LR, Ahlmann ER, Falkinstein Y, Allison DC. Periacetabular reconstruction with a new endoprosthesis. *Clin Orthop Relat Res.* 2009;467(11):2831–2837. doi:10.1007/s11999-009-1043-z
10. Ji T, Guo W, Yang RL, Tang XD, Wang YF. Modular hemipelvic endoprosthesis reconstruction--experience in 100 patients with mid-term follow-up results. *Eur J Surg Oncol.* 2013;39(1):53–60. doi:10.1016/j.ejso.2012.10.002
11. Oyem PC, Burke ZD, Mesko NW, Nystrom LM. Custom three-dimensional printed implants for reconstruction of oncologic pelvic defects. *J Surg Oncol.* 2024;129(2):424–435. doi:10.1002/jso.27465
12. Wang J, Min L, Lu M, et al. What are the complications of three-dimensionally printed, custom-made, integrative hemipelvic endoprostheses in patients with primary malignancies involving the acetabulum, and what is the function of these patients?. *Clin Orthop Relat Res.* 2020;478(11):2487–2501. doi:10.1097/CORR.0000000000001297
13. Delloye C, Banse X, Brichard B, Docquier PL, Cornu O. Pelvic reconstruction with a structural pelvic allograft after resection of a malignant bone tumor. *J Bone Joint Surg Am.* 2007;89(3):579–587. doi:10.2106/JBJS.E.00943
14. Beadel GP, McLaughlin CE, Wunder JS, Griffin AM, Ferguson PC, Bell RS. Outcome in two groups of patients with allograft-prosthetic reconstruction of pelvic tumor defects. *Clin Orthop Relat Res.* 2005;438:30–35. doi:10.1097/01.blo.0000180048.43208.2f
15. Ayvaz M, Bekmez S, Mermerkaya MU, Caglar O, Acaroglu E, Tokgozoglu AM. Long-term results of reconstruction with pelvic allografts after wide resection of pelvic sarcomas. *ScientificWorldJournal.* 2014;2014:605019. Published 2014 Jan 27. doi:10.1155/2014/605019
16. Jeon DG, Kim MS, Cho WH, Song WS, Lee SY. Reconstruction with pasteurized autograft-total hip prosthesis composite for periacetabular tumors. *J Surg Oncol.* 2007;96(6):493–502. doi:10.1002/jso.20834
17. Wafa H, Grimer RJ, Jeys L, Abudu AT, Carter SR, Tillman RM. The use of extracorporeally irradiated autografts in pelvic reconstruction following tumour resection. *Bone Joint J.* 2014;96-B(10):1404–1410. doi:10.1302/0301-620X.96B10.33470
18. Wilson RJ, Freeman TH Jr, Halpern JL, Schwartz HS, Holt GE. Surgical outcomes after limb-sparing resection and reconstruction for pelvic sarcoma: a systematic review. *JBJS Rev.* 2018;6(4):e10. doi:10.2106/JBJS.RVW.17.00072
19. Hoffmann C, Gosheger G, Gebert C, Jürgens H, Winkelmann W. Functional results and quality of life after treatment of pelvic sarcomas involving the acetabulum. *J Bone Joint Surg Am.* 2006;88(3):575–582. doi:10.2106/JBJS.D.02488
20. Hillmann A, Hoffmann C, Gosheger G, Rödl R, Winkelmann W, Ozaki T. Tumors of the pelvis: complications after reconstruction. *Arch Orthop Trauma Surg.* 2003;123(7c):340–344. doi:10.1007/s00402-003-0543-7
21. Gebert C, Wessling M, Hoffmann C, et al. Hip transposition as a limb salvage procedure following the resection of periacetabular tumors. *J Surg Oncol.* 2011;103(3):269–275. doi:10.1002/jso.21820
22. Pring ME, Weber KL, Unni KK, Sim FH. Chondrosarcoma of the pelvis. A review of sixty-four cases. *J Bone Joint Surg Am.* 2001;83(11):1630–1642.
23. Gouin F, Paul L, Odri GA, Cartiaux O. Computer-assisted planning and patient-specific instruments for bone tumor resection within the pelvis: a series of 11 patients. *Sarcoma.* 2014;2014:842709. doi:10.1155/2014/842709

15 Sacral Resection and Reconstruction

INTRODUCTION

Sacral tumors represent a rare and heterogeneous group of neoplasms that pose significant challenges in diagnosis, planning, and surgical management. They account for less than 7% of all spinal tumors, and their insidious onset and deep anatomical location often result in delayed clinical detection and substantial tumor growth before diagnosis is established [1]. These tumors may arise from various tissues, including notochordal remnants (chordomas), bone (osteosarcoma, giant cell tumor), nerve sheath (schwannoma, malignant peripheral nerve sheath tumor), or may represent metastatic disease from other primary sites such as breast, prostate, or lung [1, 2].

The sacrum's unique anatomical positioning at the confluence of the spinal axis and pelvic ring, adjacent to critical neurovascular and visceral structures, makes resection of sacral tumors particularly demanding. The sacral nerve roots play a pivotal role in lower limb function and control of bowel, bladder, and sexual functions. Consequently, surgical management aims to achieve oncological clearance while preserving neurological function wherever possible [2].

Sacral resections, or sacrectomies, are indicated predominantly for the curative treatment of primary malignant tumors such as chordomas, chondrosarcomas, or high-grade sarcomas. They may also be considered in benign but locally aggressive tumors such as giant cell tumors or aneurysmal bone cysts, especially when these recur or compromise neurological function [3]. En bloc resection with wide margins remains the cornerstone of curative treatment, given the high rates of local recurrence associated with intralesional excision or incomplete margins [2, 3].

The complexity of sacrectomy mandates a multidisciplinary approach. This involves coordinated planning between orthopedic oncologists, spine surgeons, general and colorectal surgeons, urologists, plastic and reconstructive teams, anesthesiologists, radiologists, and pathologists [3]. Such collaboration ensures not only safe resection with optimal oncologic outcomes but also effective reconstruction and rehabilitation post-surgery. Advancements in imaging, biopsy techniques, preoperative embolization, and reconstructive strategies have significantly improved the safety and efficacy of sacral resections. However, the risks of substantial blood loss, postoperative neurological deficits, wound complications, and functional impairment remain considerable [1–3].

ANATOMY AND BIOMECHANICS OF THE LUMBOSACROPELVIC JUNCTION

The lumbosacropelvic junction is a structurally complex and biomechanically demanding region where the mobile lumbar spine transitions into the rigid pelvic ring. This junction comprises the fifth lumbar vertebra (L5), the sacrum, coccyx, sacroiliac joints, and the surrounding ligamentous and muscular stabilizers. It plays a pivotal role in axial load transmission, postural support, and pelvic-lumbar articulation.

ANATOMICAL OVERVIEW

The sacrum articulates:

- Superiorly with L5 at the lumbosacral joint
- Inferiorly with the coccyx at the sacrococcygeal joint and
- Laterally with the ilium at the sacroiliac joints.

Because of the anterior tilt of the sacral base, weight transmitted through the spine exerts a rotatory force on the sacrum—pushing the promontory forward and apex posteriorly. The axis of this rotation is believed to pass through the S2 vertebral segment. This tendency is biomechanically restrained by several ligamentous structures:

- Interosseous and posterior sacroiliac ligaments, the strongest in the region, counteract anterior tilt of the sacral base.
- Sacrotuberous and sacrospinous ligaments stabilize the caudal sacrum and coccyx by resisting posterior displacement.
- Iliolumbar ligaments limit anterior migration of L5 on the sacral promontory.

The sacroiliac joint (SIJ) is a synovial articulation characterized by complementary irregularities of its articulating surfaces, which enhance mechanical interlocking. The sacral surface is lined by thick hyaline cartilage, while the iliac surface is covered by a thinner fibrocartilage. The joint extends up to S2, which has critical implications for surgical resection planning. Tumors confined to the lower sacral segments (below S2) can often be excised without compromising pelvic stability, as the SIJ and its posterior ligaments remain uninvolved.

BIOMECHANICAL CONSIDERATIONS

Biomechanically, the lumbosacropelvic junction transmits axial loads from the spine to the pelvis and resists multidirectional stresses during motion and weight-bearing. In both standing and sitting postures, weight is transmitted through L5 to the sacrum and then dispersed bilaterally across the SIJs. The SIJs thus function as critical force-transmitting interfaces between the spine and pelvis.

DOI: 10.1201/9780367822002-19

Disruption of this junction, especially through high sacral resections involving S1 or above, results in both vertical and rotational instability, necessitating reconstructive intervention. Conversely, resection of the lower sacrum (S3 and below) typically spares pelvic stability due to preservation of SIJs and associated ligamentous attachments.

A cadaveric study by Gunterberg et al. [4] experimentally validated this principle, concluding that pelvic stability is maintained if at least 50% of one or both SI joints remain intact after resection. This foundational biomechanical insight underscores the critical role of preserving SIJ integrity in sacrectomy planning. Total sacrectomy, particularly when it involves bilateral SIJs and portions of the iliac wings, disconnects the spine from the pelvis. This results in the loss of spinopelvic continuity, leading to impaired ambulation, inability to bear axial load, and chronic instability unless corrected via surgical reconstruction (e.g., spinopelvic fixation).

Understanding these complex relationships is essential for planning oncologic resections that aim to balance oncological clearance with the preservation or restoration of mechanical stability and function.

VASCULAR ANATOMY OF THE SACRAL REGION

A comprehensive understanding of the vascular anatomy of the sacral region is critical for the safe and effective execution of anterior sacral resections and for the planning of preoperative embolization. The intricate network of arteries and veins in this area, closely related to vital neural and visceral structures, presents both technical challenges and opportunities for control during oncologic surgery.

The vascular supply to the sacral region originates primarily from the abdominal aorta, which typically bifurcates at the level of the L4 vertebral body, just left of the midline, into the right and left common iliac arteries (CIAs). The right CIA, usually longer (approx. 5 cm) than the left (approx. 4 cm), courses in proximity to several key structures. Anteriorly, it is crossed by the ureter and ovarian artery (in females), along with descending branches of the sympathetic chain. Medially and laterally, it is bordered by the inferior vena cava, the termination of the right common iliac vein, the left common iliac vein, the superior hypogastric plexus, and the psoas muscle.

The left CIA, being shorter, is also crossed anteriorly by the ureter, ovarian artery, sympathetic nerve branches, and the terminal portion of the inferior mesenteric artery (IMA). It lies adjacent to the psoas muscle laterally and the middle sacral artery medially. This spatial relationship must be appreciated, especially during mobilization and dissection in the presacral space.

The internal iliac arteries (IIAs) branch off from the CIAs and dive caudally and posteriorly into the pelvis. These arteries give rise to several critical branches relevant to sacral resections:

- The iliolumbar artery emerges dorsally and courses rostro-laterally, crossing over the lumbosacral trunk.
- The lateral sacral arteries, often one or more in number, run a paramedian course over the piriformis muscle and in proximity to the anterior sacral foramina. These vessels are major contributors to the vascular supply of presacral tumors and are frequently targeted during embolization.
- The superior gluteal artery, the largest branch of the IIA, exits the pelvis through the greater sciatic foramen above the piriformis and traverses the upper sacral plexus.
- The inferior gluteal artery passes between the piriformis and coccygeal muscles, intersecting the lower sacral plexus en route to the gluteal region.

Additionally, the middle sacral artery, a small midline vessel arising from the posterior aorta near its bifurcation, courses along the anterior surface of the sacrum and coccyx, and may also contribute to tumor vascularity.

These arteries are frequently encountered during anterior sacral resections. Injuries to them, particularly the lateral sacral and middle sacral arteries, can result in significant intraoperative hemorrhage. Preoperative embolization of these vessels, especially in hypervascular tumors, has been shown to reduce intraoperative blood loss.

The venous anatomy of the sacral region largely parallels the arterial layout but is notably more variable and complex. Key venous structures include:

- The presacral venous plexus, a fragile, valveless network located anterior to the sacrum that communicates with the lateral sacral veins, basivertebral veins, and pelvic venous plexuses. It poses a significant bleeding risk during anterior dissection and tumor mobilization.
- The middle sacral vein, unlike its arterial counterpart, typically drains into the left common iliac vein rather than directly into the inferior vena cava.
- The iliolumbar veins, which often drain into the common iliac veins instead of the internal iliac veins, are at risk during dissection in the lateral pelvic wall.

Because of their thin walls and lack of valves, presacral veins cannot constrict effectively to stop bleeding. This makes control of venous hemorrhage particularly challenging, especially in narrow operative fields where tamponade is limited. Surgical strategies such as the application of hemostatic agents, bipolar cautery, and ligation clips are routinely employed to manage this bleeding. Moreover, precise knowledge of the venous course helps avoid inadvertent injury during retraction or tumor dissection.

The vascular complexity of the sacral region necessitates precise preoperative imaging and planning. Advanced imaging modalities such as contrast-enhanced computed tomography (CT) angiography and MR angiography can delineate arterial anatomy and identify anomalous vessels. In large or hypervascular tumors, selective preoperative embolization of the middle and lateral sacral arteries significantly reduces intraoperative blood loss and facilitates a cleaner dissection plane.

Surgeons must be acutely aware of the intimate relationship between the sacral vasculature and adjacent neural, visceral, and muscular structures. Mobilization of vascular bundles should be done with extreme caution to avoid iatrogenic injury, particularly during anterior approaches to tumors that encroach upon the lumbosacral junction or involve the presacral area.

SACRAL NEURAL ANATOMY

A detailed understanding of sacral neural anatomy is critical for planning sacral resections, as the preservation or sacrifice of sacral nerve roots significantly impacts lower limb function, sphincter control, and sexual function. The sacral plexus, located in the pelvis anterior to the piriformis muscle, is formed by the union of the lumbosacral trunk (L4–L5) and the anterior rami of S1–S3, with contributions from S4. This union occurs over the sacroiliac joint, typically at the level of the S2 sacral foramina.

The sciatic nerve, the largest branch of the plexus and a key structure in lower limb function, forms near the S3 level and exits the pelvis via the greater sciatic foramen. The superior and inferior gluteal nerves, the most proximal branches of the plexus, also exit through the greater sciatic foramen and innervate gluteal musculature. Motor branches to the quadratus femoris, gemelli, and obturator internus muscles arise from this plexus. Sensory branches such as the posterior femoral cutaneous nerve and perforating cutaneous nerve also exit the pelvis via the greater sciatic foramen.

Medial and inferior to the main sacral plexus, branches of S2–S4 form the pudendal nerve, which uniquely exits the greater sciatic foramen and reenters through the lesser sciatic foramen after looping around the sacrospinous ligament. It innervates the levator ani, coccygeus, and external anal sphincter, and provides key perineal sensory input. The coccygeal plexus, formed by S4, S5, and coccygeal nerves, contributes to perianal sensation.

The sympathetic trunks course caudally along the anterior sacral surface, contributing gray rami communicantes to sacral nerves and forming the superior hypogastric plexus. At S1–S2, this divides into two inferior hypogastric (pelvic) plexi, positioned over the obturator internus muscles at S2–S4. The parasympathetic fibers, from S2 to S4 anterior roots, form the pelvic splanchnic nerves, which integrate into the pelvic plexi and innervate pelvic organs. The sympathetic system governs ejaculation and visceral motility, while the parasympathetic system primarily mediates erectile reflexes and bladder contraction.

Functional loss following sacral resections correlates directly with the level and laterality of nerve root sacrifice:

- **Unilateral root loss**, particularly below S2, often preserves most functions.
- **Bilateral S2–S4 resections** result in neurogenic bladder and bowel, sexual dysfunction, and perineal sensory loss.
- Preserving **at least one S2 root** can retain partial autonomic control.

In oncologic sacral surgery, every effort should be made to preserve **S2–S4 nerve roots**, especially unilaterally, to maintain sphincter and sexual function. Preoperative counseling and postoperative neurorehabilitation are crucial when sacrifice of these roots is unavoidable.

CLASSIFICATION AND LEVELS OF SACRECTOMY

Sacrectomies are most commonly classified according to the highest sacral nerve root or vertebral level resected. This classification reflects both the potential neurological compromise and the degree of mechanical destabilization of the pelvic ring and spine. Partial sacrectomy refers to resections involving the sacral segments below the S3 level, typically preserving the S1 and S2 nerve roots, as well as the sacroiliac joints. In such cases, pelvic stability is usually maintained, and neurological deficits, if present, are often mild and limited to minor disturbances in perineal sensation or bowel function, especially if only the unilateral S3 root is resected (Figure 15.1).

Subtotal sacrectomy involves resection extending up to the S2 level. Although S1 is preserved, bilateral resection of the S2 roots can result in partial loss of bowel and bladder control, and depending on the extent of bone resection around the sacroiliac joints, pelvic stability may be compromised. These cases often require reconstruction if the integrity of the sacroiliac articulation is significantly altered.

Total or high sacrectomy entails resection at or above the S1 level, resulting in complete disconnection between the spine and pelvis. This procedure is associated with profound functional consequences, including complete loss of voluntary bladder and bowel control, major motor deficits, and the necessity for spinopelvic fixation due to severe biomechanical instability. The S1 vertebral segment is of particular importance, as it serves as a critical conduit for axial load transmission between the spine and pelvis. Its removal mandates rigid spinopelvic stabilization using instrumentation such as iliac screws and rod constructs to restore continuity and allow ambulation.

PREOPERATIVE EVALUATION AND PLANNING

Preoperative evaluation and planning are paramount in the management of sacral tumors, given the anatomical complexity of the region and the high risk of functional and mechanical compromise. A meticulous multidisciplinary

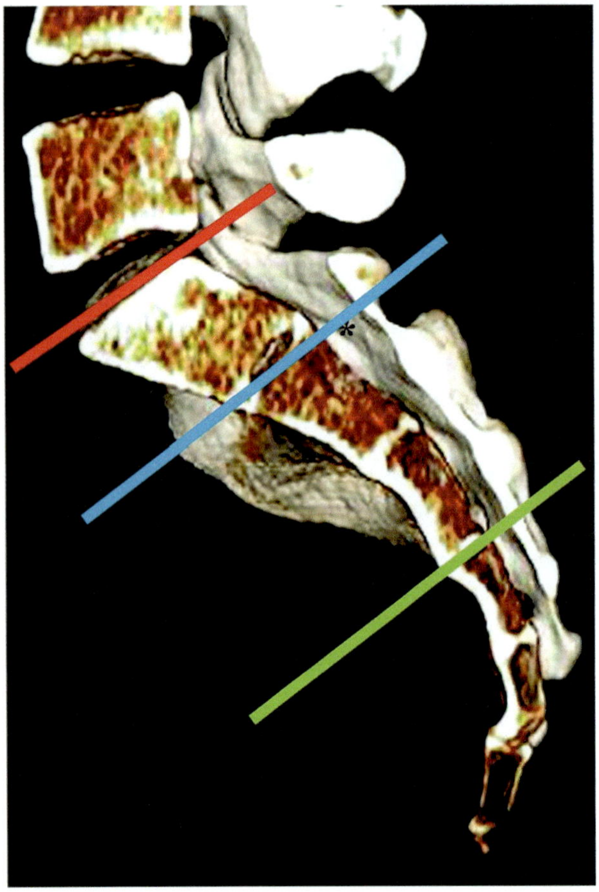

FIGURE 15.1 Illustration of levels of sacrectomy. The green line depicts a partial sacrectomy, in which resection is performed below the S3 level, preserving the S1 and S2 roots as well as the sacroiliac joints. The blue line indicates a subtotal sacrectomy, extending up to the S2 level with sparing of S1. The red line represents a total or high sacrectomy, involving resection at or above the S1 level, which results in complete disconnection of the spine from the pelvis.

approach, incorporating clinical assessment, advanced imaging, oncologic staging, and surgical planning, is essential to achieving oncological control while minimizing morbidity.

The initial step involves a comprehensive clinical evaluation, including a detailed neurological examination to assess motor and sensory deficits, bowel and bladder function, and gait stability. These findings are critical in predicting the impact of potential nerve root sacrifice and help in counseling the patient regarding functional outcomes. Pain characteristics—particularly sacral, radicular, or visceral—also guide localization and assessment of neural involvement. A digital rectal examination (DRE) serves as a valuable adjunct in preoperative decision-making. If the surgeon can palpate above the superior margin of the lesion during DRE, a posterior-only approach is often sufficient. Additionally, this examination helps assess the involvement of the rectal mucosa, offering insight into potential tumor adherence or invasion.

Radiological imaging plays a central role in delineating tumor extent, involvement of critical structures, and planning resection margins. Magnetic resonance imaging (MRI) is the modality of choice for local staging (Figure 15.2). It provides superior soft tissue contrast, allowing precise evaluation of tumor extension into the sacral canal, neural foramina, pelvic viscera, and musculature. Contrast-enhanced MRI is beneficial for assessing vascular encasement and peritumoral inflammation. CT complements MRI by offering detailed visualization of cortical bone involvement, sacroiliac joint erosion, and for preoperative planning of osteotomies and instrumentation.

CT angiography or MR angiography is recommended in cases where tumors abut or encase major vascular structures. These studies help map arterial anatomy and identify anomalous branches, which is crucial if preoperative embolization is planned to minimize intraoperative blood loss in hypervascular tumors.

Biopsy must be performed with utmost care, typically under imaging guidance, ensuring that the tract is placed along a line that can be excised en bloc with the tumor. A multidisciplinary tumor board review should confirm the diagnosis and guide treatment sequencing.

Functional and oncologic assessment, including chest imaging (CT thorax) and whole-body bone scans or PET-CT, are necessary for staging and to exclude metastatic disease, particularly in high-grade sarcomas.

From a surgical standpoint, preoperative planning should incorporate decisions regarding the level of sacral resection, expected neurological deficits, and the need for spinopelvic reconstruction. When high sacrectomy is anticipated, preoperative discussions with plastic surgeons may be warranted to address soft tissue coverage (pedicled vertical rectus abdominis myocutaneous [VRAM] and/or gluteal flaps) and assistance with vascularized fibular transfer (as needed for spinopelvic reconstruction). Similarly, urology and colorectal teams may need to be involved if adjacent organs are involved or displaced. Ureteral stents may be required for tumors with large ventral extension or anatomic distortion. Colorectal surgeons can provide useful assistance with anterior vascular and visceral mobilization, and also with potential colostomy or meso-rectal dissection. Importantly, patient counseling must be thorough and realistic. Discussions should include anticipated neurological deficits, possible loss of bowel/bladder control, sexual dysfunction, need for colostomy or urinary diversion, and the protracted recovery process. Psychological support and prehabilitation should be initiated early.

In select cases, particularly for large, low-grade, or slow-growing tumors, neoadjuvant therapy—including embolization, radiation, or chemotherapy—may be utilized to downsize the lesion or devascularize the tumor, improving the surgical field and reducing intraoperative bleeding. Ultimately, a well-coordinated, multidisciplinary preoperative plan ensures optimal surgical outcomes, facilitates complete oncological resection, and minimizes intraoperative and postoperative complications.

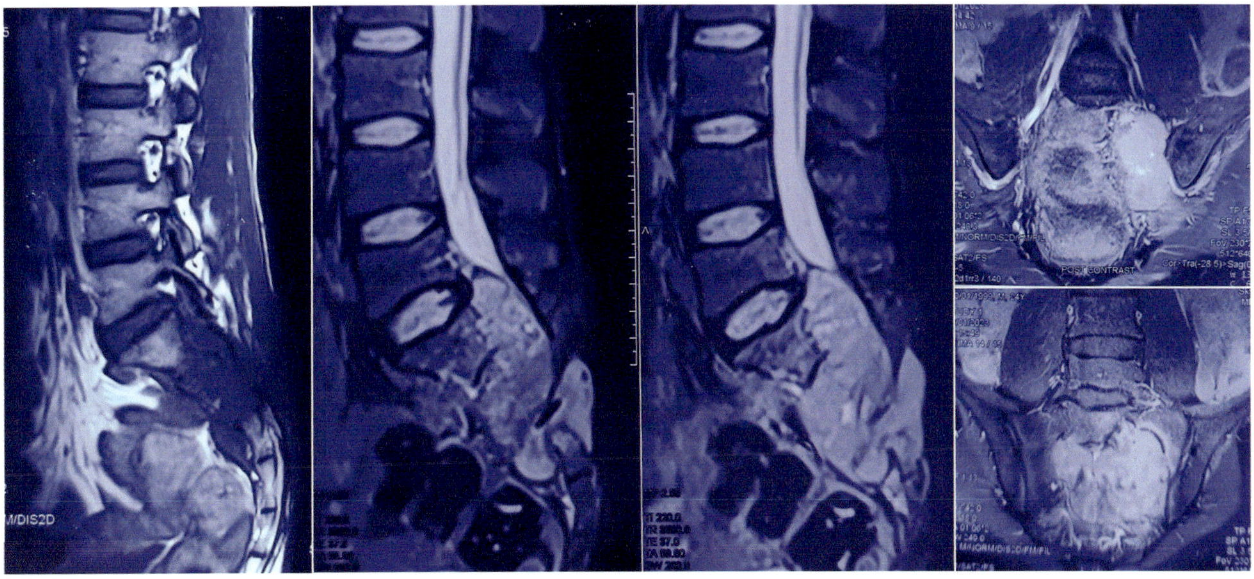

FIGURE 15.2 MRI of the pelvis and lumbosacral spine showing a chordoma involving the sacrum from S1 to S4. A large prevertebral soft tissue mass is seen displacing the rectum anteriorly, with extension into the spinal canal up to the level of L5. The sacroiliac joints are preserved bilaterally. Chordomas typically present as destructive midline sacral lesions with prominent soft tissue extension, and MRI is essential in delineating tumor extent, neural involvement, and surgical planning.

SURGICAL APPROACHES TO SACRAL RESECTION

The cranial extent of a sacral tumor plays a pivotal role in determining the optimal surgical approach for wide excision. While institutional protocols may vary, a posterior-only approach is generally sufficient for tumors located at or below the S2–S3 junction, provided the anticipated soft tissue defect is manageable with local gluteal flap coverage. However, for tumors that extend cranially beyond this level or are associated with extensive soft tissue involvement, a combined anterior and posterior approach is typically warranted. This preference is guided by multiple surgical priorities, including the need to optimize patient safety, achieve adequate oncologic margins, evaluate the requirement for colostomy, and ensure effective soft tissue closure [2, 3].

ANTERIOR PROCEDURE (INTRAPERITONEAL APPROACH)

The anterior intraperitoneal approach is an essential component of high sacral resections, particularly for tumors involving the anterior sacrum or in proximity to pelvic viscera and major vessels. Although technically demanding, it provides unparalleled access to anterior sacral pathology and critical vascular structures, setting the stage for safe and effective oncologic resection. This stage is often performed first in a staged anterior-posterior resection and plays a critical role in tumor mobilization, vascular control, and preparation for posterior osteotomy.

The patient is positioned supine with careful padding at all contact points. A midline vertical laparotomy incision is made from approximately 2–3 cm above the umbilicus to the symphysis pubis. Access to the retroperitoneal tumor can be achieved via either a transperitoneal or bilateral extraperitoneal route, depending on tumor extent and involvement. Once the bowel is packed away, the posterior parietal peritoneum is opened unilaterally to allow entry into the presacral space. The ureters are identified bilaterally, and the iliac vessels are carefully dissected. Preoperative ureteric stenting may assist in visual identification. If the rectum is uninvolved, it is mobilized anteriorly following incision of the retrorectal peritoneal reflection, allowing exposure of the tumor capsule.

A key objective of this approach is early vascular control. The internal iliac and middle sacral arteries and veins, along with any direct tumor-feeding vessels, are ligated. The external iliac arteries are preserved. Mobilization of the iliac veins medially and laterally is often required to facilitate anterior sacral osteotomy. Despite the frequent anterior extension of sacral tumors into the pelvic cavity, the sacral periosteum and presacral fascia commonly act as effective barriers, preserving a dissection plane between the tumor and rectum. These structures often prevent direct rectal infiltration, even in cases where the tumor has breached the cortical boundary of the sacrum, thereby enabling safe mobilization of the rectum during resection. The peritoneal investment and periosteum are incised caudally, sometimes down to the greater sciatic notch, to expose the anterior cortex of the sacrum. Scoring the cortex anteriorly facilitates subsequent posterior osteotomies.

The anterior sacral foramina serve as anatomical landmarks for guiding osteotomy planes. The lumbosacral trunk (L4–5) is identified over the sacral ala. The sacroiliac joint is approached lateral to the nerve roots, and a bilateral partial anterior sacroiliac osteotomy is performed using chisels or drills. The L5–S1 disc is exposed and excised with the anterior annulus. If not obscured by tumor, S1–S3 nerve roots are divided at their foramina under direct vision, with osteotomy cuts waxed to minimize bleeding and improve visualization.

A flexible silastic sheath is placed posterior to the rectum and vascular structures to prevent adhesions and facilitate the second-stage posterior dissection. Closure is performed in layers, with placement of a suction drain. Importantly, autonomic nerve disruption during this stage can lead to a transient postoperative ileus, typically resolving over several days.

In cases of extensive sacral resection, pedicled rectus abdominis myocutaneous flaps are often harvested during the anterior stage to facilitate soft tissue closure during the posterior procedure. This technique has substantially reduced complications related to wound breakdown and prolonged drainage.

When the posterior procedure follows the anterior stage in the same sitting, a rectus abdominis myocutaneous flap is prepared during the anterior exposure and based on the inferior epigastric vessels. The skin island of the flap is sealed with an iodine-impregnated adhesive dressing, wrapped in an antibiotic-soaked laparotomy pad, and temporarily stowed within the pelvis. Large gelatin sponges may be inserted between the tumor mass and critical structures like the iliac vessels, sacral plexus, or pelvic organs to aid hemostasis and guide subsequent dissection. The abdomen is then closed, and if required, colostomy formation is deferred until after sacrectomy and reconstruction to minimize infection risk.

POSTERIOR APPROACH

The posterior approach is a principal component of sacral resections, offering direct access to the dorsal sacrum, sacral nerve roots, and posterior pelvic elements. It is employed either alone in low sacral tumors or as part of a staged procedure in combination with the anterior approach for high sacrectomies. Importantly, it also facilitates the creation and transposition of vascularized myocutaneous flaps for reconstruction.

After repositioning the patient in the prone position, a longitudinal midline incision is made extending from L2 to below the coccyx. Skin, subcutaneous tissue, and musculature overlying the sacrum are preserved for en bloc excision. Tumor- or biopsy-compromised skin and any irradiated or previously incised tissue are included in the resection specimen. A lumbosacral myocutaneous flap is elevated and retracted cranially, offering wide exposure without retractor-induced injury.

The dissection deepens in a conical fashion, accommodating posterior tumor extension. The posterior iliac crests, greater sciatic notches, sciatic nerves, L3–L5 spinous processes, and facet joints are exposed bilaterally. L5 and subtotal S1 laminectomy facilitates exposure of the thecal sac and cauda equina. The posterior sacral foramina and sacral nerve roots (S1–S5) are identified. Preservation or sacrifice of these roots is guided by preoperative neurological assessment and the extent of tumor involvement. Whenever possible, bilateral preservation of the S2 roots is attempted to maintain partial bowel, bladder, and sexual function. Laminectomy and nerve root dissection are carried out meticulously. The laminae and spinous processes of the involved sacral segments are removed en bloc or piecemeal, depending on tumor location and margins. Sacral nerve roots are identified and divided at their foramina according to oncologic and functional goals. The dural sac is closed with double-layer watertight sutures to prevent cerebrospinal fluid (CSF) leakage (Figure 15.3).

Key ligamentous and muscular attachments are then divided: the sacrospinalis muscles, posterior sacroiliac ligaments, gluteal musculature, piriformis muscles, superior and inferior gluteal vessels and nerves, and sciatic, pudendal, and posterior femoral cutaneous nerves are identified and preserved when possible. If rectal preservation is

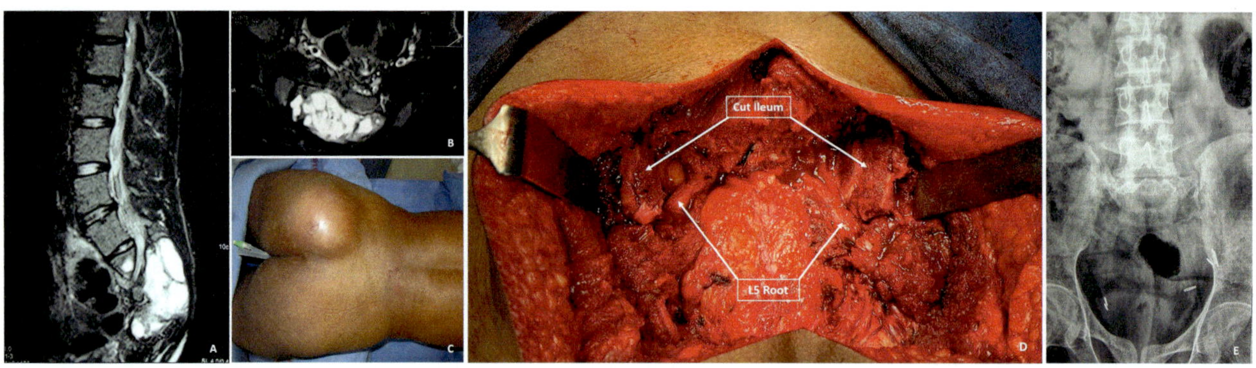

FIGURE 15.3 Chondrosarcoma of the sacrum in a 44-year-old male. (A, B) MRI showing a large sacral mass with heterogeneous signal intensity and extensive soft tissue component, arising from the sacrum and extending into the presacral space, with displacement of adjacent structures. (C) Preoperative clinical photograph demonstrating a large lumbosacral swelling with stretched, shiny overlying skin. Patient underwent total sacrectomy without reconstruction. (D) Intraoperative image of the surgical bed after tumor resection, with the cut ilium and exposed L5 root marked. (E) Postoperative radiograph at 18 months follow-up.

planned, the anococcygeal ligament, coccygeal muscles, and sacrotuberous and sacrospinous ligaments are transected. In cases requiring rectal resection, the anus and levator muscles are dissected circumferentially.

The previously placed silastic sheath from the anterior approach serves as a critical anatomical guide for safe osteotomy completion. Once the posterior bony elements are exposed and decompression is completed, the sacral osteotomy is performed using osteotomes, drills, or ultrasonic bone scalpels. In cases where an anterior stage has been completed, the anterior scoring of the cortex guides posterior osteotomy placement. Care must be taken during osteotomy to avoid injuring the presacral structures, and osteotomy surfaces are often waxed to control bleeding. The posterior sacral osteotomies are then performed along the ilium, potentially entering the sciatic notch either medial or lateral to the ischial spine. Once osteotomies are completed, tumor delivery is facilitated by mobilizing the remaining attachments circumferentially, followed by en bloc extraction. Sacral nerve roots are divided as they exit the foramina, and the sciatic nerves are preserved. Hemostasis is achieved using bipolar cautery, bone wax, tamponade, and hemostatic agents.

This approach not only permits oncologically sound resection but also sets the stage for soft tissue coverage using previously prepared or regional flaps, reducing wound complications, and enhancing functional outcomes.

OPERATIVE TECHNIQUES OF SPINOPELVIC RECONSTRUCTION

Reconstructing the spinopelvic junction after partial or total sacrectomy is a technically demanding and biomechanically complex procedure. The operative approach must address both the immediate mechanical stability of the spinal column and pelvis, and long-term fusion and function, especially in ambulatory patients. The extent of sacral resection, preservation or sacrifice of the sacroiliac joints, and involvement of nerve roots and surrounding musculature largely determines the choice of reconstruction technique.

The key biomechanical objectives of reconstruction include:

- Reestablish axial load transmission from the spine to the pelvis.
- Restore pelvic ring integrity.
- Minimize motion at the lumbopelvic junction to facilitate fusion.
- Prevent construct failure due to high mechanical stress.

INDICATIONS FOR RECONSTRUCTION AFTER SACRECTOMY

Reconstruction following sacrectomy is primarily guided by the level of resection and its biomechanical impact on spinopelvic stability. The sacrum serves as the vital structural interface between the spine and pelvis. Sacrectomies, particularly those extending into the upper sacral segments, may disrupt this load-bearing continuity, necessitating reconstructive stabilization.

In a cadaveric biomechanical study, Hugate et al. [5] examined the mechanical effects of high transverse partial sacrectomies at two levels—just below and just above the S1 neural foramina. Their findings revealed a significant decrease in load-bearing capacity with more cephalad resections. Resections above the S1 foramen exhibited markedly reduced stiffness and lower failure loads, which were below physiological loads encountered during daily activities such as standing and sitting with flexion. In contrast, resections just below the S1 foramen maintained relatively higher load-bearing capability, sufficient to tolerate standard postoperative mobilization without immediate reconstruction in select cases.

Further clinical and anatomical evidence also refines these indications. Structural sacral integrity can be preserved if the sacral body above the S1 neural foramina and the sacral ilia remain intact. In such cases, adequate stability is maintained through the preservation of the sacral ala and the lumbopelvic ligaments (Figure 15.4). Some authors have reported no instability following resection at the S1–S2 interspace or S2-level resection in patients with sacrococcygeal chordoma [6].

Nevertheless, spinopelvic reconstruction becomes necessary under specific conditions. Based on Gunterberg's seminal work [4], the absolute indications for reconstruction are total sacrectomy involving complete removal of the sacroiliac joints bilaterally, and partial sacrectomy where more than 50% of the sacroiliac joint is resected on either side.

Thus, the key indications for reconstruction after sacrectomy include:

- **High sacral resection involving or above the S1 body**: These resections compromise pelvic ring integrity and exhibit failure under physiological loading conditions, warranting immediate spinopelvic reconstruction.
- Significant sacroiliac joint resection
- **Planned early weight-bearing**: Reconstruction is critical to prevent pathologic fractures and ensure safe mobilization.
- **Fracture risk or pre-existing instability**: Especially in patients with poor bone quality or prior pelvic surgery/radiation.

Reconstruction Strategies: The key reconstruction strategies include:

1. Spinopelvic Fixation (SPF): Connects the lumbar spine to the ilium.
2. Posterior Pelvic Ring Fixation (PPRF): Stabilizes the bilateral iliac bones.
3. Anterior Spinal Column Fixation (ASCF): Links the lumbar vertebrae to the pelvis.

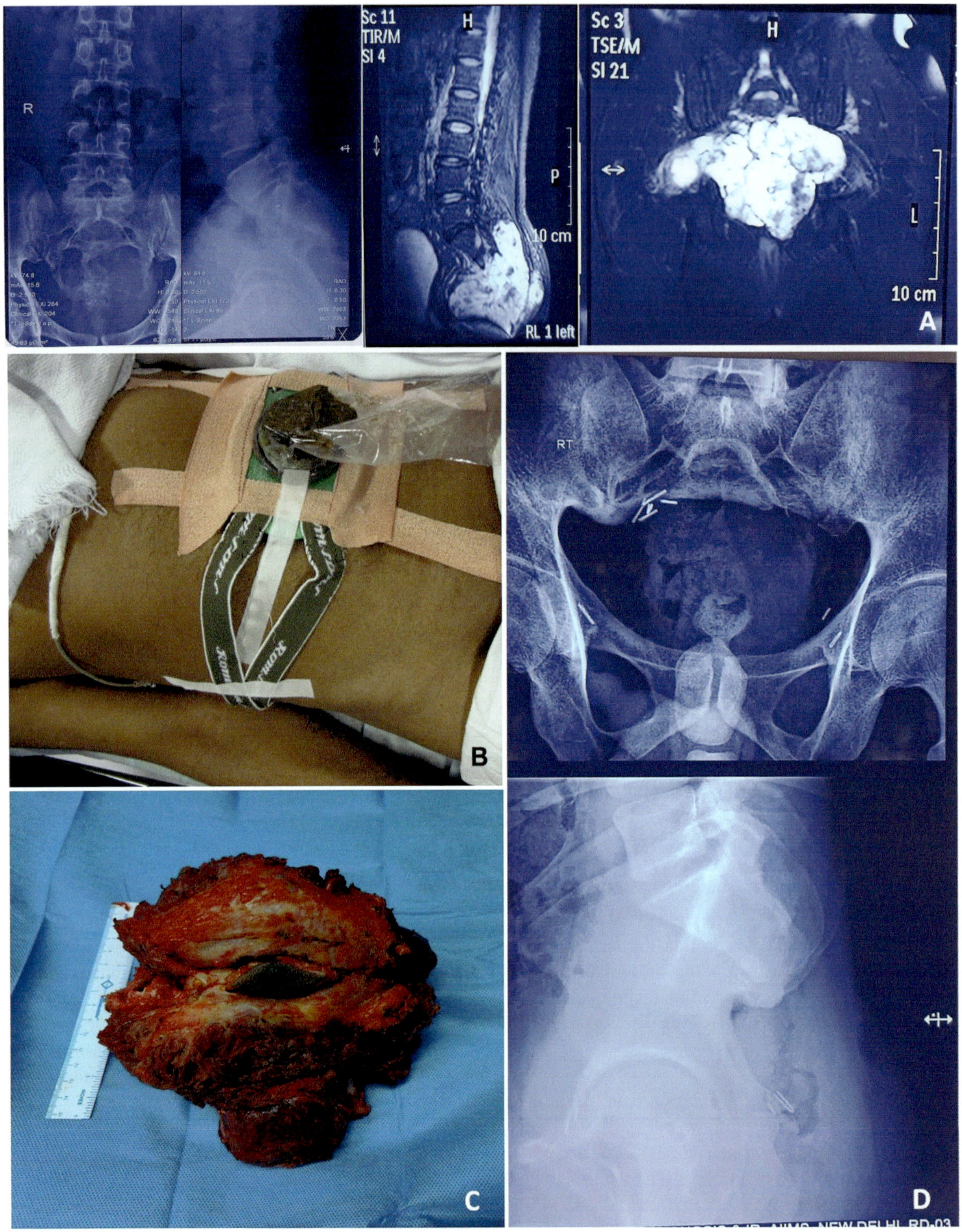

FIGURE 15.4 Chordoma of the sacrum in a 58-year-old male. (A) Radiographs and MRI showing a destructive sacral lesion with a large soft tissue component occupying the presacral space, extending superiorly up to S2 while sparing S1. (B) Preoperative clinical photograph showing a diversion colostomy performed before tumor resection. (C) Gross specimen of the resected tumor following subtotal sacrectomy (up to S2 level). (D) Postoperative radiographs confirm the extent of sacral resection. Subtotal sacrectomy up to the S2 level allows preservation of S1 roots and sacroiliac joints.

SPINOPELVIC FIXATION (SPF) TECHNIQUES

Early efforts at lumbopelvic stabilization involved the use of Harrington hook-rod constructs and Cotrel-Dubousset instrumentation. However, these constructs demonstrated poor mechanical stability and high failure rates due to inadequate resistance to axial and torsional forces. Fusion failures and implant breakage were frequent, owing to excessive stress at the hook-lumbar interface and motion at the fusion site [6].

The evolution of spinopelvic fixation saw a major advancement with the introduction of pedicle screw-rod systems and iliac fixation. Originally, the rod was used in conjunction with sublaminar wiring of the lumbar spine. These constructs, however, did not provide substantial torsional stability or resistance to extension. Gokaslan and colleagues [7] pioneered the use of pedicle screws in the lumbar spine combined with iliac rods, thus significantly improving construct rigidity and reducing failure rates. This modified Galveston technique remains a cornerstone in spinopelvic reconstruction, particularly in cases involving high sacral resection or total sacrectomy.

These modern SPF constructs typically involve multilevel pedicle fixation with pedicle screws placed from L3 to L5 using fluoroscopic or navigation guidance, with larger diameter screws at the lower lumbar vertebrae to counter cantilever forces. Bilateral dual iliac screws (typically 7.5–8.5 mm in diameter, 80–100 mm in length) are inserted from the posterior superior iliac spine toward the anterior inferior iliac spine, securing purchase in the dense cancellous bone. Cross-linking transverse connectors placed between rods significantly enhances torsional rigidity.

Bone grafts, including autologous iliac crest bone, allograft chips, and demineralized bone matrix, are placed around the posterior elements to enhance fusion. This construct functions as a cantilever beam, counteracting the flexion and shearing forces exerted across the lumbosacral junction. It is particularly useful when the sacral alar or promontory is compromised, as in total sacrectomies or when sacroiliac integrity is lost.

POSTERIOR PELVIC RING FIXATION

The posterior pelvic ring plays a key role in distributing loads and maintaining transverse stability after sacral resection. Several techniques are used to reestablish posterior ring integrity:

- **Iliac-Iliac Rod Constructs**: Titanium rods (5.5–6.0 mm) connecting bilateral iliac screws restore up to 89% of native stiffness.
- **Posterior Iliosacral Plating**: In patients with partial sacral preservation, plates bridging the iliac wings and residual sacrum can provide stability, particularly in low-demand patients.
- **Structural Grafts**: Tricortical iliac crest autografts or femoral shaft allografts help bridge defects and promote biological fusion.
- **Titanium Cages**: These can be packed with autograft or allograft bone and placed anteriorly to provide vertical load support and facilitate fusion.

Load-sharing concepts such as the closed-loop technique have demonstrated improved biomechanical profiles in finite element analyses.

ANTERIOR SPINAL COLUMN FIXATION

ASCF is a pivotal component in restoring flexion-extension stability after high sacral resections. This anterior support is particularly vital when the S1 vertebral body or sacroiliac joints are resected. Techniques include:

- **Structural Allografts**: Vertical femoral or tibial allografts can provide immediate axial support, although supplemental fixation is required.
- **Expandable Titanium Cages**: These allow intraoperative adjustment and better endplate interface, reducing the risk of subsidence.
- **Triangular Frame Constructs**: A hybrid of anterior, posterior, and transverse elements that replicates the three-dimensional load-bearing capacity of the native lumbopelvic junction.

ASCF offers the advantage of lower hardware failure and complication rates when combined with SPF/PPRF [8].

COMBINED ANTERIOR-POSTERIOR INSTRUMENTATION

For extensive defects involving the anterior column, such as when the L5–S1 vertebral body is compromised, anterior support using strut grafts (fibular or tibial allograft) or titanium cages may be necessary. These are combined with posterior rod-and-screw constructs to restore height and maintain sagittal balance.

Anterior support is typically placed after tumor resection via the anterior approach and prior to the posterior phase. Biomechanically, the combined construct provides superior stability and distributes axial loads more effectively than posterior constructs alone.

SOFT TISSUE COVERAGE AND MYOCUTANEOUS FLAPS

Effective soft tissue reconstruction is integral to reducing wound complications and ensuring long-term implant viability. Common strategies include:

- **Rectus Abdominis Myocutaneous Flap**: Harvested during the anterior approach and rotated into the posterior sacral defect after resection.
- **Gluteal Advancement or Gracilis Flaps**: Preferred when prior surgeries or radiation preclude rectus use.

- **Free Flaps**: Reserved for complex or previously operated fields, often involving microvascular anastomosis.

These flaps obliterate dead space, protect underlying instrumentation, and reduce infection risks.

POSTOPERATIVE MANAGEMENT AND REHABILITATION

Patients are usually monitored in a high-dependency or ICU setting in the immediate postoperative period. Key priorities include pain control, neurovascular assessment, wound monitoring, and deep vein thrombosis (DVT) prophylaxis. Broad-spectrum antibiotics are continued for 48–72 hours, and negative pressure wound therapy may be used for large or complex wounds. Multimodal analgesia is employed. Sacral nerve root sacrifice often results in neurogenic bowel and bladder, requiring intermittent catheterization and structured bowel regimens.

Early mobilization (within 48–72 hours) is encouraged with physiotherapy support. TLSO (thoraco-lumbo-sacral orthosis) or lumbopelvic braces may be used for 8–12 weeks. Weight-bearing depends on construct stability—robust fixations allow earlier mobilization. Physiotherapy focuses on progressive mobility, core strengthening, and gait training. Occupational therapy supports adaptation to daily activities. Functional outcomes are closely tied to preserved nerve roots, especially L5 and S1.

Flaps (e.g., rectus abdominis or gluteal) must be monitored for viability. Frequent sterile wound inspection is essential. Infections or hardware exposure may necessitate debridement or revision.

BIOMECHANICAL CONSIDERATIONS

Biomechanical studies indicate that constructs extending anterior to the pivot point of the lumbosacral junction (i.e., posterior annulus of the L5–S1 disc) provide the most effective stabilization. Dual iliac screw constructs provide superior fatigue resistance and mitigate rod breakage, especially in long fusion constructs, when compared to single iliac rod systems. Cross-links between rods enhance rigidity and minimize rod toggling. Longer constructs spanning from the thoracolumbar junction may be warranted in osteoporotic bone or when additional spinal segments are destabilized during resection.

A comparative biomechanical study by Mindea et al. [9] evaluated four reconstruction techniques following total sacrectomy: double-rod double iliac screw (DDS), double iliac screw (DIS), single-rod single iliac screw (SSS), and the modified Galveston technique (MGT). All constructs significantly reduced spinal motion post-sacrectomy. Among them, the DDS construct demonstrated the highest stiffness across all motion planes—flexion-extension, lateral bending, and axial rotation—showing 55%–60% superior motion control over the other methods. DIS provided improved stability compared to SSS and MGT, attributed to the biomechanical advantage of a triangular support from dual iliac screws. While MGT offered some stabilization, it was biomechanically inferior and better suited for select partial sacrectomy cases.

Key features contributing to construct stability include the use of multiple iliac screws to enhance load distribution and rotational control, the incorporation of cross-links and trans-iliac bars for torsional rigidity, and the adoption of four-rod constructs, which further improve multi-planar stiffness. Clinically, dual iliac screw systems have reduced rod breakage and improved pelvic tilt correction, though failure may still occur in osteoporotic bone or with suboptimal hardware placement. Overall, biomechanical evidence favors the use of dual iliac screws with multi-rod configurations in total sacrectomy reconstruction to optimize stability, promote early mobilization, and minimize complications.

A finite element study compared four sacrectomy reconstruction techniques: sacral-rod (SRR), four-rod (FRR), bilateral fibular flaps (BFFR), and improved compound (ICR). ICR demonstrated superior stability (minimal L5 motion ≤1°/1mm) and lowest implant stresses by combining anterior fibular flaps with posterior fixation. FRR showed poor stability (64° rotation) and high failure risk. BFFR provided intermediate stability. While ICR is biomechanically optimal, its complexity may limit use. The findings emphasize anterior load-sharing to reduce posterior implant failure [10].

COMPLICATIONS

Spinopelvic reconstruction following total or partial sacrectomy is a high-risk procedure associated with a substantial complication rate. These include wound-related issues, instrumentation failure, non-union, and persistent neurological deficits. Several systematic reviews [11, 12] have consolidated data from numerous case series and institutional experiences, helping to quantify these risks and highlight factors influencing functional outcomes (Table 15.1).

A study identified a 25% incidence of spinopelvic fixation mechanical failure after total sacrectomy, with the primary risk factors being the non-use of the four-rod technique (FRT) for spinopelvic fixation (SPF), absence of ASCF, and female gender. To minimize failure, the authors recommend adopting FRT and ASCF during reconstruction, particularly in female patients [13].

OUTCOMES

Functional outcomes following sacrectomy are primarily determined by the extent of nerve root preservation, particularly the S1–S3 segments. Systematic reviews [11, 12] consistently highlight that ambulation is best preserved when the S1 nerve roots are intact bilaterally, with up to 90% of such patients walking independently. Even in cases where bilateral S1 roots are sacrificed, ambulation remains possible in approximately 60%–70% of patients using assistive devices or orthoses. However, resections involving nerve roots

TABLE 15.1
Complications Following Sacrectomy

Complication/Outcome	Incidence
Deep infections	21%–44%, reduced by flap coverage
Implant failure	15%–30%
Pseudarthrosis	16%–20%
Permanent neurological deficits	Up to 90% in total sacrectomy
Local recurrence	12%–35%, varies by tumor type
Independent ambulation	~35%–45%
Reoperation for complications	20%–30%
30-day mortality	1%–6%

above S1 markedly reduce independent mobility. While ambulation outcomes were similar between reconstructed and non-reconstructed groups, reconstruction significantly reduced wound complications and hospital stay [14].

Bladder and bowel dysfunction are common, especially when bilateral S2–S4 roots are resected, with up to 80% of patients experiencing incontinence or requiring catheterization and bowel regimens. Unilateral preservation of these roots significantly improves continence outcomes. Sexual dysfunction is frequently observed but less consistently reported, typically correlating with injury to parasympathetic sacral nerves.

Pain relief is often achieved postoperatively due to tumor debulking, although neuropathic pain may persist. Functional scores such as the Musculoskeletal Tumor Society (MSTS) and Karnofsky Performance Status generally reflect acceptable outcomes, particularly when stable biomechanical reconstruction and timely rehabilitation are achieved. While no reconstruction technique has shown clear superiority in terms of functional restoration, constructs offering enhanced stability facilitate earlier mobilization and better overall recovery.

SUMMARY

- Sacral tumors pose complex diagnostic and surgical challenges due to their deep anatomical location and proximity to neurovascular and pelvic structures, requiring a multidisciplinary approach for optimal outcomes.
- Spinopelvic reconstruction becomes essential after high sacral resections or bilateral sacroiliac joint compromise to restore axial load transfer and maintain structural integrity.
- Modern spinopelvic fixation constructs, especially those using dual iliac screws, four-rod configurations, and anterior column support, provide superior biomechanical stability and reduce implant failure.
- Despite the high complication rate, comprehensive preoperative planning, meticulous surgical technique, and structured rehabilitation can yield favorable functional and oncological outcomes.

REFERENCES

1. Fiani B, Runnels J, Rose A, Kondilis A, Wong A, Musch BL. Clinical manifestations, classification, and surgical management of sacral tumors and the need for personalized approach to sacrectomy. *Surg Neurol Int.* 2021;12:209. doi:10.25259/SNI_133_2021
2. Puri A, Agarwal MG, Shah M, et al. Decision making in primary sacral tumors. *Spine J.* 2009;9(5):396–403. doi:10.1016/j.spinee.2008.10.001
3. Rose PS, Houdek MT. Team approach: oncologic sacrectomy. *JBJS Rev.* 2020;8(9):e1900226. doi:10.2106/JBJS.RVW.19.00226
4. Gunterberg B, Romanus B, Stener B. Pelvic strength after major amputation of the sacrum. *An experimental study. Acta Orthop Scand.* 1976;47(6):635–642. doi:10.3109/17453677608988751
5. Hugate RR Jr, Dickey ID, Phimolsarnti R, Yaszemski MJ, Sim FH. Mechanical effects of partial sacrectomy: when is reconstruction necessary? *Clin Orthop Relat Res.* 2006;450:82–88. doi:10.1097/01.blo.0000229331.14029.44
6. Zhang HY, Thongtrangan I, Balabhadra RS, Murovic JA, Kim DH. Surgical techniques for total sacrectomy and spinopelvic reconstruction. *Neurosurg Focus.* 2003;15(2):E5. doi:10.3171/foc.2003.15.2.5
7. Jackson RJ, Gokaslan ZL. Spinal-pelvic fixation in patients with lumbosacral neoplasms. *J Neurosurg.* 2000;92(1 Suppl):61–70. doi:10.3171/spi.2000.92.1.0061
8. Bederman SS, Shah KN, Hassan JM, Hoang BH, Kiester PD, Bhatia NN. Surgical techniques for spinopelvic reconstruction following total sacrectomy: a systematic review. *Eur Spine J.* 2014;23(2):305–319. doi:10.1007/s00586-013-3075-z
9. Mindea SA, Chinthakunta S, Moldavsky M, Gudipally M, Khalil S. Biomechanical comparison of spinopelvic reconstruction techniques in the setting of total sacrectomy. *Spine (Phila Pa 1976).* 2012;37(26):E1622–E1627. doi:10.1097/BRS.0b013e31827619d3
10. Zhu R, Cheng LM, Yu Y, Zander T, Chen B, Rohlmann A. Comparison of four reconstruction methods after total sacrectomy: a finite element study. *Clin Biomech (Bristol).* 2012;27(8):771–776. doi:10.1016/j.clinbiomech.2012.05.008
11. Branco E Silva M, Branco E, Silva M, Conceição Maia Martins S, Voltan Garofo K, Eduardo Hideo Hanasilo C, Etchebehere M. Analysis of morbidity and mortality in patients with primary bone tumors who underwent sacrectomy: A systematic review. *J Bone Oncol.* 2022;35:100445. doi:10.1016/j.jbo.2022.100445
12. Zoccali C, Skoch J, Patel AS, Walter CM, Maykowski P, Baaj AA. Residual neurological function after sacral root resection during en-bloc sacrectomy: a systematic review. *Eur Spine J.* 2016;25(12):3925–3931. doi:10.1007/s00586-016-4450-3
13. Tang X, Yang R, Qu H, Cai Z, Guo W. Factors associated with spinopelvic fixation mechanical failure after total sacrectomy. *Spine (Phila Pa 1976).* 2018;43(18):1268–1274. doi:10.1097/BRS.0000000000002635
14. Reynolds JJ, Khundkar R, Boriani S, et al. Soft tissue and bone defect management in total sacrectomy for primary sacral tumors: a systematic review with expert recommendations. *Spine (Phila Pa 1976).* 2016;41(Suppl 20):S199–S204. doi:10.1097/BRS.0000000000001834

Section V

Miscellaneous

16 Resections and Reconstructions in Skeletally Immature

INTRODUCTION

Primary malignant bone tumors, notably osteosarcoma and Ewing sarcoma, are among the most challenging oncologic diagnoses encountered in children. The vast majority of these lesions occur in the metaphyseal regions of long bones, particularly around the knee, where the physis plays a vital role in longitudinal skeletal growth. Surgical management in this demographic must therefore strike a balance between effective oncologic clearance and preservation of future growth potential and function.

Limb salvage in skeletally immature patients remains a controversial topic. The developing skeleton introduces unique complexities, including the risk of leg-length discrepancies due to physeal sacrifice, the need for durable reconstructions that can accommodate growth, and the long-term burden of multiple revision surgeries. In some cases, these challenges have prompted a reevaluation of amputation or rotationplasty as preferred surgical options, especially in very young patients or those with extensive soft tissue involvement [1].

Nevertheless, limb salvage options have expanded significantly, with innovations such as expandable endoprostheses, allograft and allograft-prosthetic composite (APC) reconstructions, vascularized fibular grafts, and devitalized autografts being applied with growing success in pediatric populations. While complication rates remain high and most studies are limited to Level IV evidence, outcomes suggest that meaningful function and growth preservation can be achieved in a substantial proportion of children undergoing limb-preserving surgeries [2].

As we delve into the detailed aspects of bone tumor resections and reconstruction strategies in skeletally immature patients, it is imperative to understand the biologic and biomechanical considerations unique to this population, alongside the evolving reconstructive modalities and their respective merits and limitations.

CHALLENGES UNIQUE TO SKELETALLY IMMATURE PATIENTS

Limb salvage in skeletally immature patients entails unique challenges, primarily due to open growth plates, smaller bone size, and the long duration over which reconstructions must function effectively.

Physeal Sacrifice and Growth Disturbance

Tumors frequently involve the distal femur and proximal tibia—sites contributing significantly to lower limb growth. Resection often requires physeal sacrifice (Figure 16.1), predisposing to leg-length discrepancies of >8 cm by maturity in younger patients [3]. While prediction methods like the arithmetic and Paley multiplier models exist, they fail to account for growth suppression due to chemotherapy or radiation, limiting their reliability in oncologic settings [3].

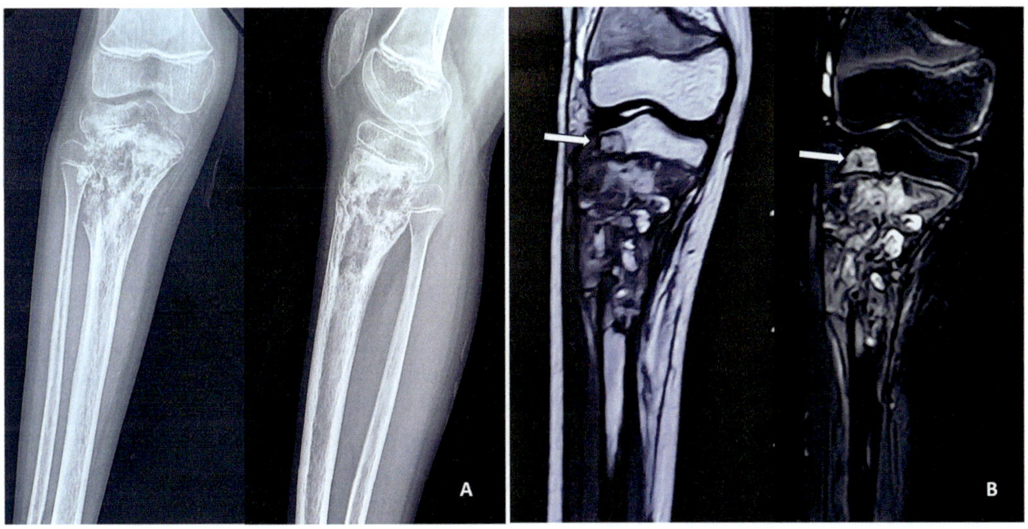

FIGURE 16.1 Plain radiographs (A) and MRI image (B) of Osteosarcoma involving the proximal tibia in a 9-year-old male, showing involvement of the proximal physes with extension of the tumor into the epiphysis (white arrows), necessitating physeal sacrifice.

DOI: 10.1201/9780367822002-21

Technical Constraints of Small Anatomy

Young children present with narrow intramedullary canals and short metaphyseal segments, making them unsuitable for standard endoprostheses. Additionally, limited soft tissue coverage increases the risk of infection and complicates soft tissue reconstruction and attachment, especially in biologic or osteoarticular reconstructions [4].

Durability and Need for Multiple Revisions

With longer expected survival, these patients face a high burden of revisions. Expandable prostheses, while growth-accommodating, have high rates of mechanical failure and infection. Biological reconstructions offer remodeling potential but are limited by delayed union, graft resorption, and infection—often worsened by chemotherapy [1, 4].

Psychosocial Implications

Aesthetic outcomes, peer acceptance, and return to activities are critical in children. While functionally equivalent to prostheses, procedures like rotationplasty may have significant psychosocial impact, especially during adolescence [1].

GROWTH AND SKELETAL MATURITY CONSIDERATIONS

The immature skeleton introduces fundamental considerations that influence both surgical planning and long-term outcomes in pediatric bone tumor management. Understanding growth patterns, the impact of oncologic therapies on the physis, and accurate prediction of limb-length discrepancy is essential for effective reconstruction.

Skeletal Growth Patterns and Timing

The distal femur and proximal tibia together contribute over two-thirds of lower limb growth, with the distal femur alone accounting for 9–10 mm/year and the proximal tibia for 6 mm/year. Girls typically reach skeletal maturity by 14 years and boys by 16 years, although variability exists [5].

Surgical resection involving these physes can result in major limb-length discrepancies (LLD) if not addressed. For example, a 6-year-old boy losing both the distal femoral and proximal tibial physes could develop a 15 cm discrepancy by maturity if uncorrected.

Impact of Chemotherapy and Radiation on the Physis

Chemotherapeutic agents such as methotrexate and doxorubicin transiently impair chondrocyte proliferation in the proliferative zone of the physis, causing temporary growth arrest. While some recovery occurs post-therapy, long-term suppression and physeal bar formation have been reported, especially with high-dose regimens [5].

Radiation therapy, particularly in Ewing sarcoma, has more permanent effects. Doses as low as 20 Gy in children under 10 years can irreversibly damage the physis, leading to asymmetric growth or premature closure. These effects are more pronounced in the axial skeleton and often necessitate close long-term monitoring [5].

Methods to Predict Limb-Length Discrepancy

Various methods exist to estimate LLD at skeletal maturity:

- **Arithmetic Method**: Assumes fixed growth rates for each physis and is suitable for children nearing skeletal maturity.
- **Growth Remaining Charts**: Based on skeletal (rather than chronological) age and growth percentiles.
- **Paley Multiplier Method**: Uses multipliers derived from large pediatric datasets to predict mature height and LLD from a single measurement.
- **Straight-Line Graph Method**: A more complex graphical tool, now embedded in digital applications for ease of use [5].

However, these models do not account for the modifying effects of cancer treatment, malnutrition, or endocrine changes, limiting their precision in oncology patients.

Clinical Relevance

For tumors near active growth plates, especially in younger children, failure to account for growth potential may result in significant LLD. Reconstruction choices such as use of expandable prostheses, contralateral epiphysiodesis, or limb overlengthening during surgery are guided by these predictions. Inaccuracy may lead to under- or overcorrection, necessitating further interventions.

Surgical Decision-Making in the Immature Skeleton

Selecting an appropriate surgical strategy for bone tumors in skeletally immature patients requires a nuanced understanding of patient age, tumor location, expected growth, reconstruction durability, and functional expectations. These considerations form the basis for a tailored, case-specific approach that balances oncologic safety with long-term musculoskeletal outcomes.

KEY DETERMINANTS OF SURGICAL STRATEGY

Several factors critically influence surgical decision-making:

- **Chronological and Skeletal Age**: Younger patients (typically <10 years) have significant residual growth potential, necessitating reconstructions that accommodate longitudinal growth. Adolescents approaching maturity (14–17 years) may be treated with adult-type implants and strategies, often obviating the need for expandable options [3].

- **Tumor Location**: Intercalary resections often permit biological reconstruction using allografts or vascularized fibular grafts. Osteoarticular resections, particularly around joints such as the distal femur or proximal tibia, require durable reconstructions that may involve modular or expandable prostheses, or allograft-prosthesis composites [2].
- **Anticipated Limb-Length Discrepancy**: Predicted LLD >2–3 cm warrants consideration of growth-accommodating reconstructions (e.g., expandable endoprostheses), overlengthening strategies, or contralateral epiphysiodesis. Younger children are more likely to benefit from expandable implants, while older adolescents may tolerate small discrepancies or be managed with contralateral procedures.
- **Patient and Family Expectations**: Functional goals, cosmetic concerns, and the willingness to undergo multiple future surgeries must be integrated into the decision-making process. For example, families prioritizing a more natural limb appearance may opt for expandable prostheses, whereas those wishing to avoid repeated interventions may prefer amputation or rotationplasty in select cases.

PROPOSED ALGORITHMIC APPROACH

Errani et al. [2] proposed an algorithm for pediatric limb reconstruction based on patient age and tumor characteristics. Key points include:

- **Children <10 years with osteoarticular resections**: Prefer allograft-prosthesis composites or rotationplasty, as modular prostheses often do not fit small anatomy.
- **Intercalary resections**: Favor biological reconstruction using massive bone allograft, vascularized fibula, or tumor-devitalized autografts.
- **Adolescents nearing maturity**: Adult-type prostheses or fixed-length APCs are typically appropriate, with or without contralateral epiphysiodesis to address minor discrepancies.

Such algorithms help standardize decision-making but must be adapted to individual patient anatomy, tumor biology, and available institutional resources.

LIMB SALVAGE AND RECONSTRUCTION STRATEGIES

Limb salvage in skeletally immature patients has evolved into a viable alternative to amputation, even in very young children. Reconstruction strategies must address the dual goals of immediate structural stability and accommodation for future growth. The choice of technique depends on tumor location, anticipated LLD, available reconstruction options, and institutional expertise. The main categories include expandable endoprostheses, allografts, APCs, vascularized fibular grafts, and tumor-devitalized autografts.

EXPANDABLE PROSTHESIS

Expandable prostheses have revolutionized limb salvage surgery in skeletally immature patients with bone tumors, addressing the critical challenge of LLD resulting from physeal resection (Figure 16.2). These implants are designed to accommodate longitudinal growth, allowing for periodic lengthening to match the contralateral limb. The development of expandable prostheses has evolved significantly, with modern designs offering minimally invasive or noninvasive lengthening mechanisms, reducing the need for repeated open surgeries [3, 6].

The development of expandable endoprostheses has undergone significant technological progression since the 1970s. The earliest documented system, the Stanmore extendible prosthesis, featured four distinct design phases between 1976 and 1992. The initial worm-drive screw mechanism (1976) was replaced in 1982 by a ball-bearing system due to manufacturing challenges. A C-collar mechanism followed in 1988, requiring open surgical lengthening, before returning to a refined screw-based design in 1992 that permitted percutaneous adjustment. A paradigm shift occurred in 2002 with the introduction of noninvasive magnetic expansion technology. This Stanmore design incorporated rare-earth magnets and an external drive unit to achieve lengthening without surgical intervention [3].

Over the past four decades, these implants have evolved through three major generations:

- **First-generation devices** (e.g., KMFTR, Howmedica Modular Resection System) required repeated surgeries.
- **Second-generation devices** introduced minimally invasive gear-driven expansion systems.
- **Third-generation systems**, such as the **Stanmore JTS**, **Repiphysis**, and **MUTARS Xpand**, enable **noninvasive magnetic expansion**, greatly improving patient comfort and reducing surgical burden.

Minimally invasive designs, such as those by Biomet and Stryker, require a small surgical incision or percutaneous access to activate the lengthening mechanism [2, 3]. Noninvasive systems, like the Stanmore magnetic prosthesis, utilize external magnetic fields to induce internal expansion, enabling outpatient lengthening without anesthesia [3, 7]. Another example, the Repiphysis prosthesis, employs a spring-loaded mechanism activated by heat induction under fluoroscopy, though its use has declined due to high complication rates, including mechanical failure and unpredictable lengthening [8, 9].

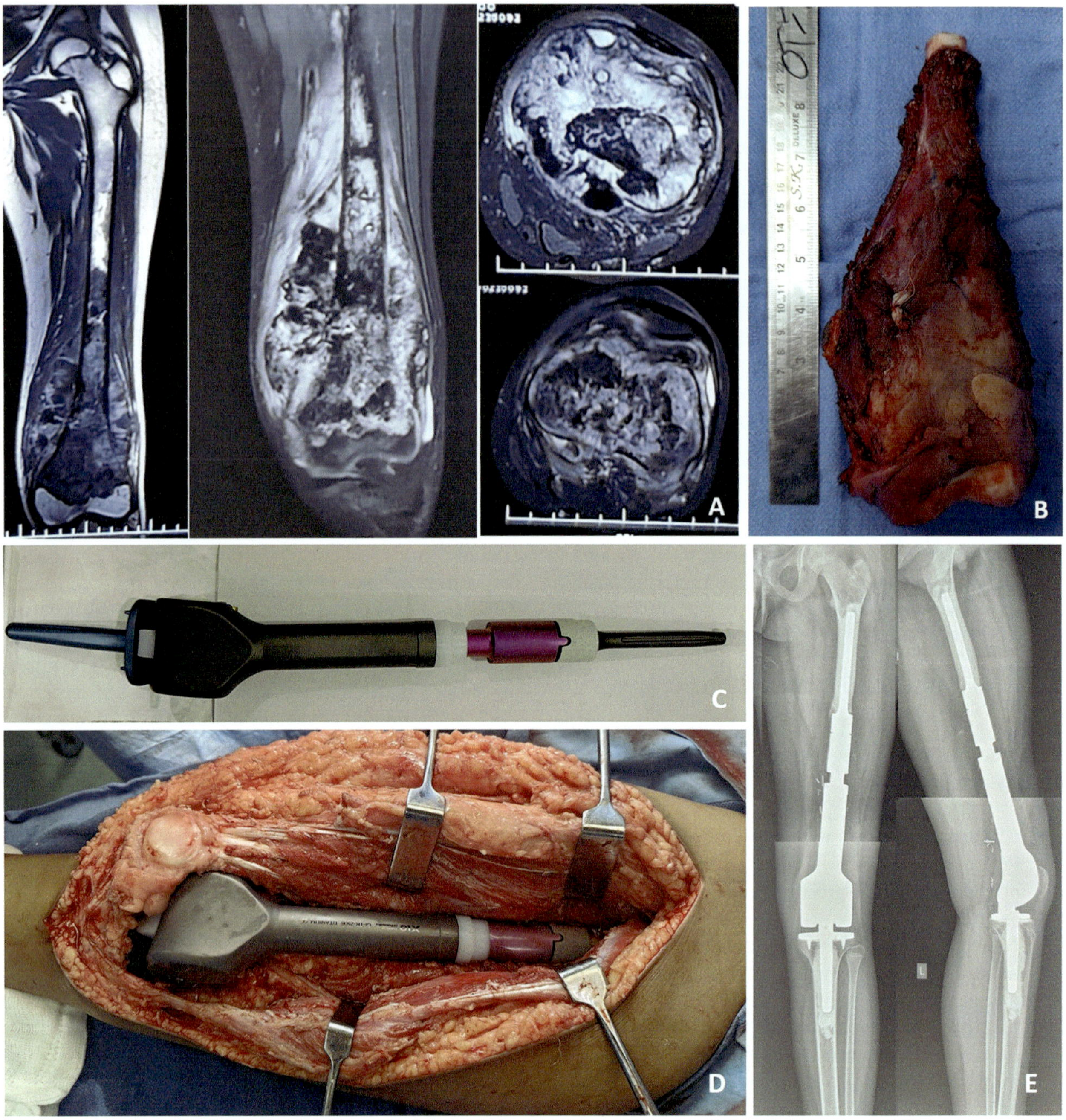

FIGURE 16.2 (A) MRI images of Osteosarcoma involving the distal femur in a 12-year-old male, showing involvement of the growth plate. An intra-articular, joint and physes-sacrificing resection was performed (B), and the skeletal defect was reconstructed with an expandable prosthesis (C & D). (E) Post-operative radiographs following resection and reconstruction.

Clinical Outcomes

Expandable prostheses are particularly advantageous for young children with significant growth potential. Studies report successful lengthening in 51%–81% of cases, with average gains of 29.9 mm in the proximal femur, 84.8 mm in total femur replacements, and 46.5 mm in distal femur reconstructions [3, 10]. However, complications such as infection, aseptic loosening, and mechanical failure (device wear, drive mechanism jamming, breakage of expansion components), remain prevalent, with failure rates ranging from 9.6% in total femur replacements to 55% in proximal femur reconstructions [3, 11]. Cortical atrophy has been noted around the stem, particularly in children under 10 years old, which may predispose to fractures or loosening [12]. The Repiphysis system, for instance, has shown failure rates exceeding 50%, often necessitating revision due to bone loss or implant breakage [8, 9].

The systematic review by Portney et al. [13] provides critical insights into the performance of expandable prostheses in skeletally immature patients undergoing limb salvage surgery for primary bone malignancies. The pooled analysis of 28 retrospective studies revealed significant findings regarding implant survival, lengthening efficacy, and functional outcomes.

The overall complication and revision rate for expandable prostheses was 43%, with a pronounced increase in failure rates over time—59% at five to ten years and 89% beyond ten years of follow-up. Kaplan-Meier survivorship analysis demonstrated a steady decline in complication-free implant survival, underscoring the challenges of long-term prosthetic durability in growing patients. Notably, noninvasive prostheses exhibited significantly higher mechanical failure rates (21%) compared to minimally invasive models (4%, P = 0.0004), primarily due to lengthening mechanism malfunctions [13].

The mean number of lengthening procedures per patient was 4.4 ± 0.3, with substantial variability depending on age and tumor location. Younger patients (<8 years) underwent more frequent expansions (5.2 ± 4.1 procedures), reflecting the necessity for ongoing growth modulation. The total cumulative lengthening achieved across the prosthesis lifespan averaged 4.5 ± 0.3 cm, though certain studies reported extensions up to 10.5 cm in cases with prolonged follow-up. Patients with distal femur reconstructions achieved a mean lengthening of 43 mm, while those with total femur replacements attained the greatest expansion 98.1 ± 57.4 mm. Despite these gains, LLD remained a persistent issue, affecting 36% of patients with discrepancies >2 cm and 50% with >1 cm, with prevalence escalating over time. The clinical significance of such discrepancies warrants consideration, as they may contribute to gait abnormalities, increased energy expenditure during ambulation, and potential long-term musculoskeletal sequelae [13].

While the meta-analysis did not explicitly report the mean time between expansions, individual studies cited in the review [14] suggested intervals of 6–12 months, aligning with physiological growth spurts in pediatric patients. The frequency of lengthening episodes correlated inversely with patient age, as younger children required more adjustments to match contralateral limb growth.

Analysis of pooled data revealed a mean MSTS score of 80.3 ± 1.3 across the study population, indicating generally favorable functional outcomes following limb salvage procedures. This finding demonstrates that expandable prostheses can effectively preserve limb function while accommodating longitudinal growth requirements. Notably, functional outcomes remained consistent across different anatomical reconstruction sites (distal femur, proximal tibia, and proximal femur) and were independent of prosthesis type (minimally invasive versus noninvasive lengthening mechanisms) [13].

Age-related analysis demonstrated significantly lower MSTS scores in the youngest patient cohort (<8 years) compared to older age groups, reflecting greater technical challenges of reconstruction in very young patients, including more extensive growth requirements and potential difficulties with rehabilitation compliance. Longitudinal assessment showed stable functional outcomes over time, suggesting durable results despite the progressive nature of skeletal growth and the associated need for multiple lengthening procedures [13].

The review found no significant differences in functional outcomes between various prosthesis designs or manufacturers. This finding suggests that while mechanical properties and failure modes may vary between devices, as evidenced by the higher complication rates in noninvasive prostheses, these differences do not necessarily translate to measurable functional deficits in surviving prostheses [13].

These findings highlight the delicate balance between achieving adequate limb elongation and mitigating mechanical complications, particularly in noninvasive devices. The high revision rates observed beyond five years emphasize the need for improved prosthetic designs to enhance longevity. Furthermore, the prevalence of LLD despite repeated expansions suggests that current lengthening protocols may not fully compensate for growth disparities, necessitating closer monitoring and potential adjunctive interventions. Innovations like the MUTARS Xpand prosthesis combine mechanical lengthening with biological growth potential via distraction osteogenesis, offering a hybrid solution [15]. Additionally, the use of smooth press-fit stems in distal femur reconstructions has demonstrated preserved growth of the adjacent tibial physis, mitigating LLD [16].

TRANSEPIPHYSEAL RESECTIONS

Transepiphyseal resection (TER) is a limb salvage technique designed to preserve the native joint in skeletally immature patients with metaphyseal bone tumors. By resecting the tumor through the epiphysis while sparing the joint, TER avoids the complications associated with endoprostheses or osteoarticular allografts, such as mechanical failure or joint degeneration [17]. A critical anatomical consideration in TER is the presence of open physes, which serve as a natural barrier to tumor invasion. The growth plate's cartilaginous structure impedes the spread of metaphyseal tumors into the epiphysis, allowing for safe oncological margins when resection is performed transepiphyseally. This biological containment, combined with meticulous preoperative imaging and chemotherapy response assessment, ensures that TER can achieve both oncological safety and functional preservation in carefully selected patients.

INDICATIONS

TER is indicated for pediatric and adolescent patients with open physes and metaphyseal tumors that do not invade the epiphysis. Key criteria include:

- **MRI-confirmed absence of epiphyseal invasion** before and after neoadjuvant chemotherapy [18].
- **Proximity to the physis**: TER is feasible for tumors near but not transgressing the growth plate, especially if post-chemotherapy MRI shows resolution of epiphyseal bone edema [17].
- **Good chemotherapy response**, as assessed on post-chemotherapy imaging which correlates with reduced local recurrence risk [17].

PREOPERATIVE EVALUATION

MRI is the gold standard for assessing tumor extent and chemotherapy response. Critical findings include:

- **Tumor-physis relationship**: Initial and post-chemotherapy MRI must confirm no epiphyseal invasion.
- **Bone edema**: Epiphyseal edema that resolves after chemotherapy suggests a favorable response and safe margins [17].

The TER procedure involves an epiphyseal osteotomy performed distal (in distal femoral tumors) or proximal (in proximal tibial tumors) to the physis, ensuring a 3–5 mm margin from the tumor boundary (Figure 16.3). Intraoperative fluoroscopy is essential to guide osteotomy placement and prevent inadvertent physeal damage. The preservation of the joint relies on the principle that the physis acts as a reliable anatomical barrier, allowing for tumor resection without compromising epiphyseal integrity [17, 19, 20].

Oncologically, TER has demonstrated excellent outcomes when strict selection criteria are followed. Studies report negative surgical margins in 100% of cases when preoperative MRI confirms the absence of epiphyseal involvement [21]. Local recurrence rates remain low (0% in some series) [17], and long-term survival parallels that of conventional wide resections, with five-year survival rates exceeding 70% [22]. The joint-preserving advantage of TER makes it a preferred option for skeletally immature patients, though long-term follow-up is necessary to assess durability and growth-related outcomes.

Transepiphyseal resection represents a sophisticated limb salvage strategy that leverages the protective role of open physes against tumor spread. By adhering to stringent imaging and histopathological criteria, surgeons can achieve safe oncological margins while preserving the native joint, offering young patients a functional and durable reconstruction alternative.

BIOLOGICAL RECONSTRUCTION OPTIONS IN CHILDREN

Biological reconstruction plays a vital role in pediatric bone tumor surgery, particularly for intercalary resections and in younger children, where expandable prostheses may not be feasible due to anatomical constraints or resource limitations. A detailed overview of biological techniques—including allografts, vascularized fibular grafts, APCs, and tumor-devitalized autografts—will be presented in Chapter 17 in this volume.

Allograft Reconstruction

Allograft reconstruction, particularly massive bone allograft, offers biological incorporation and excellent bone stock preservation. It is preferred in intercalary defects where joint surfaces can be preserved.

Advantages:
- Anatomical matching
- Allows soft tissue reattachment
- Preserves host bone stock for future revisions

Limitations:
- Risk of nonunion, infection, and graft fracture
- Limited availability in regions without bone banks
- Slow revascularization, particularly in chemotherapy-treated patients

Use of allografts is especially favored in older children or adolescents with intercalary resections of the femur or tibia. Studies report graft survival of up to 70% at ten years but highlight higher failure rates in reconstructions >15 cm or in femoral sites [2].

Allograft-Prosthetic Composite

The APC combines the structural support of a prosthesis with the biological benefits of an allograft. It is particularly suitable for osteoarticular reconstructions in small children where endoprosthetic fixation alone is not feasible.

Advantages:
- Provides attachment site for ligaments and tendons
- Offers immediate stability and potential for integration
- Useful when prosthetic size mismatch limits implant use

Limitations:
- Technical complexity of achieving stable graft-prosthesis-host integration
- Risk of graft resorption, infection, or junctional failure

APCs are commonly used for reconstruction of the proximal humerus and proximal tibia in very young patients [2].

Vascularized or Free Fibular Autografts

The vascularized fibular graft (VFG) is a versatile biological option for intercalary reconstruction, particularly in long diaphyseal defects (Figure 16.4). It can be used alone or in combination with an allograft (composite technique).

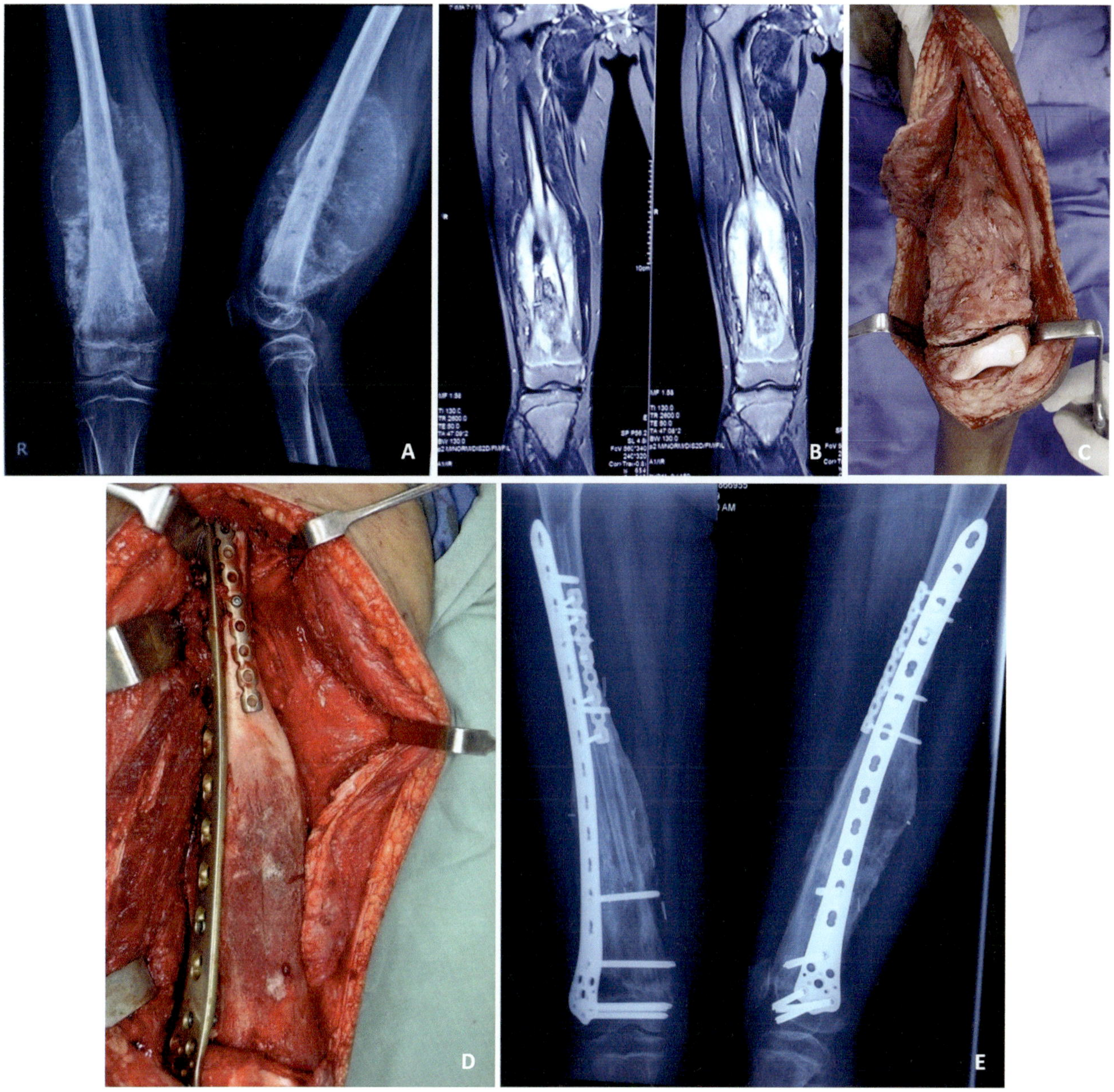

FIGURE 16.3 Plain radiographs (A) and MRI images (B) of Osteosarcoma involving the distal femur, sparing the distal physes in a 11-year-old male. A transepiphyseal, joint-sparing resection was performed through the distal physes (C). The resected tumor-bearing segment was devitalized with irradiation and re-implanted (D). (E) Post-operative radiographs following resection reconstruction with irradiated autograft.

Advantages:

- Provides living bone capable of hypertrophy and remodeling
- Faster union compared to nonvascularized grafts
- Can be harvested ipsilaterally to reduce operative time

Limitations:

- Donor site morbidity (ankle valgus, toe flexion deformity)
- Technical demand of microsurgical anastomosis
- Risk of graft fracture, especially in long reconstructions

When used with allografts, VFGs have been shown to reduce nonunion rates in defects >15 cm. However, their use also prolongs operative time and may increase infection risk in immunocompromised children [2].

Tumor-Devitalized Autografts

This technique involves resection of the tumor-bearing bone segment followed by devitalization (via irradiation, freezing, autoclaving, or pasteurization) and reimplantation (Figure 16.5).

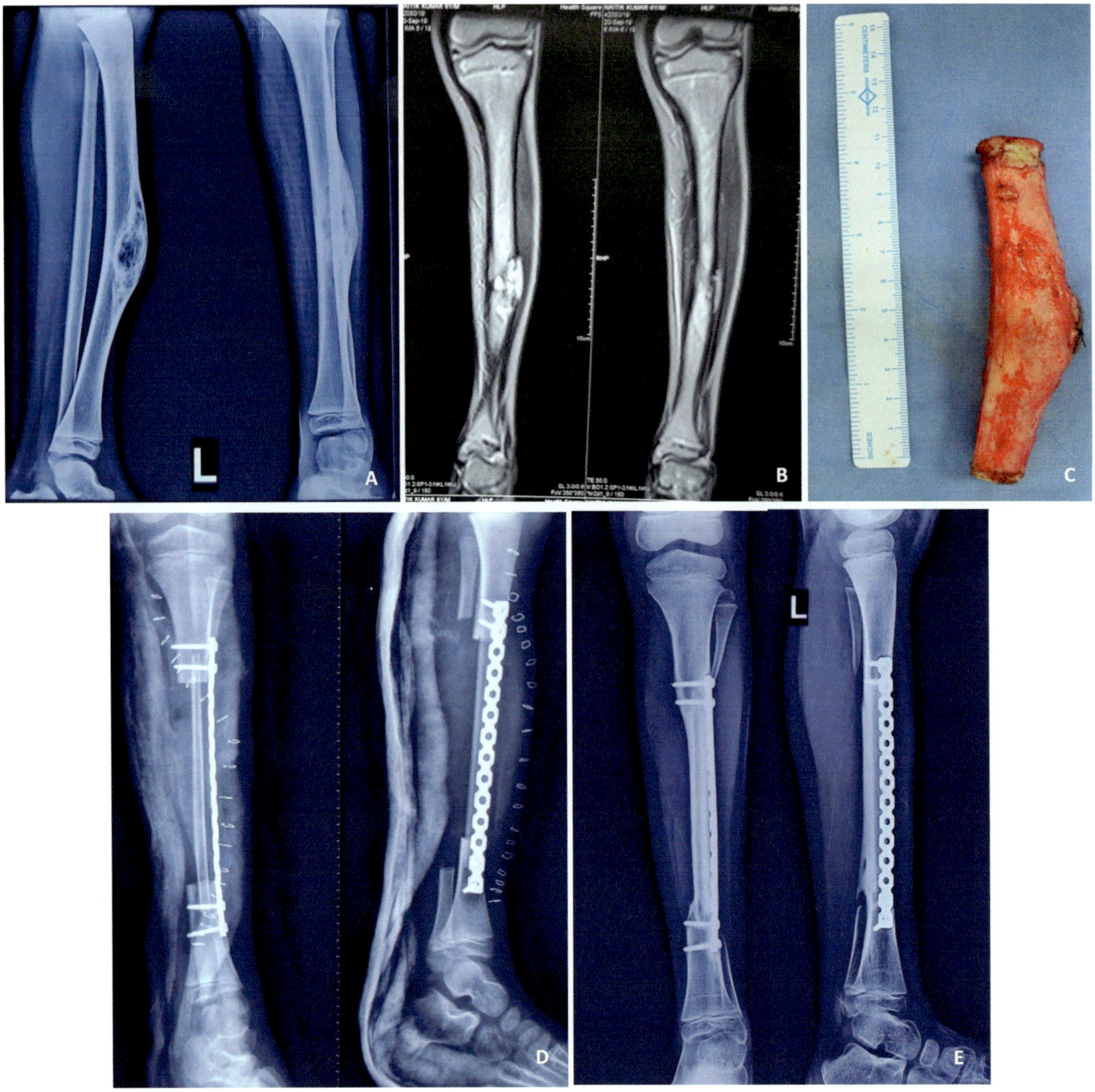

FIGURE 16.4 Plain radiographs (A) and MRI images (B) of Adamantinoma involving the tibial diaphysis in a 9-year-old male. Wide resection was performed (C). The skeletal defect was reconstructed using the ipsilateral fibula translocated into the defect. (D) Immediate post-operative radiographs following resection and translocation of the ipsilateral fibula. (E) Post-operative radiographs at 24 months follow-up showed hypertrophy and incorporation of the translocated fibula.

Advantages:

- Perfect anatomical match
- Cost-effective and suitable for low-resource settings
- Preserves ligament and tendon insertion sites

Limitations:

- Inability to assess true surgical margins post-reimplantation
- Poor incorporation if extensive cortical destruction is present
- Risk of infection, nonunion, and fracture similar to allografts

Frozen autografts have shown superior histological integration compared to autoclaved or pasteurized grafts. Their use is most appropriate in intercalary reconstructions where joint preservation is feasible [2].

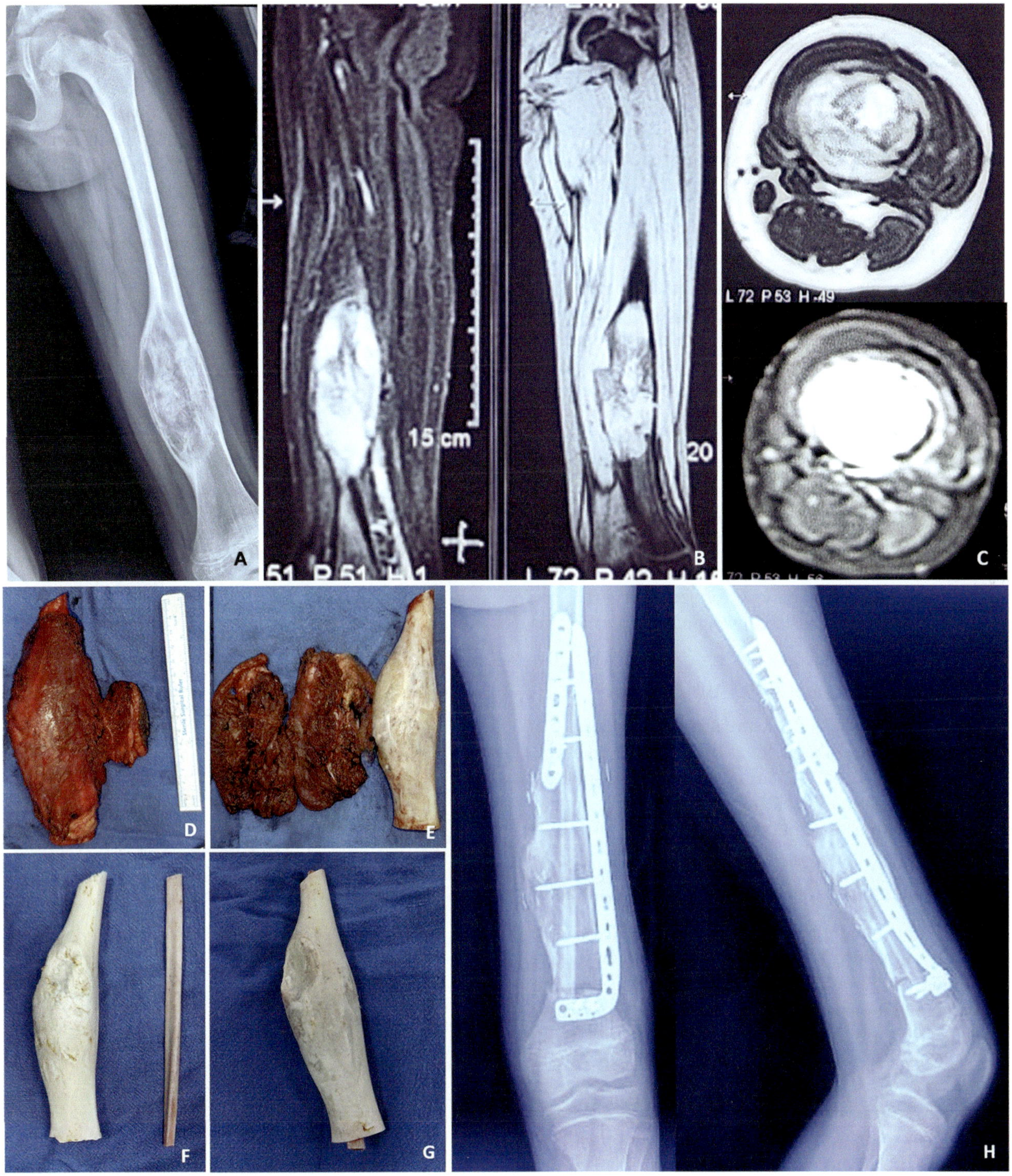

FIGURE 16.5 Plain radiographs (A) and MRI images (B & C) of Osteosarcoma involving the femur diaphysis in a 10-year-old female. Wide resection was performed (D). Soft tissue, including periosteum, is stripped off the tumor-bearing segment on a separate table (E), and the bone is prepared, washed, sterile packed, and treated with 50Gy radiation. The irradiated, sterilized bone is washed thoroughly, and the harvested free fibula is placed intramedullary (F, G). The construct is then re-implanted into the defect and secured with internal fixation (H).

MODALITIES FOR MANAGING LIMB-LENGTH DISCREPANCIES

LLD is a common sequela in skeletally immature patients undergoing tumor resection involving the physis. The choice of modality for managing LLD is influenced by patient age, predicted discrepancy at maturity, reconstruction type, and institutional expertise.

Expandable Endoprostheses

As discussed in detail earlier, expandable prostheses remain the mainstay for managing LLD in children requiring osteoarticular resections with significant remaining growth. They allow controlled lengthening over time, reduce the need for contralateral interventions, and preserve joint mobility when feasible.

Contralateral Epiphysiodesis

For predicted discrepancies of 2–5 cm, contralateral epiphysiodesis may be employed to equalize limb lengths at maturity. It is most suitable in older children nearing skeletal maturity and is commonly performed using either percutaneous drill or physeal stapling techniques.

Limb Overlengthening at Index Surgery

In some cases, particularly with intercalary allograft or APC reconstructions, the affected limb may be intentionally overlengthened by 1–2 cm to compensate for future growth loss. This is best applied in children near the end of growth or in conjunction with close follow-up.

External Fixation and Distraction Osteogenesis

In patients not suited for prosthetic expansion, Ilizarov or hexapod-based external fixation may be used for gradual lengthening of the residual limb. Although effective, this method entails prolonged treatment time and carries risks of pin-site infection and joint stiffness.

Shoe Lifts or Nonsurgical Compensation

For small discrepancies (<2 cm), nonsurgical interventions such as shoe lifts often provide sufficient functional correction without surgical morbidity.

Each modality should be individualized based on growth potential, expected discrepancy, psychosocial considerations, and feasibility of long-term follow-up. Multidisciplinary planning is essential to optimize both functional and cosmetic outcomes.

The use of vascularized fibula epiphyseal transfer as a reconstructive option for longitudinal growth after oncologic resection of the proximal humerus in pediatric patients has been an area of interest among orthopedic oncologists. It provides a reliable oncologic reconstruction of proximal humerus in children. It not only offers the ability of longitudinal growth, hypertrophy, and osseous union but also diminishes reconstructive complications and improves shoulder function. Lu et al. retrospectively investigated five children (three osteosarcoma and two Ewing's sarcoma) who underwent biological reconstruction with combination of vascularized fibula epiphyseal transfer and massive bone allograft after oncologic resection of the proximal humerus. They reported no graft fracture, hardware failure, or infection. In the meantime, osseous union was 2.9 months at fibula-humerus junction and 6.2 months at allograft-humerus junction. Hypertrophy and axial growth were evident in all, except one patient who has avascular necrosis of the fibula head, with a mean hypertrophy index of 51.5%, mean growth of 4.4 mm per annum, and mean arm discrepancy of 4.6 cm [23].

SUMMARY

- Limb salvage in children must balance oncologic clearance with preservation of growth and long-term function.
- Expandable prostheses are the preferred modality for managing LLD in growing children but have high complication and revision rates.
- Biological reconstructions—including allografts, vascularized fibular grafts, and devitalized autografts—remain essential, especially in intercalary/transepiphyseal resections and resource-limited settings.
- Growth prediction tools guide reconstruction planning but are limited by the effects of chemotherapy and radiation.
- Site-specific anatomy, patient age, and residual growth potential heavily influence reconstruction strategy.

REFERENCES

1. Groundland JS, Ambler SB, Houskamp LDJ, Orriola JJ, Binitie OT, Letson GD. Surgical and functional outcomes after limb-preservation surgery for tumor in pediatric patients: a systematic review. *JBJS Rev.* 2016;4(2):e2. doi:10.2106/JBJS.RVW.O.00013
2. Errani C, Atherley O'Meally A, Tsukamoto S, Mavrogenis AF, Tanaka Y, Manfrini M. An algorithm for surgical treatment of children with bone sarcomas of the extremities. *SICOT J.* 2024;10:38. doi:10.1051/sicotj/2024033
3. Groundland JS, Binitie O. Reconstruction after tumor resection in the growing child. *Orthop Clin North Am.* 2016;47(1):265–281. doi:10.1016/j.ocl.2015.08.027
4. Errani C, Aiba H, Atherley A, et al. What is the revision-free survival of resurfaced allograft-prosthesis composites for proximal humerus reconstruction in children with bone tumors?. *Clin Orthop Relat Res.* January 23, 2024. doi:10.1097/CORR.0000000000002969
5. Lindberg M, Conrad EU, Punt SE, et al. (2014). Surgical management of sarcomas in skeletally immature patients. In: Conrad EU (ed), *Orthopaedic Knowledge Update: Musculoskeletal Tumors 3.* American Academy of Orthopaedic Surgeons, pp. 444–459.

6. Gupta A, Meswania J, Pollock R, et al. Non-invasive distal femoral expandable endoprosthesis for limb-salvage surgery in paediatric tumours. *J Bone Joint Surg Br.* 2006;88(5):649–654.
7. Neel MD, Wilkins RM, Rao BN, et al. Early multicenter experience with a noninvasive expandable prosthesis. *Clin Orthop Relat Res.* 2003;(415):72–81.
8. Cipriano CA, Gruzinova IS, Frank RM, et al. Frequent complications and severe bone loss associated with the Repiphysis expandable distal femoral prosthesis. *Clin Orthop Relat Res.* 2015;473(3):831–838.
9. Staals EL, Colangeli M, Ali N, et al. Are complications associated with the Repiphysis expandable distal femoral prosthesis acceptable for its continued use? *Clin Orthop Relat Res.* 2015;473(9):3003–3013.
10. Henderson ER, Pepper AM, Marulanda G, et al. Outcome of lower-limb preservation with an expandable endoprosthesis after bone tumor resection in children. *J Bone Joint Surg Am.* 2012;94(6):537–547.
11. Ruggieri P, Mavrogenis AF, Pala E, et al. Outcome of expandable prostheses in children. *J Pediatr Orthop.* 2013;33(3):244–253.
12. Kim W, Han I, Cho H-S, et al. Cortical atrophy related to tumor prosthesis in skeletally immature osteosarcoma patients. *J Pediatr Orthop.* 2018;38(1):60–68.
13. Portney DA, Bi AS, Christian RA, Butler BA, Peabody TD. Outcomes of expandable prostheses for primary bone malignancies in skeletally immature patients: a systematic review and pooled data analysis. *J Pediatr Orthop.* 2020;40(6):e487–e497. doi:10.1097/BPO.0000000000001459
14. Schindler OS, Cannon SR, Briggs TW, Blunn GW. Stanmore custom-made extendible distal femoral replacements. Clinical experience in children with primary malignant bone tumours [published correction appears in J Bone Joint Surg Br 1998 May;80(3):562]. *J Bone Joint Surg Br.* 1997;79(6):927–937. doi:10.1302/0301-620x.79b6.7164
15. Torner F, Segur JM, Ullot R, et al. Non-invasive expandable prosthesis in musculoskeletal oncology paediatric patients for the distal and proximal femur. *Int Orthop.* 2016;40(8):1683–1688.
16. Neel MD, Heck R, Britton L, et al. Use of a smooth press-fit stem preserves physeal growth after tumor resection. *Clin Orthop Relat Res.* 2004;(426):125–128.
17. Kim Y, Jang WY, Park JW, et al. Transepiphyseal resection for osteosarcoma in patients with open physes using MRI assessment. *Bone Joint J.* 2020;102-B(6):772–778. doi:10.1302/0301-620X.102B6.BJJ-2019-1141.R2
18. San-Julian M, Aquerreta JD, Benito A, Cañadell J. Indications for epiphyseal preservation in metaphyseal malignant bone tumors of children: relationship between image methods and histological findings. *J Pediatr Orthop.* 1999;19(4): 543–548. doi:10.1097/00004694-199907000-00025
19. Kawaguchi N, Ahmed AR, Matsumoto S, Manabe J, Matsushita Y. The concept of curative margin in surgery for bone and soft tissue sarcoma. *Clin Orthop Relat Res.* 2004;(419): 165–172. doi:10.1097/00003086-200402000-00027
20. Li X, Moretti VM, Ashana AO, Lackman RD. Impact of close surgical margin on local recurrence and survival in osteosarcoma. *Int Orthop.* 2012;36(1):131–137. doi:10.1007/s00264-011-1230-x
21. Muscolo DL, Ayerza MA, Aponte-Tinao LA, Ranalletta M. Partial epiphyseal preservation and intercalary allograft reconstruction in high- grade metaphyseal osteosarcoma of the knee. *J Bone Joint Surg Am.* 2004;86-A(12):2686–2693.
22. Schrager J, Patzer RE, Mink PJ, Ward KC, Goodman M. Survival outcomes of pediatric osteosarcoma and Ewing's sarcoma: a comparison of surgery type within the SEER database, 1988–2007. *J Registry Manag.* 2011;38(3): 153–161.
23. Lu Y, Xiao X, Li M, Chen G, Huang M, Ji C, Wang Z, Li J. Use of vascularized fibular epiphyseal transfer with massive bone allograft for proximal humeral reconstruction in children with bone sarcoma. *Ann Surg Oncol.* 2021 Nov;28(12):7834–7841. doi:10.1245/s10434-021-10032-y. Epub 2021 May 11. PMID: 33974195.

17 Intercalary Resection and Reconstruction

INTRODUCTION

Limb salvage surgery has become the preferred treatment for malignant bone tumors, largely replacing amputation due to advances in imaging, neoadjuvant chemotherapy, and surgical techniques. When tumors are confined to the diaphyseal or metaphyseo-diaphyseal regions, **intercalary resection**—a segmental resection that preserves adjacent joints—offers the opportunity to maintain near-normal limb function [1].

Reconstructing the resultant intercalary defect is technically demanding, requiring restoration of limb length, alignment, and stability while ensuring oncological safety. Reconstruction methods are broadly classified into the following:

- **Biological techniques**: massive allografts, vascularized/non-vascularized fibular autografts, and recycled tumor-bearing autografts sterilized by extracorporeal irradiation, pasteurization, autoclaving, or freezing [2].
- **Nonbiological techniques**: modular intercalary endoprostheses, increasingly used in elderly patients or those with metastatic disease [1].

Selection of the optimal technique depends on patient age, tumor location, defect size, biomechanical demands, bone quality, and surgical expertise. This chapter reviews the various intercalary reconstruction options, discussing indications, surgical principles, outcomes, and complications.

INDICATIONS AND PATIENT SELECTION

The decision to perform intercalary reconstruction after diaphyseal tumor resection is determined by patient-specific and tumor-specific factors. This approach is most feasible when the tumor spares the epiphysis and articular surface, allowing joint preservation—critical for optimizing function and quality of life [1, 2].

TUMOR LOCATION AND EXTENT

Intercalary reconstruction is most applicable to tumors in the diaphysis of long bones—commonly the femur, tibia, or humerus—including high-grade malignancies (e.g., osteosarcoma, Ewing sarcoma), low-grade lesions (e.g., adamantinoma), and selected metastatic deposits in patients with good prognosis [1, 3] (Figure 17.1).

A safe oncological margin between the tumor and the planned osteotomy site is essential. In skeletally immature patients, preserving the physis not only retains function but also contributes to continued limb growth [4]. Preoperative MRI is critical for assessing the intraosseous extent and proximity to the joint. When tumors abut the growth plate, barrier concepts such as those described by Kawaguchi et al. can allow transphyseal resections while maintaining joint integrity [5].

PATIENT AGE AND FUNCTIONAL DEMAND

Age and functional expectations are pivotal in determining reconstruction type.

- **Younger patients** with longer life expectancy and higher activity levels are generally best served by biological reconstructions (allografts, vascularized fibula, or recycled autografts), which offer potential for long-term durability and avoid complications related to prosthetic wear [2].
- **Elderly patients** or those with limited survival expectancy—such as individuals with metastatic disease or poor performance status—may benefit from nonbiological methods like modular intercalary endoprostheses, which enable immediate weight-bearing and faster rehabilitation [1].

The use of endoprostheses in young patients remains controversial due to higher revision rates and long-term implant complications [6].

BONE QUALITY AND DEFECT SIZE

Host bone quality and defect length influence reconstruction choice.

- **Poor cortical integrity** (e.g., extensive osteolysis, pathological fractures) may preclude recycled autografts, which require adequate cortical structure for strength [2, 7].
- **Large segmental defects** (>15 cm) carry increased risks of nonunion and graft fracture with biological methods [8]. In such cases, composite reconstructions—such as allograft combined with vascularized fibula—offer both structural support and biological integration [3].
- Osteoporotic bone may require enhanced fixation techniques, including double plating or hybrid constructs, to improve stability [4].

DOI: 10.1201/9780367822002-22

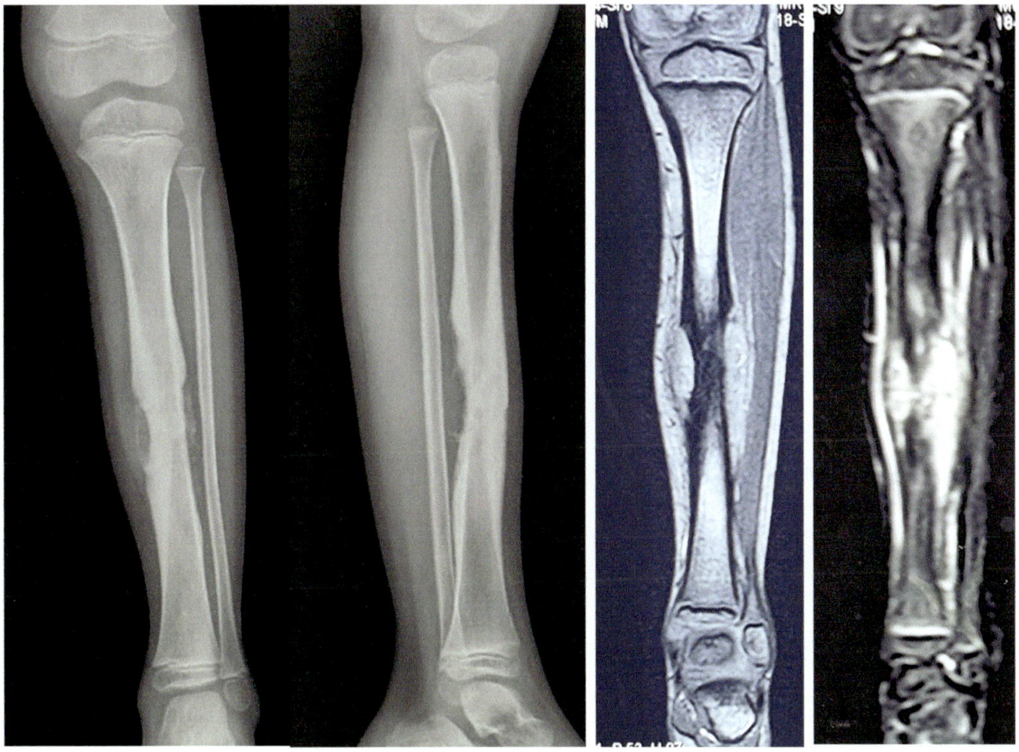

FIGURE 17.1 Plain radiographs and MRI images of a 6-year-old female with Ewing sarcoma involving the diaphysis of the tibia. The lesion shows cortical destruction and intramedullary involvement, with soft tissue extension evident on MRI. The location and extent of the disease make it suitable for intercalary resection.

ONCOLOGICAL CONSIDERATIONS

Oncological safety takes precedence over joint preservation. Adequate margins must not be compromised; in cases of ambiguous margins or skip metastases, more radical resection with joint sacrifice may be required, rendering intercalary reconstruction unsuitable. Patients with poor histological response to neoadjuvant chemotherapy are at higher risk for local recurrence and may require wider excision [4].

Intercalary reconstruction offers the potential for excellent functional preservation in appropriately selected patients, provided oncological principles are upheld. Careful preoperative planning—integrating tumor location, patient factors, bone quality, and available expertise—is critical to achieving durable, functional, and safe outcomes.

ALLOGRAFT RECONSTRUCTION

Allograft reconstruction is a well-established biological method for managing intercalary bone defects following tumor resection. It uses a size-matched cadaveric graft to restore limb length, alignment, and mechanical stability, while preserving host bone stock and avoiding donor site morbidity associated with autografts [2]. This approach is more prevalent in regions with organized bone banking systems, such as Europe and North America.

The procedure entails en bloc tumor resection with clear margins, followed by implantation of a contoured and osteotomized allograft matched to the defect. Stable fixation—using plates, screws, or intramedullary nails—is essential to promote union and prevent mechanical failure. Additional strategies, such as incorporating an intramedullary fibular autograft or bone graft substitutes, enhance biological healing at graft-host interfaces. Fixation should span the entire defect, with overlapping plates and compression at junctions to reduce nonunion risk [1, 2].

Outcomes

Reported union rates vary considerably, with nonunion occurring in 6%–43% of cases, influenced by host bone type, fixation method, and adjuvant therapy [9]. Fracture rates range from 7% to 45%, often at stress points near screw holes [2]. Infection occurs in up to 28%, typically within the first two to three years [9]. Despite these challenges, functional results are generally satisfactory, with systematic reviews citing mean Musculoskeletal Tumor Society (MSTS) scores of 67%–92%, comparable to prosthetic and recycled graft reconstructions [9] (Table 17.1).

TABLE 17.1
Allograft Reconstruction: Outcomes and Complications

Author	Year	No. of Patients	Mean/ Median Age	Follow-Up (Months)	% Nonunion	% Graft Fractures	% Implant Failures	% Infections	Oncological Outcome	MSTS Score
Albergo et al. [6]	2020	71	Median 16/19	Mean 129	6	24	0	6	Local recurrence (3)	Mean 92%
Aponte-Tinao et al. [10]	2012	83	Mean 26	Median 61	27	17	0	1	Local recurrence (3)	Mean 90%
Bus et al. [8]	2014	87	Median 17	Median 84	40	29	26	14	Local recurrence (2)	NR
Deijkers et al. [11]	2005	35	Median 24	Median 86	9	34	0	9	Local recurrence (4)	77%–80%
Frisoni et al. [12]	2012	101	Mean 20	Median 112	27	31	25	NR	Local recurrence (NR)	NR
Houdek et al. [13]	2018	29	Mean 12	Mean 156	34	45	17	18	Local recurrence (2)	Mean 90%
Houdek et al. [14]	2016	18	Mean 11	Mean 96	33	39	0	0	Local recurrence (1)	Mean 93%
Muscolo et al. [15]	2004	59	Mean 35	Mean 60	19	7	0	5	Local recurrence (6)	NR

Complications

Key complications include:

- **Nonunion**, particularly at diaphyseal junctions lacking metaphyseal cancellous bone; worsened by chemotherapy or inadequate fixation [16].
- **Fracture**, usually at junctions or screw sites, due to fatigue and remodeling-related weakening [8].
- **Infection**, more common in immunosuppressed or chemotherapy-treated patients, occasionally requiring graft removal [1].
- **Resorption or collapse**, especially in younger, active patients [16].

  Outcomes may be improved by augmenting the construct with vascularized fibular autografts [3], employing double plating or overlapping fixation [4], or using intramedullary cement augmentation for enhanced screw hold [17].

Limitations

Drawbacks include dependence on certified bone banks, risks of immune rejection or rare disease transmission, prolonged protected weight-bearing, and potential delays in surgery due to graft size-matching requirements.

In appropriately selected patients, intercalary allografts provide durable reconstruction with acceptable complication rates, especially when meticulous surgical technique and biological augmentation are employed.

VASCULARIZED OR FREE FIBULAR AUTOGRAFTS

Free fibular autografts (FFAs), particularly when harvested with their vascular pedicle intact as vascularized fibular grafts (VFGs), are an established biological option for intercalary reconstruction after tumor resection. Introduced by Weiland in 1977, VFGs retain intrinsic osteogenic potential, resist infection, and integrate biologically, making them especially suitable for younger patients with high functional demands [18].

Unlike non-vascularized grafts, VFGs remain viable post-transfer, enabling rapid union with host bone and hypertrophy in response to load [2]. The fibula is harvested with the peroneal vessels and contoured to bridge the defect, followed by microvascular anastomosis to local recipient vessels. Reconstruction options include:

- **Single fibula** for narrow, low-load diaphyseal defects (Figure 17.2)
- **Double-barrel fibula** to increase diameter for load-bearing bones like the femur [2] (Figure 17.3)
- **Combination constructs** with allografts or recycled autografts (Capanna technique) for enhanced stability and biology [3]

Fixation is typically with plates, ensuring pedicle protection during instrumentation.

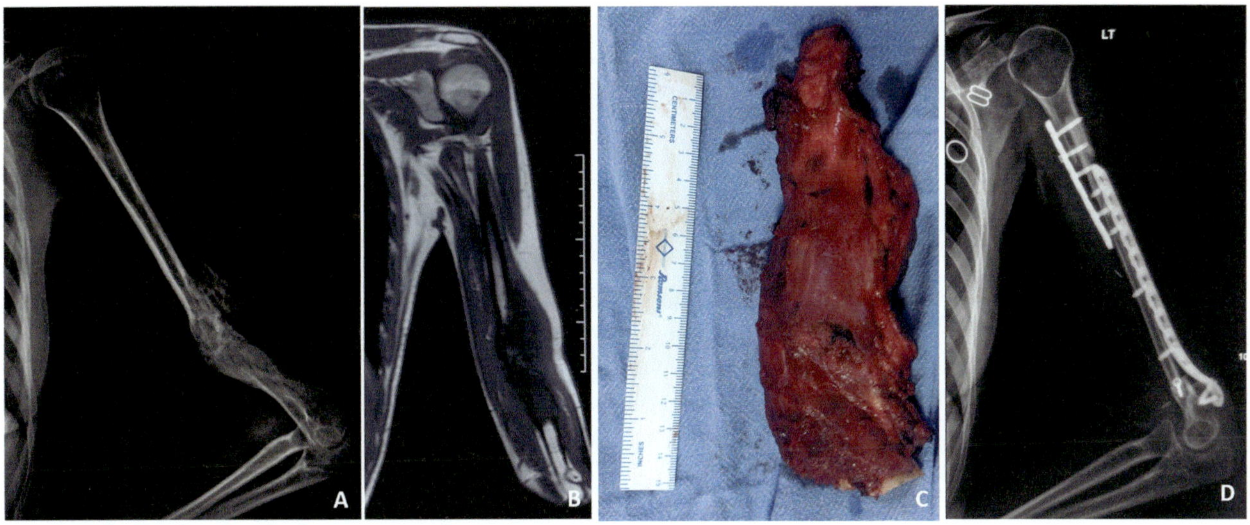

FIGURE 17.2 Plain radiographs (A) and MRI images (B) of Osteosarcoma involving the distal humerus diaphysis in a 22-year-old female. (C) An intercalary wide resection was performed. The skeletal defect was reconstructed using the free fibular strut graft, secured proximally and distally, to the residual humerus (D).

Outcomes

Union rates are high, especially in metaphyseal osteotomies. Campanacci et al. reported 100% union in 12 VFG patients with mean MSTS scores of 90% [19]. Studies of combined VFG–allograft constructs show nonunion rates of 0%–33% and fracture rates of 0%–44%, influenced by defect size and fixation method. Progressive fibular hypertrophy improves long-term mechanical performance, with mean MSTS scores of 86%–94% reported across series [1, 20]. Structural strategies—such as double-barrel fibula or the Capanna technique—enhance early mechanical stability and long-term function [3, 16] (Table 17.2).

Complications

- **Fatigue fractures**, particularly in the early phase before hypertrophy [1, 16]
- **Donor site morbidity**—peroneal nerve palsy, ankle instability, contracture, or valgus deformity, more common in children [1, 16]
- **Microvascular failure**—flap loss or thrombosis
- **Delayed union**, especially at diaphyseal interfaces or with inadequate fixation

  Infection is rare but possible in immunocompromised or chemotherapy-treated patients.

Limitations

- Technically demanding and time-intensive, requiring microsurgical expertise
- Limited initial strength in large or high-load reconstructions
- Prolonged protected weight-bearing (≥6 months)
- Potential donor site functional loss with extensive fibular harvests

VFGs remain a durable, biologically active reconstruction choice, offering high union rates and excellent long-term function when applied in appropriately selected patients with skilled microsurgical support.

RECYCLED TUMOR-BEARING AUTOGRAFTS

Recycled tumor-bearing autografts involve reimplantation of the resected tumor-bearing bone segment after devitalization through a sterilization method. This approach preserves the patient's native bone geometry, ensures anatomical fit, and eliminates the need for a bone bank or secondary donor site. It is particularly valuable in resource-limited settings or when precise anatomical reconstruction is a priority. The devitalized graft serves as a biological scaffold, allowing creeping substitution and gradual incorporation into host bone.

TECHNIQUES OF DEVITALIZATION

1. **Extracorporeal Irradiation (ECRT)**
   The resected segment is exposed to a single high dose (typically 50 Gy) of external beam irradiation, effectively sterilizing the specimen while maintaining its structural form. ECRT is widely used and oncologically safe [7]. However, biomechanical studies have shown reduced stiffness, increased plastic deformation, and lower mineral content, predisposing to resorption, fracture, or construct failure [23].
2. **Autoclaving**
   Heating the bone to 120°C for 10–15 minutes ensures sterilization but significantly weakens mechanical properties and removes osteoinductive proteins [24].

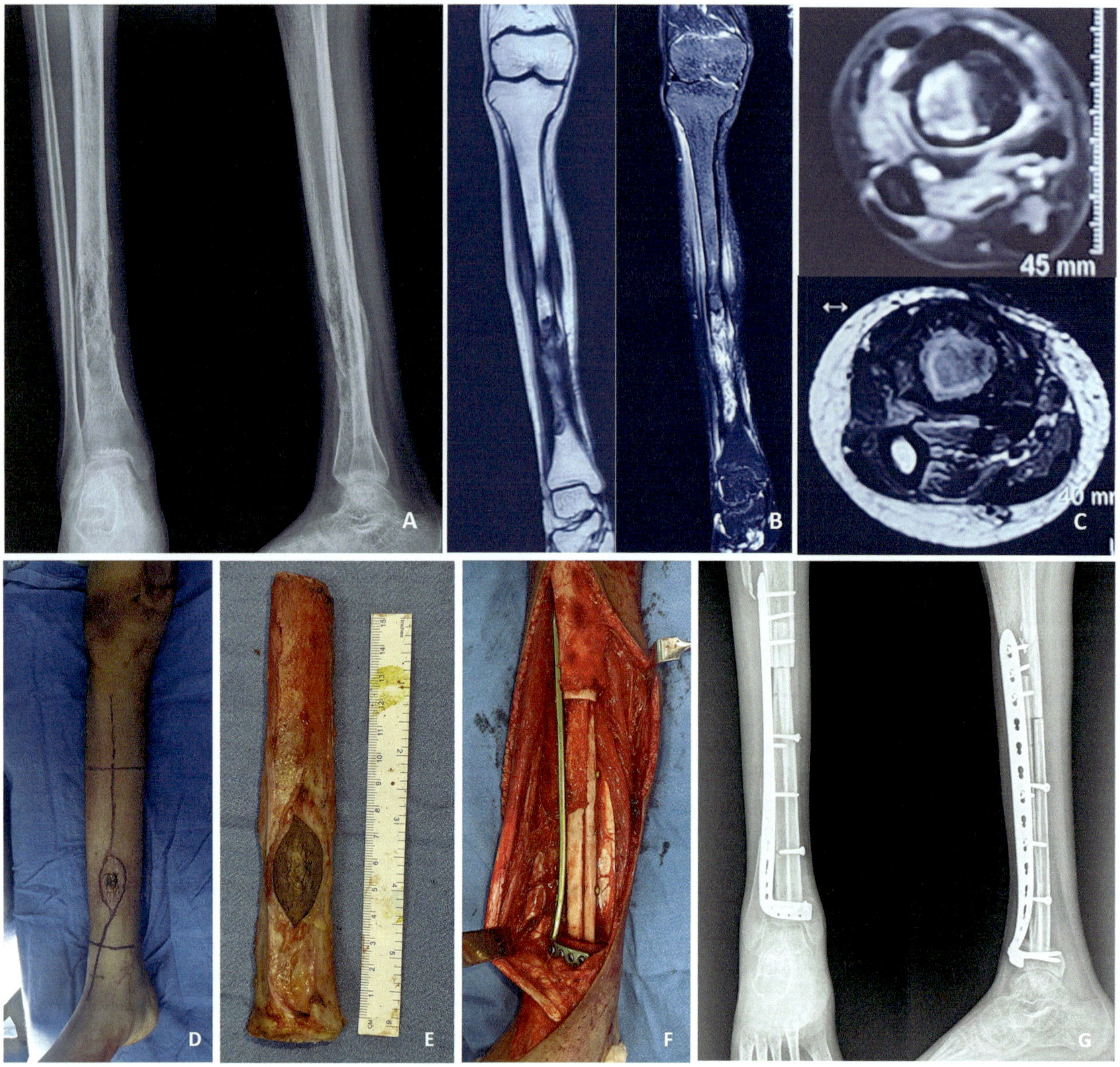

FIGURE 17.3 Plain radiographs (A) and MRI images (B & C) of Osteosarcoma involving the distal tibial diaphysis in a 16-year-old female. (D) Longitudinal skin incision incorporating the previous surgical scar. An ankle-sparing intercalary wide resection was performed (E). The skeletal defect was reconstructed using the ipsilateral fibula translocated intramedullary, proximally and distally, into the residual tibia. The reconstruction was supplemented with free fibular strut harvested from the contralateral limb and secured with a plate (F). (G) Post-operative radiographs following resection reconstruction with a double strut fibula graft.

3. **Pasteurization**
   Heating to 60°C for 30 minutes preserves more bone morphogenetic proteins than autoclaving, potentially improving biological incorporation [25, 26].
4. **Liquid Nitrogen Freezing**
   Immersion in liquid nitrogen (−196°C) followed by thawing maintains collagen architecture and osteoconductivity, with encouraging biological outcomes [27, 28].

Surgical Technique

After wide tumor resection, the bone is stripped of soft tissues, curetted, and processed via the chosen devitalization method. The sterilized segment is then reimplanted and stabilized using plates or intramedullary nails. Augmentation with an intramedullary fibula or bone cement is often employed to enhance early mechanical stability (Figures 17.4 and 17.5). Weight-bearing is delayed until radiographic union, which is typically slower than with vascularized grafts or endoprosthetic reconstructions.

Outcomes

Recycled autografts yield good functional results, with MSTS scores ranging from 70% to 93% [9]. In ECRT-based reconstructions, the mean union time in patients under 20

TABLE 17.2
Allograft with Vascularized Fibular Graft Reconstruction: Outcomes and Complications

Author et al.	Year	No. of Patients	Mean/ Median Age	Follow-Up (Months)	% Nonunion	% Graft Fractures	% Implant Failures	% Infections	Oncological Outcome	MSTS Score
Campanacci et al. [19]	2014	12	Mean 23	Mean 147	0	8	8	8	Local recurrence (0)	Mean 90%
Campanacci et al. [21]	2018	23	Mean 16	Mean 141	13	22	0	0	Local recurrence (0)	Mean 94%
Errani et al. [1]	2019	81	Mean 13	Mean 96	NR	23	NR	6	Local recurrence (7)	Good to excellent in 91%
Errani et al. [20]	2020	25	Mean 11	Median 123	16	28	5	16	Local recurrence (2)	Mean 86%
Frisoni et al. [12]	2012	30	Mean 20	NR	27	31	25	NR	Local recurrence (NR)	NR
Houdek [14]	2016	18	Mean 11	Mean 96	33	39	0	0	Local recurrence (1)	Mean 93%
Li et al. [22]	2010	11	Mean 19	Mean 34	9	0	9	0	Local recurrence (2)	Mean 92%

years was 9.2 months, with V-shaped osteotomies and supplemental plate fixation facilitating earlier union [7]. Union rates are generally higher in metaphyseal than in diaphyseal osteotomies due to superior vascularity.

Complication rates vary with the devitalization technique:

- **Nonunion**: 7%–31%, particularly in diaphyseal sites [9]
- **Fracture**: 6%–20%, influenced by method and fixation quality [29, 30]
- **Infection**: 5%–20%, more frequent in irradiated and autoclaved grafts [9]
- **Resorption/Collapse**: Especially with autoclaved grafts lacking osteoinductive capacity [9]

Oike et al. reported nonunion in 37.5% and infection in 16.6% of ECRT cases [31]. Hayashi et al. [29] noted fracture in 11%, while Puri et al. observed 6% [30] (Table 17.3).

Strategies to Improve Outcomes

- **ECRT + Fibula**: Intramedullary or onlay fibular augmentation enhances biological activity and mechanical strength [7].
- **Cement Augmentation**: PMMA within the medullary canal improves screw purchase and load sharing [30].
- **Modified Osteotomies**: Chevron or V-shaped cuts increase surface area for union [7].

Recycled autografts remain a versatile, cost-effective, and anatomically precise reconstruction method, particularly in settings without allograft availability, provided mechanical weaknesses are addressed through augmentation techniques and robust fixation.

MODULAR INTERCALARY ENDOPROSTHESIS

Modular intercalary endoprostheses are mechanical reconstruction systems used for diaphyseal or metaphyseo-diaphyseal bone defects following tumor resection. Comprising prefabricated titanium or cobalt–chrome alloy components, these implants can be assembled intraoperatively to restore bone continuity while preserving adjacent native joints. They offer immediate structural stability, allow early weight-bearing, and enable rapid rehabilitation—making them particularly suitable for patients with limited biological potential for graft incorporation [9, 16].

Originally favored for elderly patients with metastatic or low-grade tumors, advances in design and fixation have broadened their application to selected younger patients with high-grade sarcomas, especially where expedited functional recovery is prioritized over long-term biological integration.

Surgical Technique

Following wide en bloc tumor resection, trial spacers determine defect length and optimal prosthetic configuration. Stems may be cemented or press-fit depending on bone quality and length of residual segments. Fluted or splined designs improve rotational stability, while porous-coated collars enhance osteointegration at the bone-implant interface. The prosthesis is assembled to restore limb length, alignment, and stability. Given limited intrinsic soft tissue attachment, synthetic meshes or muscle flaps are often used to augment coverage and rotational control [16].

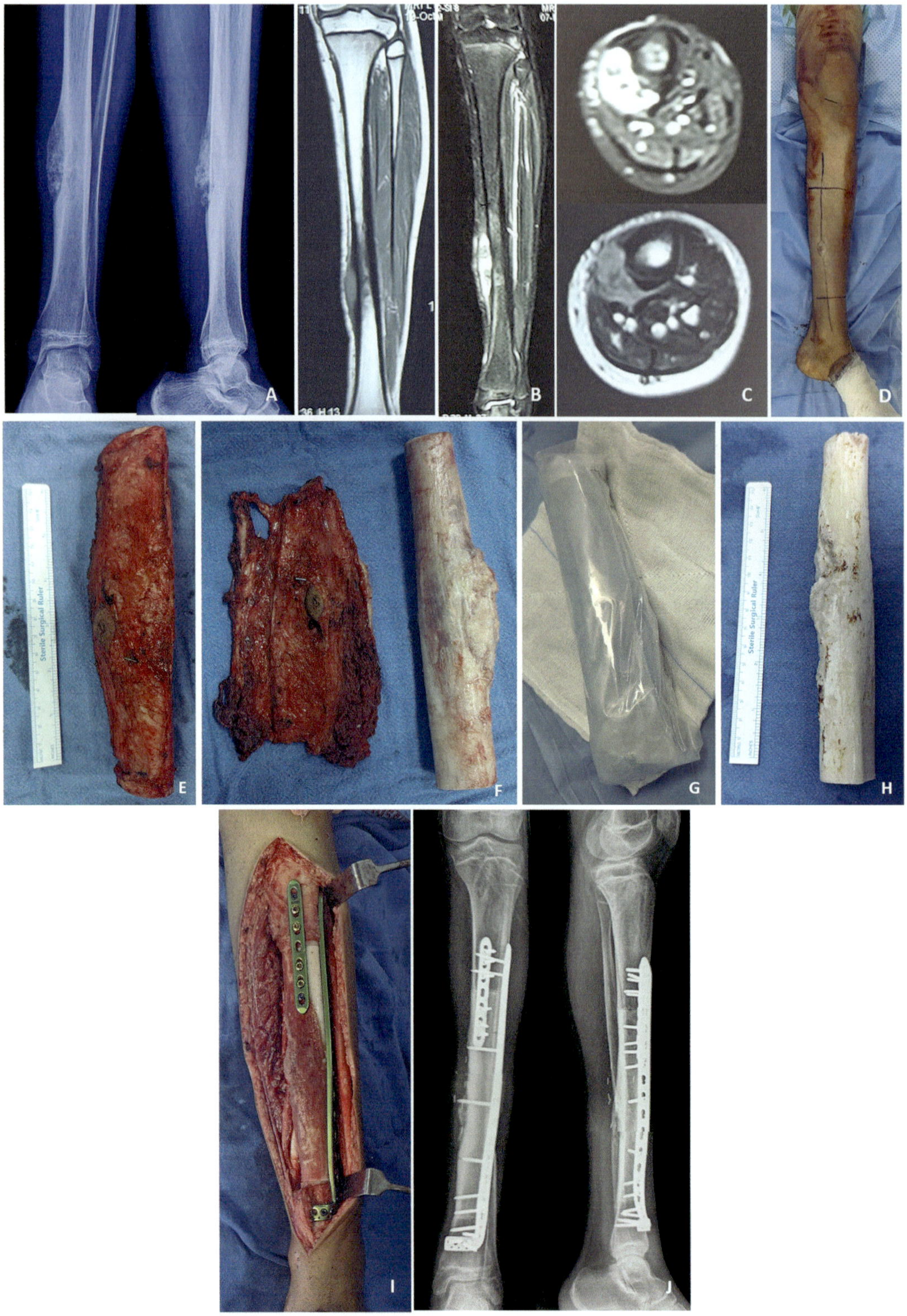

FIGURE 17.4 Plain radiographs (A) and MRI images (B & C) of Ewing sarcoma involving the tibial diaphysis in a 13-year-old male. (D) Planned skin incision incorporating the biopsy scar. An intercalary wide resection was performed (E). Soft tissue, including periosteum, is stripped off the tumor-bearing segment on a separate table (F), and the bone is prepared, washed, sterile packed (G), and treated with 50Gy radiation. The sterilized bone segment (H) is then reimplanted in the defect and stabilized using plates (I). (J) Post-operative radiographs at 7 months follow-up showed incorporation of the re-cycled autograft.

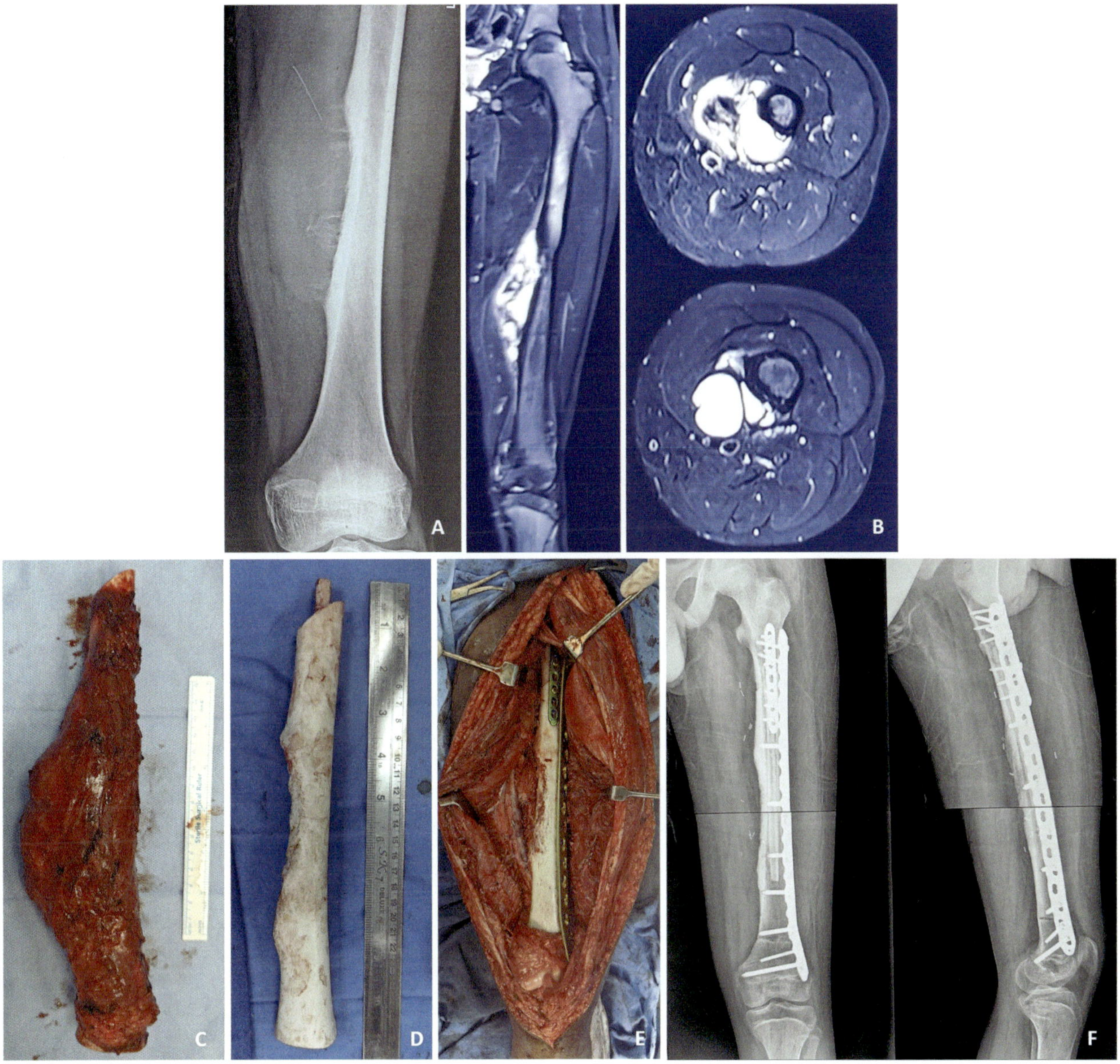

FIGURE 17.5 Plain radiographs (A) and MRI images (B) of Ewing sarcoma involving the femur diaphysis in a 15-year-old male. An intercalary wide resection was performed (C). The tumor-bearing bone is stripped of soft tissues, curetted, washed, sterile packed, and sterilized with a single high dose (typically 50 Gy) of external beam irradiation (D). The sterilized bone segment is then augmented with an intramedullary fibula and reimplanted and stabilized using plates (E). (F) Post-operative radiographs at 8 months follow-up showed bridging across the osteotomy sites.

Outcomes

Modern series report good short- and mid-term functional results, with mean MSTS scores ranging from 77% to 92% [9]. Early mobilization—often within six weeks—is a major advantage. One-year implant survival rates approach 92%, declining to approximately 72% at five years, with superior outcomes in the femur (83%) compared to the humerus (55%) [36]. Long-term follow-up reveals higher mechanical failure rates: Aldlyami et al. [37] reported 63% survival at ten years. These data highlight the greater durability of biological reconstructions in younger patients, as prosthetic devices remain susceptible to mechanical complications over time.

Complications

Common failure modes include:

- **Aseptic loosening** (0%–33%), more frequent in cemented designs and long-term survivors [9]
- **Mechanical failure** at stems or modular junctions, particularly in active patients or high-stress locations [9]
- **Infection** (5%–18%), sometimes necessitating implant removal [9]
- **Periprosthetic fracture** near the stem tip
- **Stress shielding and osteolysis** in long-term cases (Table 17.4)

TABLE 17.3
Recycled Tumor-Bearing Autografts: Outcomes and Complications

Author et al.	Year	Devitalization Technique	No. of Patients	Mean/ Median Age	Follow-Up (Months)	% Nonunion	% Graft Fractures	% Implant Failures	% Infections	Oncological Outcome	MSTS Score
Kapoor et al. [7]	2023	ECRT	46	Mean 15.8	Mean 42.1	14	NR	NR	12.5	Local recurrence (14.5%)	Mean 63%
Chen et al. [32]	2005	ECRT	15	9–74	Mean 71	7	20	0	0.0	Local recurrence (2)	Mean 87%
Davidson et al. [33]	2005	ECRT + VFG	16	Mean 19	Mean 45	31	6	25	6.0	Local recurrence (0)	Mean 93%
Krieg et al. [34]	2007	ECRT ± VFG	16	Mean 17	Mean 50	31	6	0	0.0	Local recurrence (0)	Mean 85%
Nakamura et al. [17]	2013	ECRT	6	Mean 10	Mean 41	17	0	0	0.0	Local recurrence (1)	40%–100%
Khattak et al. [24]	2006	Autoclaving	19	Mean 21	Mean 49	5	0	5	11.0	Local recurrence (2)	Mean 70%
Jeon et al. [26]	2006	Pasteurization	21	Mean 35	Mean 74	24	10	0	14.0	Local recurrence (2)	Mean 88%
Higuchi et al. [27]	2017	Frozen Autograft	18	Mean 12	Mean 46	11	17	0	11.0	Local recurrence (3)	Mean 90%
Lu et al. [28]	2020	Frozen Autograft + VFG	8	Mean 14	Mean 43	0	0	0	0.0	Local recurrence (1)	Mean 90%
Puri et al. [30]	2012	ECRT	32	Mean 15	Mean 34	16	0	16	13	Local recurrence (3)	Mean 87%
Zekry et al. [35]	2017	Frozen Autograft	34	Mean 35	Mean 62	15	18	0	6	Local recurrence (4)	Mean 90%

TABLE 17.4
Modular Prosthesis: Outcomes and Complications

Author et al.	Year	No. of Patients	Mean/ Median Age	Follow-Up (Months)	% Aseptic Loosening	% Fractures	% Implant Failures	% Infections	Oncological Outcome	MSTS Score
Agarwal et al. [38]	2010	6	2–43	Median 34	0	4	16	8	Local recurrence (2)	90%
Albergo et al. [6]	2020	36	Median 16, 19	Mean 129, 114	33	0	11	3	Local recurrence (3)	Mean 92%, 91%
Aldlyami et al. [37]	2005	35	Median 29	Mean 107	20	3	6	3	Local recurrence (5)	NR
Benevenia et al. [39]	2016	41	Mean 63	Mean 14	12	0	15	2	Local recurrence (1)	Mean 77%
Liu et al. [40]	2020	12	Mean 37	Mean 23	0	0	0	0	Local recurrence (1)	Mean 93%
Hanna et al. [41]	2010	23	Mean 41	Mean 97	4	4	4	4	Local recurrence (1)	Mean 87%
Lun et al. [42]	2018	16	Mean 65	Mean 7	6	6	NR	6	Local recurrence (2)	Mean, 90%
Sewell et al. [43]	2011	18	Mean 43	Mean 59	22	0	11	6	Local recurrence (1)	Mean 77%

Strategies to Improve Longevity

- Porous-coated collars for bone on growth and junctional stability
- Cementless press-fit stems to reduce loosening risk
- Modular taper junctions for intraoperative flexibility, with secure locking to prevent dissociation
- Expandable stems and offset connectors for improved alignment

LIMITATIONS

These devices lack biological remodeling potential, are challenging to revise, and may not achieve secure fixation in short residual bone segments. Mechanical failure risk is significant in younger, high-demand patients, limiting their role as a first-line option in such cases.

SEGMENTAL TRANSPORT

Segmental transport, based on distraction osteogenesis principles, provides a biological option for reconstructing large intercalary defects, particularly in skeletally immature patients or those with high regenerative capacity. First described by Tsuchiya et al. [44], it involves gradual transport of a bone segment across the defect using an external fixator or a fixator–intramedullary nail combination. Variants include conventional bone transport, shortening–distraction, and hybrid methods with internal stabilization. The regenerate bone is biologically active, capable of remodeling and hypertrophy. Limitations include prolonged treatment duration, high patient compliance demands, and complications such as pin tract infection, docking site nonunion, delayed consolidation, and axial deviation [44].

BONE CEMENT SPACER AND INDUCED-MEMBRANE TECHNIQUE

The Masquelet (induced-membrane) technique is a two-stage approach for segmental bone loss. In stage one, a polymethylmethacrylate (PMMA) spacer induces a vascularized membrane rich in osteoinductive factors (VEGF, BMP-2). In stage two, typically after 6–8 weeks, the spacer is replaced with cancellous autograft or a bone substitute [45]. While extensively used in post-traumatic and septic nonunions, oncologic applications are limited to small defects or upper limb reconstructions due to low mechanical demands. Advantages include technical simplicity, low morbidity, and biological potential. Drawbacks in lower limb oncology include limited early load-bearing capacity and the need for prolonged immobilization [16].

SUMMARY

- **Intercalary reconstruction** enables joint preservation and functional restoration following diaphyseal tumor resections.
- **Biological options** such as allografts, VFGs, and recycled autografts offer long-term durability but carry risks of nonunion and fracture.
- **Modular intercalary endoprostheses** provide immediate stability and early weight-bearing but have higher long-term failure rates, especially in younger patients.
- **Hybrid techniques**, combining biological and mechanical constructs (e.g., allograft + VFG), optimize both strength and incorporation.
- **Extracorporeally irradiated autografts (ECRT)** are cost-effective, anatomically precise, and oncologically safe in well-selected patients.
- Individualized reconstruction planning, based on patient age, tumor biology, defect size, and available resources, is essential for optimal outcomes.

REFERENCES

1. Errani C, Ceruso M, Donati DM, Manfrini M. Microsurgical reconstruction with vascularized fibula and massive bone allograft for bone tumors. *Eur J Orthop Surg Traumatol.* 2019;29(2):307–311. doi:10.1007/s00590-018-2360-2
2. Fuchs B, Ossendorf C, Leerapun T, et al. Intercalary segmental reconstruction after bone tumor resection. *Eur J Surg Oncol.* 2008;34:1271–1276.
3. Capanna R, Campanacci DA, Belot N, et al. A new reconstructive technique for intercalary defects of long bones: the association of massive allograft with vascularized fibular autograft. Long-term results and comparison with alternative techniques. *Orthop Clin North Am.* 2007;38:51–60.
4. Ikuta K, Nishida Y, Sugiura H, Tsukushi S, Yamada K, Urakawa H, et al. Predictors of complications in heat-treated autograft reconstruction after intercalary resection for malignant musculoskeletal tumors of the extremity. *J Surg Oncol.* 2018;117(7):1469–1478. doi:10.1002/jso.25028
5. Kawaguchi N, Ahmed AR, Matsumoto S, Manabe J, Matsushita Y. The concept of curative margin in surgery for bone and soft tissue sarcoma. *Clin Orthop Relat Res.* 2004;419: 165–172. doi:10.1097/00003086-200402000-00027
6. Albergo JI, Gaston LC, Farfalli GL, et al. Failure rates and functional results for intercalary femur reconstructions after tumour resection. *Musculoskelet Surg.* 2020;104(1):59–65. doi:10.1007/s12306-019-00595-1
7. Kapoor L, Singh H, Sahoo B, et al. Factors affecting the incorporation of extracorporeally irradiated autograft for the treatment of bone tumours-a retrospective analysis from a tertiary referral centre. *Int Orthop.* 2023;47(5):1361–1372. doi:10.1007/s00264-023-05730-z
8. Bus MPA, Dijkstra PDS, Van de Sande MAJ, et al. Intercalary allograft reconstructions following resection of primary bone tumors. *J Bone Joint Surg Am.* 2014;96:e26.
9. Errani C, Tsukamoto S, Almunhaisen N, Mavrogenis A, Donati D. Intercalary reconstruction following resection of diaphyseal bone tumors: A systematic review. *J Clin Orthop Trauma.* 2021;19:1–10. doi:10.1016/j.jcot.2021.04.033
10. Aponte-Tinao L, Farfalli GL, Ritacco LE, et al. Intercalary femur allografts are an acceptable alternative after tumor resection. *Clin Orthop Relat Res.* 2012;470:728–734.
11. Deijkers RLM, Bloem RM, Kroon HM, Van Lent JB, Brand R, Taminiau AHM. Epidiaphyseal versus other intercalary allografts for tumors of the lower limb. *Clin Orthop Relat Res.* 2005;(439):151–160.

12. Frisoni T, Cevolani L, Giorgini A, Dozza B, Donati DM. Factors affecting outcome of massive intercalary bone allografts in the treatment of tumours of the femur. *J Bone Joint Surg Br.* 2012;94(6):836–841. doi:10.1302/0301-620X.94B6.28680
13. Houdek MT, Rose PS, Milbrandt TA, Stans AA, Moran SL, Sim FH. Comparison of pediatric intercalary allograft reconstructions with and without a free vascularized fibula. *Plast Reconstr Surg.* 2018;142(4):1065–1071. doi:10.1097/PRS.0000000000004794
14. Houdek MT, Wagner ER, Stans AA, et al. What is the outcome of allograft and intramedullary free fibula (Capanna technique) in pediatric and adolescent patients with bone tumors? *Clin Orthop Relat Res.* 2016;474(3):660–668. doi:10.1007/s11999-015-4204-2
15. Muscolo DL, Ayerza MA, Aponte-Tinao L, Ranalletta M, Abalo E. Intercalary femur and tibia segmental allografts provide an acceptable alternative in reconstructing tumor resections. *Clin Orthop Relat Res.* 2004;426:97–102.
16. Zekry KM, Yamamoto N, Hayashi K, et al. Reconstruction of intercalary bone defect after resection of malignant bone tumor. *J Orthop Surg (Hong Kong).* 2019;27(1):2309499019832970. doi:10.1177/2309499019832970
17. Nakamura T, Abudu A, Grimer RJ, et al. The clinical outcomes of extracorporeal irradiated and re-implanted cemented autologous bone graft of femoral diaphysis after tumour resection. *Int Orthop.* 2013;37:647–651.
18. Weiland AJ, Daniel RK, Riley LH. Application of the free vascularized bone graft in the treatment of malignant or aggressive bone tumors. *Johns Hopkins Med J.* 1977;140:85–96.
19. Campanacci DA, Puccini S, Caff G, et al. Vascularised fibular grafts as a salvage procedure in failed intercalary reconstructions after bone tumour resection of the femur. *Injury.* 2014;45(2):399–404. doi:10.1016/j.injury.2013.10.012
20. Errani C, Alfaro PA, Ponz V, Colangeli M, Donati DM, Manfrini M. Does the addition of a vascularized fibula improve the results of a massive bone allograft alone for intercalary femur reconstruction of malignant bone tumors in children?. *Clin Orthop Relat Res.* 2021;479(6):1296–1308. doi:10.1097/CORR.0000000000001639
21. Campanacci DA, Totti F, Puccini S, et al. Intercalary reconstruction of femur after tumour resection: is a vascularized fibular autograft plus allograft a long lasting solution? *Bone Joint J.* 2018;100-B(3):378–386.
22. Li J, Wang Z, Guo Z, Chen GJ, Fu J, Pei GX. The use of allograft shell with intramedullary vascularized fibula graft for intercalary reconstruction after diaphyseal resection for lower extremity bony malignancy. *J Surg Oncol.* 2010;102(5):368–374.
23. Chauhan S, Manoj K, Rastogi S, Khan SA, Prasad A. Biomechanical investigation of the effect of extracorporeal irradiation on resected human bone. *J Mech Behav Biomed Mater.* 2017;65:791–800.
24. Khattak MJ, Umer M, Haroon-ur-Rasheed, Umar M. Autoclaved tumor bone for reconstruction: an alternative in developing countries. *Clin Orthop Relat Res.* 2006;447:138–144.
25. Lee SY, Jeon DG, Cho WH, Song WS, Kim BS. Are pasteurized autografts durable for reconstructions after bone tumor resections? *Clin Orthop Relat Res.* 2018;476(9):1728–1737.
26. Jeon DG, Kim MS, Cho WH, Song WS, Lee SY. Pasteurized autograft for intercalary reconstruction: an alternative to allograft. *Clin Orthop Relat Res.* 2007;(456):203–210.
27. Higuchi T, Yamamoto N, Nishida H, et al. Knee joint preservation surgery in osteosarcoma using tumour-bearing bone treated with liquid nitrogen. *Int Orthop.* 2017;41(10):2189–2197.
28. Lu Y, Zhu H, Huang M, et al. Is frozen tumour-bearing autograft with concurrent vascularized fibula an alternative to the Capanna technique for the intercalary reconstruction after resection of osteosarcoma in the lower limb? *Bone Joint J.* 2020;102-B(5):646–652.
29. Hayashi K, Araki N, Koizumi M, et al. Long-term results of intraoperative extracorporeal irradiation of autogenous bone grafts on primary bone and soft tissue malignancies. *Acta Oncol.* 2015;54(1):138–141.
30. Puri A, Gulia A, Jambhekar N, Laskar S. The outcome of the treatment of diaphyseal primary bone sarcoma by resection, irradiation and re-implantation of the host bone: extracorporeal irradiation as an option for reconstruction in diaphyseal bone sarcomas. *J Bone Joint Surg Br.* 2012;94(7):982–988.
31. Oike N, Kawashima H, Ogose A, et al. Long-term outcomes of an extracorporeal irradiated autograft for limb salvage operations in musculoskeletal tumours: over ten years' observation. *Bone Joint J.* 2019;101-B(9):1151–1159.
32. Chen TH, Chen WM, Huang CK. Reconstruction after intercalary resection of malignant bone tumours: comparison between segmental allograft and extracorporeally-irradiated autograft. *J Bone Joint Surg Br.* 2005;87(5):704–709. doi:10.1302/0301-620X.87B5.15491
33. Davidson AW, Hong A, McCarthy SW, Stalley PD. En-bloc resection, extracorporeal irradiation, and re-implantation in limb salvage for bony malignancies. *J Bone Joint Surg Br.* 2005;87(6):851–857.
34. Krieg AH, Davidson AW, Stalley PD. Intercalary femoral reconstruction with extracorporeal irradiated autogenous bone graft in limb-salvage surgery. *J Bone Joint Surg Br.* 2007;89(3):366–371. doi:10.1302/0301-620X.89B3.18508
35. Zekry KM, Yamamoto N, Hayashi K, et al. Intercalary frozen autograft for reconstruction of malignant bone and soft tissue tumours. *Int Orthop.* 2017;41(7):1481–1487.
36. Mahdal M, Pazourek L, Apostolopoulos V, Adámková Krákorová D, Staniczková Zambo I, Tomáš T. Outcomes of intercalary endoprostheses as a treatment for metastases in the femoral and humeral diaphysis. *Curr Oncol.* 2022;29(5):3519–3530. doi:10.3390/curroncol29050284
37. Aldlyami E, Abudu A, Grimer RJ, Carter SR, Tillman RM. Endoprosthetic replacement of diaphyseal bone defects. *Long-term results. Int Orthop.* 2005;29:25–29.
38. Agarwal M, Puri A, Gulia A, Reddy K. Joint-sparing or physeal-sparing diaphyseal resections: the challenge of holding small fragments. *Clin Orthop Relat Res.* 2010;468(11):2924–2932. doi:10.1007/s11999-010-1458-6
39. Benevenia J, Kirchner R, Patterson F, et al. Outcomes of a modular intercalary endoprosthesis as treatment for segmental defects of the femur, tibia, and humerus. *Clin Orthop Relat Res.* 2016;474(2):539–548.
40. Liu W, Shao Z, Rai S, et al. Three-dimensional-printed intercalary prosthesis for the reconstruction of large bone defect after joint-preserving tumor resection. *J Surg Oncol.* 2020;121(3):570–577.

41. Hanna SA, Sewell MD, Aston WJS, et al. Femoral diaphyseal endoprosthetic reconstruction after segmental resection of primary bone tumours. *J Bone Joint Surg Br.* 2010;92(6):867–874.
42. Lun DX, Hu YC, Yang XG, Wang F, Xu ZW. Short-term outcomes of reconstruction subsequent to intercalary resection of femoral diaphyseal metastatic tumor with pathological fracture: comparison between segmental allograft and intercalary prosthesis. *Oncol Lett.* 2018; 15(3):3508–3517.
43. Sewell MD, Hanna SA, McGrath A, et al. Intercalary diaphyseal endoprosthetic reconstruction for malignant tibial bone tumours. *J Bone Joint Surg Br.* 2011;93(8):1111–1117.
44. Tsuchiya H, Abdel-Wanis ME, Sakurakichi K, et al. Osteosarcoma around the knee. Intraepiphyseal excision and biological reconstruction with distraction osteogenesis. *J Bone Joint Surg Br.* 2002;84:1162–1166.
45. Masquelet AC, Begue T. The concept of induced membrane for reconstruction of long bone defects. *Orthop Clin North Am.* 2010;41:27–37.

18 Partial Limb Salvage in Extensive Extremity Sarcomas

INTRODUCTION

The evolution of limb salvage surgery has revolutionized the management of extremity sarcomas by enabling oncologically safe resections while maintaining or restoring function. However, in certain clinical scenarios involving extensive soft tissue or skeletal involvement, conventional reconstruction techniques—such as endoprosthetic replacement, allografts, or biological reconstruction—may be unfeasible or prone to unacceptably high complication rates. In such instances, partial limb salvage procedures, including **rotationplasty** and **surgical phocomelia**, offer an innovative solution, balancing oncological control with functional preservation.

By redefining anatomical relationships and reconfiguring the residual limb, these techniques allow prosthetic integration and functional rehabilitation that often surpass the outcomes of traditional amputation or endoprosthesis in select patients. While more technically demanding and associated with different rehabilitative considerations, these surgical techniques provide an alternative in extreme cases where conventional limb salvage may not be possible.

ROTATIONPLASTY

Rotationplasty is a functional biological reconstruction, widely accepted as an alternative to amputation in extensive lower limb sarcomas, especially in skeletally immature patients. The procedure entails intercalary resection (commonly distal femur or proximal tibia), 180° external rotation of the distal limb, and fixation in reversed orientation. This repositions the ankle to function as the knee, enabling efficient gait with a below-knee prosthesis [1, 2].

First described by Borggreve in 1930 for a tubercular stiff knee [3] and popularized by Van Nes for proximal femoral focal deficiency [4], its oncologic application was pioneered by Salzer et al. in the 1980s [5]. It is indicated when conventional limb salvage is unfeasible due to extensive soft tissue involvement, recurrence, or failed reconstruction [1, 6].

Advantages include preservation of an active, innervated distal limb with intact proprioception, improved prosthetic control, reduced infection risk, and long-term durability without multiple revisions [1, 6–8]. Cosmetic concerns from the backward foot position are mitigated by high patient satisfaction, functional independence, and psychosocial adaptation when thorough preoperative counseling is provided [1, 9].

Indications have expanded to congenital deficiencies, failed arthroplasty, severe trauma, and salvage after prosthetic infection or tumor recurrence.

PREREQUISITES AND INDICATIONS

Successful rotationplasty requires careful patient selection, comprehensive preoperative evaluation, and strict adherence to anatomical and oncological principles. Suitability is determined by functional prerequisites, oncologic safety, and psychosocial readiness.

Prerequisites

1. **Intact Neurovascular Structures** – Preservation of the sciatic nerve, with functional tibial and peroneal divisions, is essential to maintain motor and sensory innervation post-rotation. The deep peroneal nerve may be sacrificed if required without significant functional compromise. While vessel resection with reconstruction is possible, intact neurovascular anatomy minimizes ischemic risk.
2. **Functional Ankle Joint** – Adequate plantarflexion, dorsiflexion, and proprioception are mandatory, as the ankle will functionally substitute for the knee. Plantarflexion simulates knee extension and dorsiflexion mimics knee flexion within the prosthesis.
3. **Skeletal Maturity Considerations** – In skeletally immature patients, loss of the distal femoral and proximal tibial physes leaves the distal tibial physis as the only growth center. Anticipated limb length discrepancy should be calculated, and planned over-lengthening of the rotated segment considered.
4. **Psychosocial Preparedness** – The reversed foot appearance necessitates thorough counseling. Preoperative interaction with prior recipients and multidisciplinary psychosocial assessment enhance acceptance and compliance.

Indications

- **Primary Tumor Indications** – Osteosarcoma or Ewing sarcoma of the distal femur, proximal tibia, or entire femur in skeletally immature patients (<10 years); tumors with extensive soft tissue involvement or pathological fractures precluding conventional limb salvage; cases requiring wide resection with neurovascular preservation.
- **Salvage Indications** – Failed endoprostheses due to infection, loosening, or nonunion; local recurrence after limb salvage; massive bone loss or poor soft tissue coverage preventing prosthetic fixation.

DOI: 10.1201/9780367822002-23

Contraindications

- **Absolute** – Tumor infiltration or loss of function of the sciatic nerve; ankle stiffness, fixed deformity, or absent motor control; profound psychosocial aversion.
- **Relative** – Bilateral limb deficiencies preventing contralateral length matching; poor general condition precluding rehabilitation and prosthetic use.

CLASSIFICATION

Rotationplasty procedures are classified according to the anatomical level of resection and the resultant functional substitution of joints. The most widely accepted classification is that proposed by **Winkelmann**, which divides cases into **Type A** and **Type B** based on the resection level and functional outcome [10]. Winkelmann's classification provides a structured framework for surgical planning in rotationplasty, distinguishing between ankle-as-knee (Type A) and knee-as-hip (Type B) reconstructions, with further subtyping by resection level.

Type A Rotationplasty (Ankle Functions as the Knee)

In Type A procedures, the ankle is repositioned to replace the functional role of the knee, most often in cases requiring resection around the distal femur or proximal tibia.

- **Type AI – Distal femoral resection**: Applied for tumors involving the distal femur. Following tumor excision, the distal tibia and foot are rotated 180° and positioned to function as the knee joint.
- **Type AII – Proximal tibial resection**: Used when the proximal tibia is involved, similarly rotating the distal tibia and foot to replace the resected knee.

Type B Rotationplasty (Knee Functions as the Hip)

Type B procedures are indicated for proximal femoral or hip joint involvement, where the knee is transposed to function as the hip and the ankle substitutes for the knee.

- **Type BI – Proximal femoral resection with intact hip joint**: The native knee is placed proximally, while the ankle functions as the new knee.
- **Type BII – Resection involving the hip joint**: Performed after extra-articular or periacetabular resection. The tibia is fixed to the pelvis; in adults, this may require an endoprosthesis.
- Type BIII – Total femoral resection:
  - **BIIIa**: Tibial condyle inserted directly into the acetabulum (used in children to allow remodeling).
  - **BIIIb**: Tibia connected to the pelvis using a custom prosthesis (common in adults or older children).

PREOPERATIVE EVALUATION AND PLANNING

Rotationplasty demands meticulous, multidisciplinary preoperative planning to achieve oncologic clearance, functional preservation, and optimal long-term outcomes.

ONCOLOGIC STAGING AND IMAGING

Complete oncologic staging is essential to confirm resectability and exclude metastases.

- **Local Imaging**: MRI defines tumor extent, joint involvement, and the relationship to neurovascular structures. CT can complement MRI for cortical bone evaluation and osteotomy planning.
- **Alignment and Skeletal Maturity**: Standing radiographs assess limb alignment and deformities.
- **Systemic Staging**: Includes CT chest, bone scintigraphy, and occasionally PET-CT to detect metastatic spread.

NEUROVASCULAR ASSESSMENT

The integrity of the **sciatic nerve** and its tibial and peroneal divisions is crucial. MRI must confirm the absence of nerve encasement. Vascular structures can be reconstructed if involved, though outcomes are best with preservation. MR angiography or conventional angiography may be indicated when vessel patency or caliber is in question [11].

GROWTH PREDICTION AND LIMB LENGTH CONSIDERATIONS

In skeletally immature patients, resection of the **distal femoral physis** (≈70% of femoral growth) and **proximal tibial physis** (≈55% of tibial growth) leaves only the **distal tibial physis** (≈43% of tibial growth) for continued lengthening [4].

- Planning:
  - Young children: Overlengthen the rotated segment by 4–6 cm.
  - Older children: Overlengthen by 1–2 cm. Growth estimation uses bone age assessment (hand radiographs), Tanner staging, and Anderson's growth charts [12, 13].

PSYCHOSOCIAL COUNSELING

Due to the unconventional appearance of the limb (foot rotated 180°), intensive preoperative counseling is vital. This includes

- reviewing photographs or meeting previous rotationplasty recipients,
- addressing body image, coping strategies, and lifestyle implications, and
- establishing realistic expectations for prosthesis use and physical activity.

  Such measures significantly enhance acceptance, compliance, and long-term satisfaction [9].

PROSTHETIC CONSULTATION

Early engagement with a prosthetics team ensures optimal postoperative outcomes.

- **Discussion Points**: Socket design, component compatibility, and expected alignment.
- **Goals**: Facilitate early weight-bearing and gait retraining.
- **Customization**: Protocols vary with resection level (knee vs. hip), extent of preserved musculature, and patient age.

SURGICAL TECHNIQUE

The surgical technique of rotationplasty is a coordinated sequence of oncologic resection, precise osteotomy planning, preservation of neurovascular structures, and functional soft tissue reconstruction. As per the Winkelmann classification, two major oncologic variants are performed: **Knee Rotationplasty (Type A)** and **Hip Rotationplasty (Type B)**.

KNEE ROTATIONPLASTY (TYPE A)

Preoperative Planning

Skin incision design must incorporate previous biopsy tracts and ensure wide oncologic resection while allowing tension-free closure. Two oblique elliptical incisions with opposing slopes are commonly used to accommodate the circumference difference between the thigh and leg. Alternatives include fish-mouth or transverse incisions with triangular extensions.

Exposure and Neurovascular Preservation

With the patient supine, the posterior thigh is exposed. The hamstrings, gastrocnemius heads, popliteal artery and vein, and tibial and common peroneal nerves are identified. Neurovascular bundles are meticulously preserved; genicular branches are ligated, and the femoral artery and sciatic nerve are mobilized proximally to the planned osteotomy site.

Bone Resection and Rotation

Femoral osteotomy is performed—usually transverse but occasionally step-cut for stability—after marking rotational alignment with Steinmann pins or cortical notches. The intercalary segment is excised, and the distal tibia osteotomized. The distal segment is rotated 180° externally, ensuring neurovascular redirection medially to avoid kinking or tension.

Fixation and Soft Tissue Reconstruction

Fixation options include compression plating, intramedullary nailing, or external fixation. The quadriceps tendon is reattached to the gastrocnemius-soleus complex, and hamstrings to tibialis anterior and peroneal muscles. The ankle is held in neutral dorsiflexion for optimal muscle tensioning. Coiled nerves and vessels are positioned in a soft tissue bed, fascia is left open to prevent compartment syndrome, and skin is closed with drains in place.

HIP ROTATIONPLASTY (TYPE B)

Positioning and Incision

The patient is supine with a roll under the ipsilateral iliac crest for lateral tilt. Two oblique elliptical skin incisions—one from below the inguinal ligament along the gluteal fold and another connecting to a posterior thigh incision—provide access to hip and thigh musculature.

Anterior and Posterior Dissection

Anteriorly, rectus femoris and sartorius are detached, and the psoas tendon divided. The quadriceps is reflected for later reattachment. Posteriorly, gluteals and abductors are detached from the femur, preserving the sciatic nerve. The femoral artery may be preserved or resected and re-anastomosed if necessary.

Joint Resection

- **Type BI**: Hip disarticulation via anterior capsulotomy.
- **Type BII**: Internal hemipelvectomy with resection margins ensuring oncologic safety.
- **Type BIII**: Total femoral resection, with tibial condyle insertion into acetabulum in children (<10 years) to allow remodeling; adults require custom endoprostheses.

Rotation and Fixation

Following segment resection, the limb is rotated 180° and fixed to the ilium in slight abduction (5°–10°). In Type BIIIa, ~5 cm of proximal fibula is removed to aid tibial seating in the acetabulum. The heel is positioned neutrally, with knee height matching the contralateral hip.

Soft Tissue Reconstruction

Iliopsoas is reattached to distal hamstrings; distal quadriceps and knee capsule are sutured to gluteals. Vascular reconstructions are performed without tension, routing vessels, and sciatic nerve subcutaneously. Wound closure is meticulous, with drains inserted based on intraoperative assessment.

POSTOPERATIVE CARE

Vascular and Limb Monitoring

Immediate postoperative care prioritizes limb perfusion assessment—checking skin color, capillary refill, temperature, pulses, and sensation. Vascular reconstructions require heightened vigilance for thrombosis. The ankle (future knee) is kept in neutral dorsiflexion, limb slightly elevated and abducted.

Wound and Drain Care

Drains are monitored and removed within 48–72 hours when output is minimal. Wounds are checked for hematoma, seroma, necrosis, or dehiscence, especially at high-tension sites.

Pain Management and Antibiotics

Multimodal analgesia (opioids, NSAIDs, regional anesthesia) is standard. Antibiotic prophylaxis is continued for 24–48 hours or longer if vascular reconstruction or significant contamination is present.

REHABILITATION AND PROSTHETIC PLANNING

Early, structured rehabilitation is essential for maximizing functional outcomes following rotationplasty. Mobilization typically begins on postoperative day one with non-weight-bearing ambulation using crutches under supervised guidance. Initial physiotherapy priorities include:

- **Ankle range-of-motion exercises** (critical as the ankle assumes the functional role of the knee)
- **Quadriceps and hamstring strengthening** to optimize limb control
- **Hip mobilization and gait training** for balanced movement patterns

In younger patients—especially those under 12 years—hip spica casting may be employed for several weeks to maintain alignment and facilitate osteosynthesis, particularly after hip rotationplasty. Older children and adults rarely require casting unless instability is evident.

Prosthetic fitting is initiated once swelling subsides and wounds are adequately healed, usually between 8 and 12 weeks postoperatively. A temporary socket allows for early ambulation; a definitive custom below-knee prosthesis is fabricated once the residual limb stabilizes. Close collaboration between the surgical team, prosthetist, and physiotherapist is essential for optimal socket fit, alignment, and gait training.

PSYCHOSOCIAL SUPPORT

Given the distinctive appearance of the rotated limb, psychological counseling is a cornerstone of care. Early and ongoing support—including peer mentoring, family counseling, and gradual reintegration into school or work—enhances coping, acceptance, and functional independence. Studies show that preoperative exposure to former rotationplasty patients improves long-term satisfaction and self-image.

COMPLICATIONS

Although rotationplasty delivers robust functional and oncological outcomes, it carries potential risks requiring prompt recognition and management.

EARLY COMPLICATIONS

1. **Vascular Compromise** – Thrombosis, kinking, or undue tension on vessels—particularly after vascular reconstruction—can precipitate limb ischemia. Urgent re-exploration is warranted; prolonged ischemia may necessitate secondary amputation [11].
2. **Compartment Syndrome** – Altered muscle orientation and vascular re-routing predispose to elevated compartment pressures. Routine avoidance of tight fascial closure mitigates risk [2].
3. **Wound Complications** – Large incisions and circumference mismatch at the proximal thigh predispose to dehiscence, necrosis, and infection. Vigilant dressing care, offloading, and drain management are essential [1].
4. **Nerve Palsy** – Transient peroneal nerve palsy can result from traction or ischemia; most cases resolve, but persistent neuropathy compromises prosthetic control. Sciatic nerve preservation is key [14].

LATE COMPLICATIONS

1. **Nonunion/Malunion** – More likely when bone contact is inadequate; step-cut osteotomies and precise perpendicular cuts improve union rates. Malrotation may require corrective osteotomy [7].
2. **Prosthetic Problems** – Poor fit may cause callosities, breakdown, or gait disturbance; regular adjustments with prosthetists are necessary [15].
3. **Growth Discrepancies** – In children, residual growth potential may cause over- or underlengthening of the rotated segment, affecting prosthetic fit [12].
4. **Joint Degeneration** – Long-term ankle arthritis is rare but should be monitored, especially in high-activity patients [15].
5. **Derotation in Children** – Seen when surgery is performed very early; careful muscle rebalancing and rotation through the knee rather than tibial osteotomy reduces risk [2].

OUTCOMES – ONCOLOGICAL AND FUNCTIONAL

Rotationplasty offers oncologic safety equivalent to amputation, while preserving superior functional potential through maintenance of neurovascular integrity and active distal muscle control.

ONCOLOGICAL OUTCOMES

Multiple series confirm that local recurrence rates are comparable to or lower than limb-sparing endoprosthetic reconstruction when margins are adequate. Gottsauner-Wolf et al. [16] reported only one recurrence; Kotz [8] observed none in 30 cases; Winkelmann [17] similarly documented no local recurrence in eight femoral tumor cases.

FUNCTIONAL OUTCOMES

Rotationplasty permits dynamic control of a below-knee prosthesis via the rotated ankle functioning as a neo-knee. This confers lower energy expenditure, enhanced proprioception, and greater mobility compared to transfemoral amputation. In a long-term cohort study by Gotta et al. [18], which included 60 patients (median follow-up 22 years), the median MSTS score was 24. Most returned to school, work, and sport. Mean Tegner activity level was 4 (moderate physical activity). Du et al. [19] in their pediatric cohort reported restoration of full muscle strength and ambulation by 12 months; performance in the 6-minute walk test and timed-up-and-go was comparable to peers and stable at a mean of 7.5 years. Gait Analysis across three comparative studies revealed that patients demonstrated slightly reduced velocity, stride length, and cadence vs. controls, but compensated through efficient prosthetic control [20]. The preservation of native musculature and proprioceptive pathways underpins these outcomes, particularly in active, growing patients.

QUALITY OF LIFE

Long-term HRQL is high and often near population norms. In the long-term series by Gotta et al. [18], SF-36 physical and mental health scores were comparable to the general population. Du et al. [19] emphasized that early rehabilitation and psychological support yield excellent social reintegration, body image acceptance, and school participation.

A recent gait study [21] highlighted that patients with pseudoknee height matching the contralateral knee achieved superior walking mechanics, whereas longer residual segments caused altered gait with increased pseudoknee flexion. Despite occasional degenerative changes in the rotated foot/ankle, adults demonstrated increased knee ROM and efficient ground reaction forces, supporting the importance of careful preoperative alignment planning.

Rotationplasty delivers durable oncologic control, high functional independence, and sustained quality of life, particularly in younger and active individuals [22]. While minor gait deviations and late orthopedic issues can arise, these are generally outweighed by the long-term biomechanical and psychosocial benefits when patient selection, surgical execution, and rehabilitation are optimized.

SURGICAL PHOCOMELIA

Introduction

Surgical phocomelia, or *phoco-reduction*, is a specialized limb salvage technique for selected upper limb sarcomas in which conventional reconstruction is not feasible. First described by Windhager et al. [23], it involves segmental resection of the diseased portion of the upper limb with preservation of the major neurovascular bundle, followed by reattachment of the distal limb to the proximal stump. This configuration resembles the congenital anomaly of phocomelia, classically associated with thalidomide embryopathy [24], but here is created surgically to preserve distal function.

Indications

Surgical phocomelia is indicated in the following:

- **Extensive upper limb sarcomas** involving bone and soft tissue where standard reconstruction is impractical
- **Preservation of the brachial artery and median nerve**, enabling continued perfusion and motor-sensory function distally
- **Oncologic resections with inadequate options for soft tissue coverage** or where critical joint involvement precludes standard reconstruction
- **Complex salvage scenarios**, such as prior unplanned surgery or tumor fungation, where amputation can be avoided

Contraindications include tumor encasement of the primary neurovascular bundle or involvement of the distal forearm to an extent where meaningful distal function cannot be preserved.

Surgical Technique (Figures 18.1 and 18.2)

Preoperative planning requires MRI/CT and angiography to map tumor extent and vessel status.

Two transverse circumferential incisions are planned above and below the involved segment, supplemented by a medial longitudinal incision for neurovascular dissection.

Key Steps:

1. Dissection and preservation of axillary and brachial vessels and major nerves.
2. Wide en bloc resection of the involved bone (partial or total humerus) with associated soft tissues, ensuring oncologic margins.
3. For total humeral resections, the proximal ulna is suspended to the acromion with nonabsorbable sutures (e.g., Mersilk) to create a pseudo-shoulder joint.
4. For isolated elbow resections, the ulna is rigidly fixed to the residual proximal humerus using plates.
5. Muscle reattachment is performed in a tension-free manner to optimize preserved function.
6. Layered closure prioritizes soft tissue coverage; immobilization for ~4 weeks precedes physiotherapy.

Complications

Windhager et al. [23] noted vascular thrombosis in cases requiring vessel resection/reconstruction. Additional reports describe restricted hand function, incomplete nerve recovery, and higher complication rates when nerve and vessel repair are needed [23, 25].

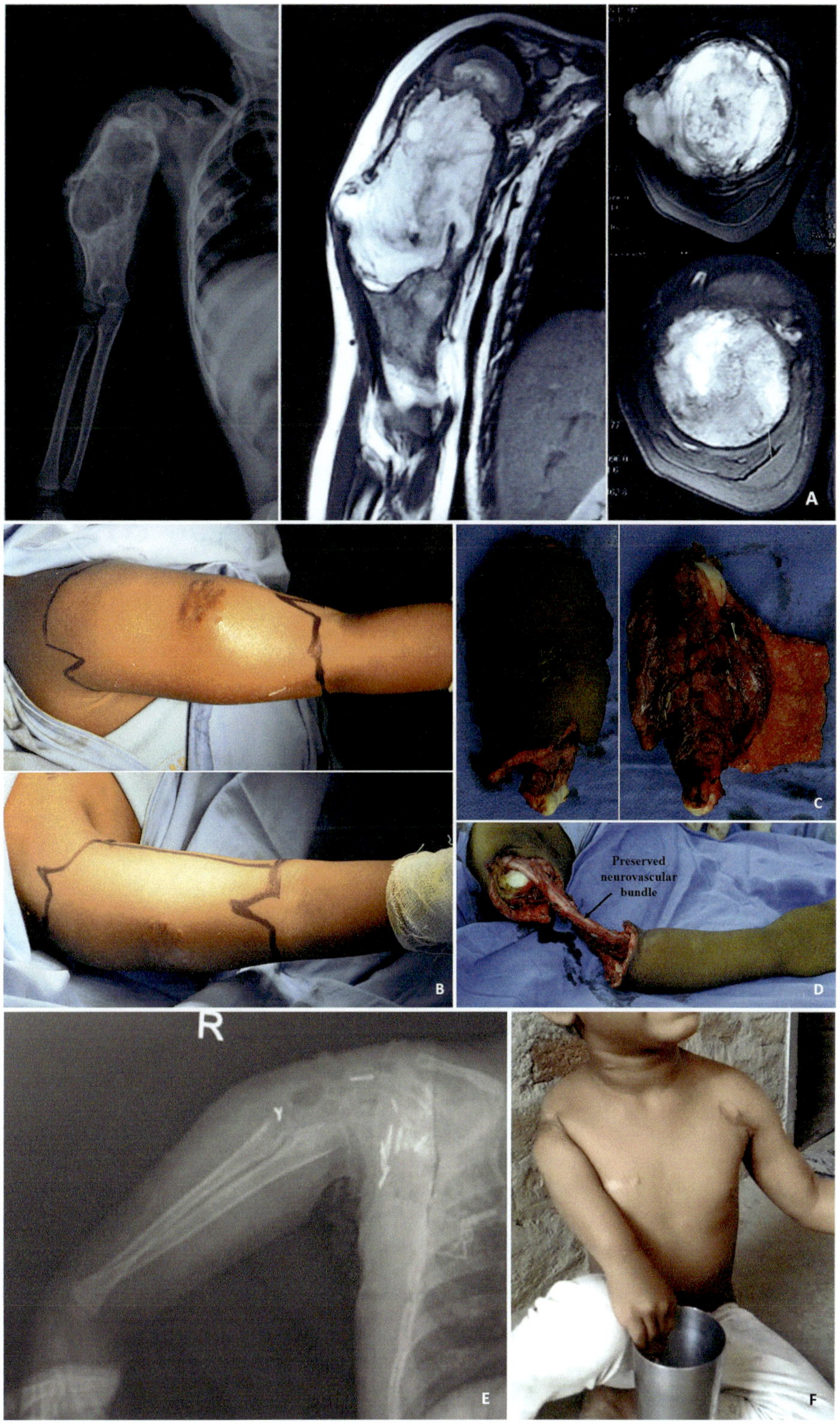

FIGURE 18.1 A case of a 4-year-old child with Ewing sarcoma of the humerus managed by surgical phocomelia. (A) Preoperative radiograph and MRI show extensive involvement of the entire humerus with cortical destruction and soft tissue extension. (B) Preoperative marking with transverse circumferential incisions above and below the diseased segment, supplemented with a medial longitudinal incision for neurovascular dissection. (C) Wide en bloc resection specimen following complete humeral excision. (D) Intraoperative image demonstrating preserved neurovascular bundle after meticulous dissection and tumor removal. (E) Postoperative follow-up radiograph and clinical photograph of the child after suspension of the proximal ulna to the acromion. (F) The reconstruction creates a functional pseudo-shoulder joint, demonstrating a satisfactory cosmetic appearance with preserved hand function.

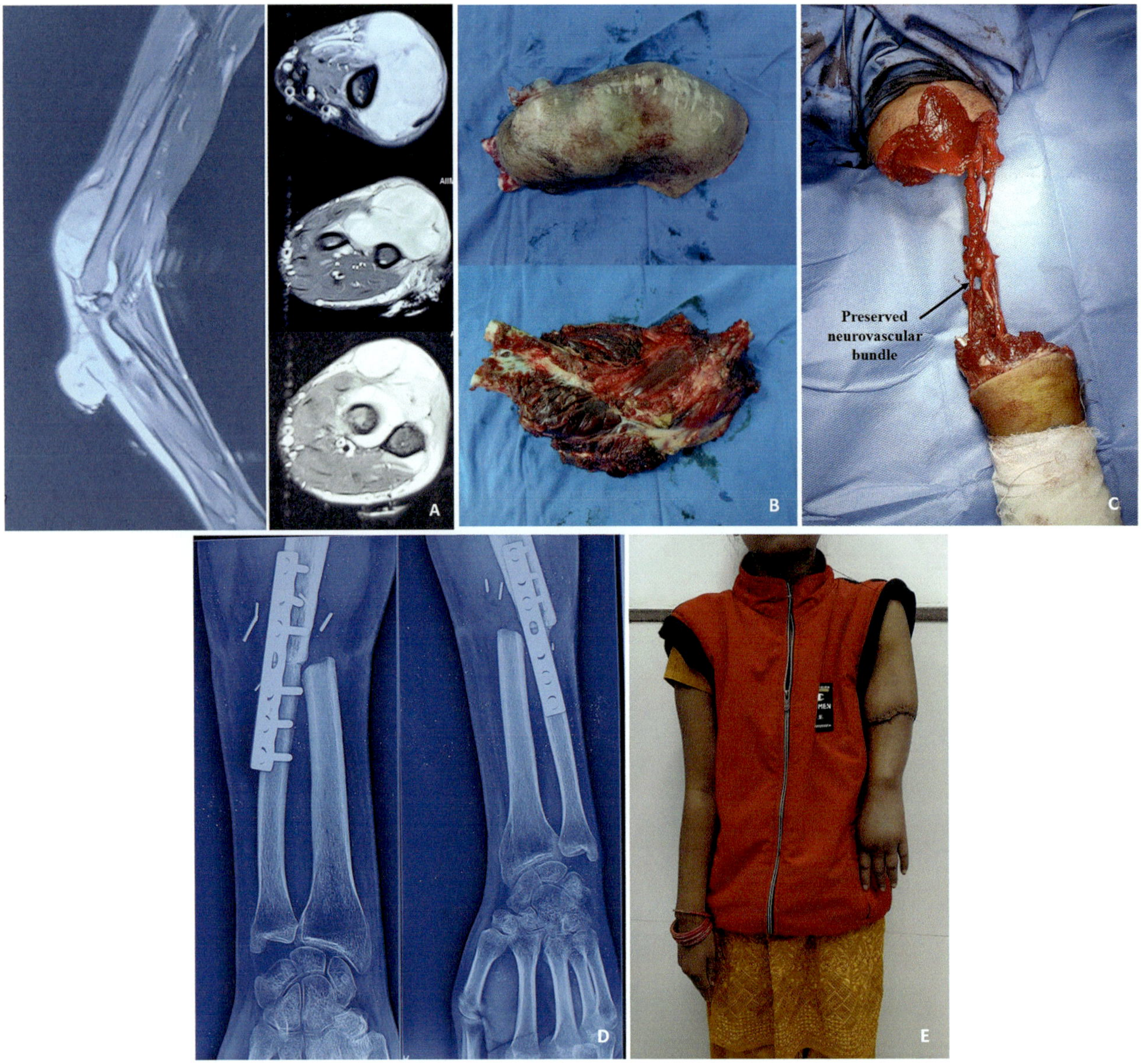

FIGURE 18.2 A case of a fungating synovial sarcoma of the forearm in a 17-year-old female. (A) MRI scan demonstrating an expansile, heterogeneous tumor of the forearm and distal arm with extensive soft tissue involvement, with extension across the elbow joint and through the skin and subcutaneous tissues. (B) Gross specimen following wide en bloc resection showing tumor mass with surrounding soft tissues. (C) Intraoperative picture showing preservation of the neurovascular bundle following tumor excision. (D) Postoperative radiographs following humero-ulnar fusion show union between the humerus and ulna. (E) Clinical photograph at follow-up demonstrating satisfactory wound healing and preserved hand function after limb salvage.

Kapoor et al. [24] documented implant failure after ulnohumeral fixation and postoperative radial nerve palsy in single cases following phoco-reduction.

Outcomes

Functional results are generally favorable. In a series of 11 patients, the mean MSTS93 score was 22/30, with handgrip strength averaging 62% of the contralateral limb [24]. Grip strength was notably higher in nerve-sparing cases, consistent with Hahn et al., who reported 66% grasp and 72% pinch power in patients with preserved peripheral nerves [26].

Patients were able to perform fine motor activities—grasping, lifting, bimanual tasks—critical for daily living. After total humeral resection with ulna–acromion suspension, mobility at the pseudo-shoulder joint allowed practical limb use for object manipulation and self-care [24].

The core aim is oncologically sound resection with maximal preservation of meaningful distal function. While the shortened limb's appearance may be unconventional, most patients prefer it to amputation due to superior physical utility and less psychological distress. A sensate, functional extremity offers greater versatility than current upper limb prostheses, especially in resource-limited settings. Unlike lower limb rotationplasty, surgical phocomelia typically eliminates the need for prosthesis, with preserved native hand function outweighing cosmetic concerns.

SUMMARY

- Rotationplasty offer durable, functional alternatives to amputation, especially in extensive sarcomas of the lower limb, by preserving proprioception, enabling active limb control, and facilitating efficient prosthetic use.
- Functional outcomes following rotationplasty are consistently high, with near-normal gait mechanics, excellent MSTS scores, and quality of life measures comparable to the general population, despite minor gait deviations and cosmetic concerns.
- Surgical phocomelia offers a limb salvage alternative to amputation in select upper limb sarcomas, ensuring oncological safety while preserving functional, sensate hand use without the need for a prosthesis.

REFERENCES

1. Fuchs B, Sim FH. Rotationplasty about the knee: surgical technique and anatomical considerations. *Clin Anat.* 2004;17(4):345–353. doi:10.1002/ca.10211
2. Gupta SK, Alassaf N, Harrop AR, Kiefer GN. Principles of rotationplasty. *J Am Acad Orthop Surg.* 2012;20(10): 657–667. doi:10.5435/JAAOS-20-10-657
3. Borggreve J: Kniegelenksersatz durch das in der Beinla ¨ngsachse um 180 Grad gedrehte Fussgelenk. *Arch Orthop Unfallchir.* 1930;28:175–178.
4. Van Nes CP: Rotation-plasty for congenital defects of the femur. *J Bone Joint Surg Br.* 1950;32(1):12–16.
5. Salzer M, Knahr K, Kotz R, Kristen H: Treatment of osteosarcomata of the distal femur by rotation-plasty. *Arch Orthop Trauma Surg.* 1981;99(2):131–136.
6. Hillmann A, Hoffmann C, Gosheger G, Krakau H, Winkelmann W. Malignant tumor of the distal part of the femur or the proximal part of the tibia: endoprosthetic replacement or rotationplasty. Functional outcome and quality-of-life measurements. *J Bone Joint Surg Am.* 1999;81(4):462–468. doi:10.2106/00004623-199904000-00003
7. Puri A, Agarwal M. Facilitating rotationplasty. *J Surg Oncol.* 2007;95(4):351–354. doi:10.1002/jso.20683
8. Kotz R. Rotationplasty. *Semin Surg Oncol.* 1997;13(1):34–40. doi:10.1002/(sici)1098-2388(199701/02)13:1<34::aid-ssu6>3.0.co;2-5
9. Rödl RW, Pohlmann U, Gosheger G, Lindner NJ, Winkelmann W. Rotationplasty--quality of life after 10 years in 22 patients. *Acta Orthop Scand.* 2002;73(1):85–88. doi:10.1080/000164702317281468
10. Winkelmann WW. Rotationplasty. *Orthop Clin North Am.* 1996;27(3):503–523.
11. Mahoney CR, Hartman CW, Simon PJ, Baxter BT, Neff JR. Vascular management in rotationplasty. *Clin Orthop Relat Res.* 2008;466(5):1210–1216. doi:10.1007/s11999-008-0197-4
12. Anderson M, Green WT, Messner MB. Growth and predictions of growth in the lower extremities. *J Bone Joint Surg Am.* 1963;45-A:1–14.
13. Merkel KD, Gebhardt M, Springfield DS. Rotationplasty as a reconstructive operation after tumor resection. *Clin Orthop Relat Res.* 1991;(270):231–236.
14. Hillmann A, Gosheger G, Hoffmann C, Ozaki T, Winkelmann W. Rotationplasty--surgical treatment modality after failed limb salvage procedure. *Arch Orthop Trauma Surg.* 2000;120(10):555–558. doi:10.1007/s004020000175
15. Gebert C, Hardes J, Vieth V, Hillmann A, Winkelmann W, Gosheger G. The effect of rotationplasty on the ankle joint: long-term results. *Prosthet Orthot Int.* 2006;30(3):316–323. doi:10.1080/03093640600863802
16. Gottsauner-Wolf F, Kotz R, Knahr K, Kristen H, Ritschl P, Salzer M. Rotationplasty for limb salvage in the treatment of malignant tumors at the knee. A follow-up study of seventy patients. *J Bone Joint Surg Am.* 1991;73(9):1365–1375.
17. Winkelmann WW. Type-B-IIIa hip rotationplasty: an alternative operation for the treatment of malignant tumors of the femur in early childhood. *J Bone Joint Surg Am.* 2000;82(6): 814–828. doi:10.2106/00004623-200006000-00008
18. Gotta J, Bielack S, Hecker-Nolting S, et al. When your ankle becomes a knee - long-term functional outcome and quality of life with a rotationplasty after resection of malignant limb tumors. Wenn der Knöchel zum Knie wird – Langzeitergebnisse und Lebensqualität mit einer Borggreve-Umkehrplastik nach Resektion maligner Knochentumore. *Klin Padiatr.* 2022;234(3):154–162. doi:10.1055/a-1681-1916
19. Du N, Zhao X, Du J, Yu JG, Xu M, Song Y. Functional rehabilitation and long term efficacy of rotationplasty in pediatrics: A retrospective study. *Oncol Lett.* 2024;28(5): 519. Published 2024 Aug 29. doi:10.3892/ol.2024.14652
20. Filis P, Varvarousis D, Ntritsos G, et al. Rotationplasty outcomes assessed by gait analysis following resection of lower extremity bone neoplasms. *Bone Jt Open.* 2023;4(11): 817–824. Published 2023 Nov 1. doi:10.1302/2633-1462.411.BJO-2023-0101.R1
21. Benedetti MG, Okita Y, Recubini E, Mariani E, Leardini A, Manfrini M. How much clinical and functional impairment do children treated with knee rotationplasty experience in adulthood?. *Clin Orthop Relat Res.* 2016;474(4):995–1004. doi:10.1007/s11999-016-4691-9
22. Hobusch GM, Hofer C, Döring K, Ellersdorfer F, Kelaridis T, Windhager R. Is rotationplasty still a reasonable reconstruction option for patients with a femoral bone sarcoma? a comparative study of patients with a minimum of 20 years of follow-up after rotationplasty and lower extremity amputation. *Clin Orthop Relat Res.* 17, 2025. doi:10.1097/CORR.0000000000003495
23 Windhager R, Millesi H, Kotz R. Resection-replantation for primary malignant tumours of the arm. An alternative to fore-quarter amputation. *J Bone Joint Surg Br.* 1995;77(2):176–184.
24. Kapoor L, Banjara R, Kumar VS, Khan SA. Surgical phocomelia or phoco-reduction as a method of limb salvage for sarcomas of the upper limb: A suitable alternative to amputation. *J Surg Oncol.* 2022;125(2):246–255. doi:10.1002/jso.26704
25. El-Gammal TA, El-Sayed A, Kotb MM. Resection replantation of the upper limb for aggressive malignant tumors. *Arch Orthop Trauma Surg.* 2002;122(3):173–176. doi:10.1007/s004020100348
26. Hahn SB, Choi YR, Kang HJ, Shin KH. Segmental resection and re plantation have a role for selected advanced sarcomas in the upper limb. *Clin Orthop Relat Res.* 2009;467(11):2918–2924.

19 Limb Salvage in Benign Bone Tumors

INTRODUCTION

Limb salvage in benign bone tumors has advanced considerably, aiming to balance oncologic safety with functional preservation. Among the available surgical strategies, intralesional curettage remains the mainstay for managing a wide spectrum of benign and low-grade malignant bone lesions (Figure 19.1). This technique removes tumor tissue from within the bone while conserving the surrounding cortex and adjacent joints—an approach particularly advantageous for lesions near articulations or in skeletally immature patients, where wide resection would cause disproportionate morbidity.

Common indications include GCT, aneurysmal bone cyst, chondroblastoma, chondromyxoid fibroma (CMF), and low-grade chondrosarcoma. Although histologically benign, several of these tumors exhibit locally aggressive behavior and significant recurrence potential. For instance, GCTs, despite their benign classification, may metastasize to the lungs in a small proportion of cases and rarely undergo malignant transformation [1, 2].

While intralesional curettage offers functional advantages over en bloc resection, it carries a higher risk of local recurrence, historically reported up to 65% with curettage alone [1]. This is largely due to the irregular internal architecture of lesion cavities, which hinders complete mechanical removal with curettes. Modern protocols therefore employ a multimodal approach: meticulous curettage, high-speed burring to extend margins, optional application of local adjuvants, and appropriate reconstruction of the osseous defect.

Mechanical (e.g., burring), thermal (e.g., cryoablation, cautery), and chemical adjuvants (e.g., phenol, ethanol, hydrogen peroxide) aim to eradicate microscopic residual tumor cells within trabecular bone. Although widely adopted, no adjuvant has proven unequivocally superior; the thoroughness of curettage and burring remains the principal determinant of local control [1].

SURGICAL TECHNIQUE OF CURETTAGE

The surgical execution of intralesional curettage in benign bone tumors is a carefully staged process designed to maximize tumor clearance while preserving adjacent anatomy. A systematic **six-step protocol** is generally followed: **(1)** surgical exposure and cortical window creation, **(2)** intralesional evacuation and curettage, **(3)** high-speed burring, **(4)** pulsatile lavage, **(5)** extended curettage with adjuvants, and **(6)** reconstruction of the defect. Each stage requires meticulous attention to detail to minimize recurrence risk.

Surgical Exposure and Cortical Window Creation

Adequate exposure is the foundation for effective curettage. A longitudinal or curvilinear incision is made in line with the involved bone, respecting anatomical planes and protecting neurovascular structures (Figure 19.2). The cortical window—serving as the entry point—must be sufficiently large to allow direct visualization and full instrument access (Figure 19.3). Evidence suggests that a window encompassing at least 50% of the lesion's longitudinal dimension improves completeness of clearance and local control [1].

Creation techniques include:

- High-speed burr sculpting through the cortex
- Multiple drill holes connected with an osteotome
- Subsequent burring to enlarge the opening and improve access to hidden recesses

Evacuation of Tumor Contents

Gross tumor removal is tailored to lesion consistency.

- **Solid tumors**: curettes, rongeurs, or pituitary forceps (Figure 19.4).
- **Cystic lesions**: aspiration followed by mechanical evacuation.

After initial clearance, suction–irrigation removes debris, followed by a systematic manual curettage to scrape the cavity walls and remove adherent tissue. To ensure completeness, different sizes and angles of curettes are used to reach all contours of the cavity.

High-Speed Burring

High-speed burring abrades the inner cavity walls, achieving:

- Removal of residual microscopic tumor nests.
- Elimination of reactive sclerotic bone.
- Smoothing of irregular contours that could harbor residual cells (Figure 19.5).

This step "opens up" trabeculated cavities, crucial for aggressive lesions such as GCT or chondroblastoma. Caution is exercised near articular cartilage and neurovascular structures to prevent iatrogenic injury. Intraoperative fluoroscopy verifies complete spatial reach, cross-referencing with preoperative imaging for accuracy (Figure 19.6).

DOI: 10.1201/9780367822002-24

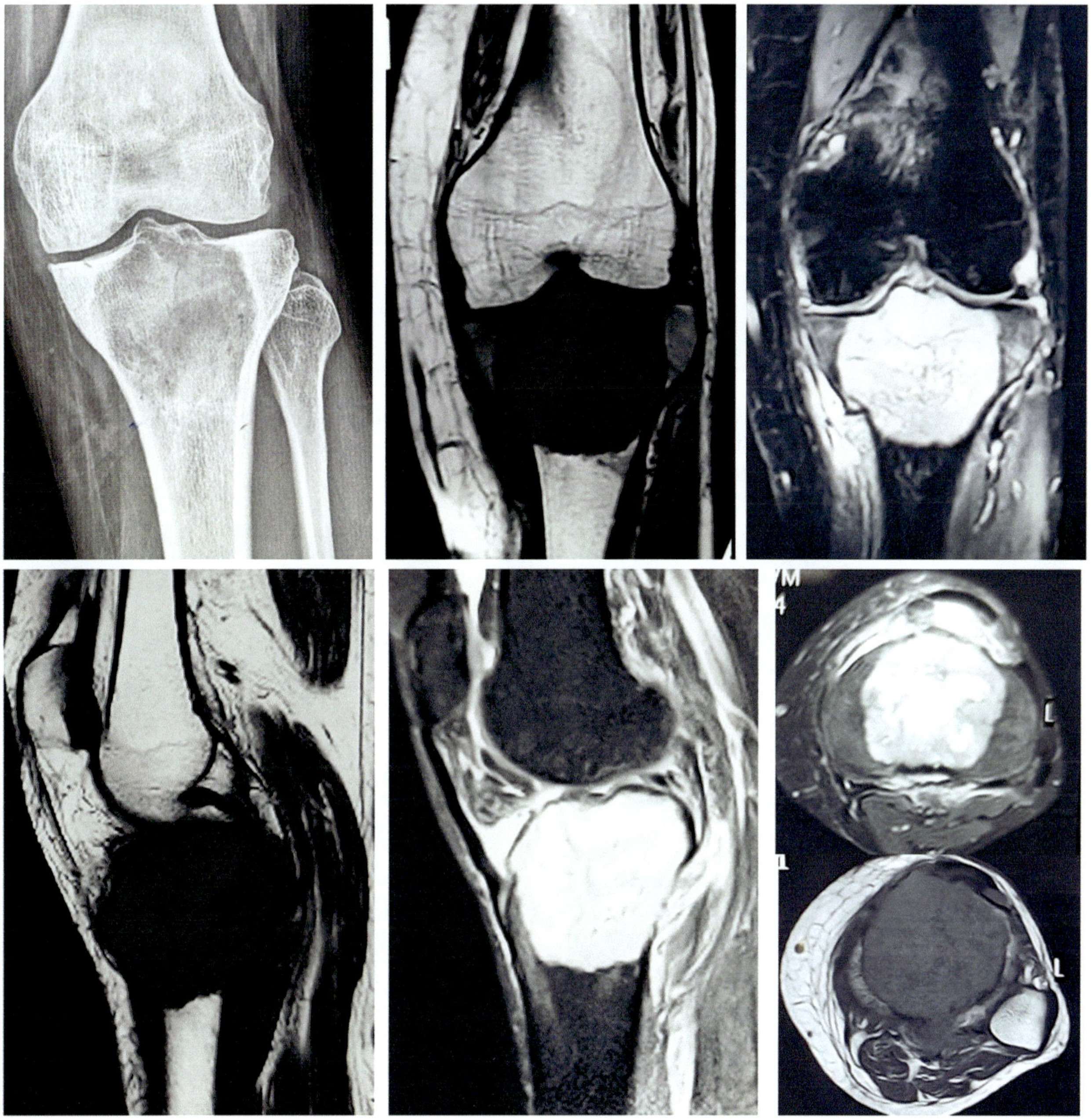

FIGURE 19.1 Radiological evaluation of a giant cell tumor of the proximal tibia in a young female. Plain radiograph reveals a well-defined, expansile lytic lesion with cortical thinning. MRI demonstrates the full extent of the lesion, including its intraosseous spread and soft tissue involvement, providing essential detail for preoperative planning of extended curettage.

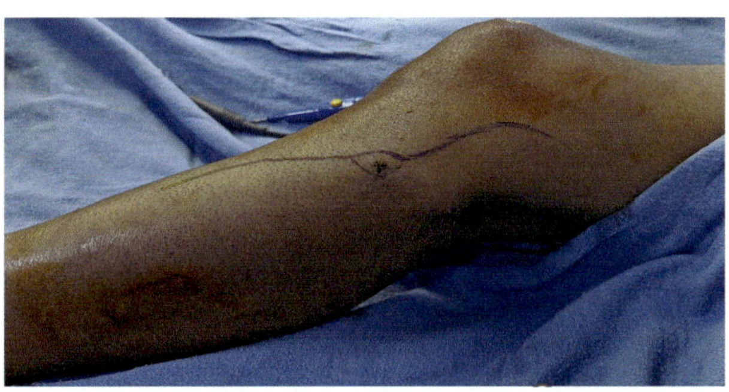

FIGURE 19.2 A longitudinal or curvilinear incision is made to approach the involved bone.

This stage is critical—microscopic remnants often reside in irregular recesses invisible to the naked eye.

Pulsatile Lavage

Before adjuvant application or reconstruction, pulsatile saline lavage is performed to:

- Remove bone dust and necrotic debris from burring.
- Flush microscopic tumor remnants from crevices.
- Create a clean bed for subsequent adjuvant treatment or grafting (Figure 19.7).

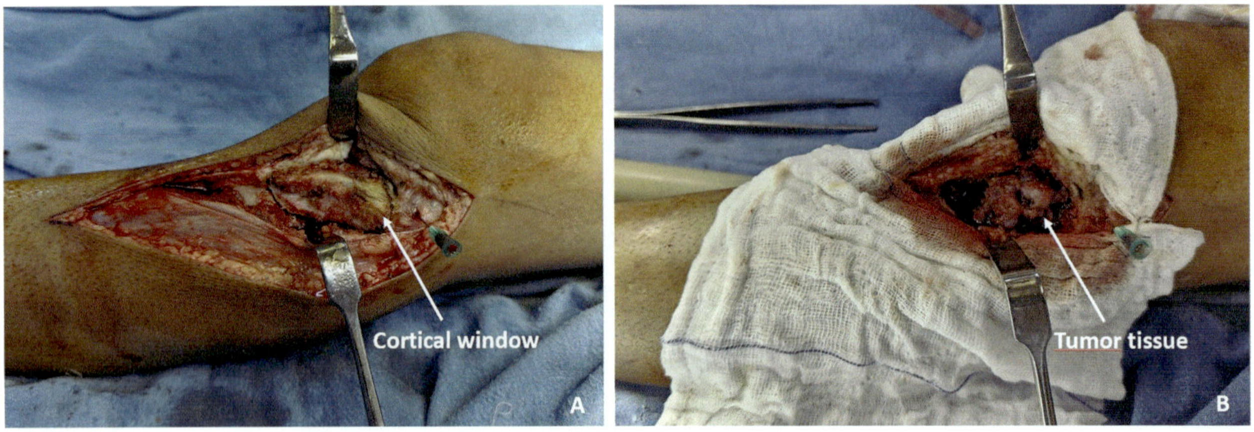

FIGURE 19.3 (A) A cortical window is marked. Wet sponges are packed around the window to avoid the spillage of tumor tissue. (B) Creation of the window provides access to the tumor tissue. The cortical window must be sufficiently large to allow direct visualization and full instrument access to ensure completeness of clearance and local control.

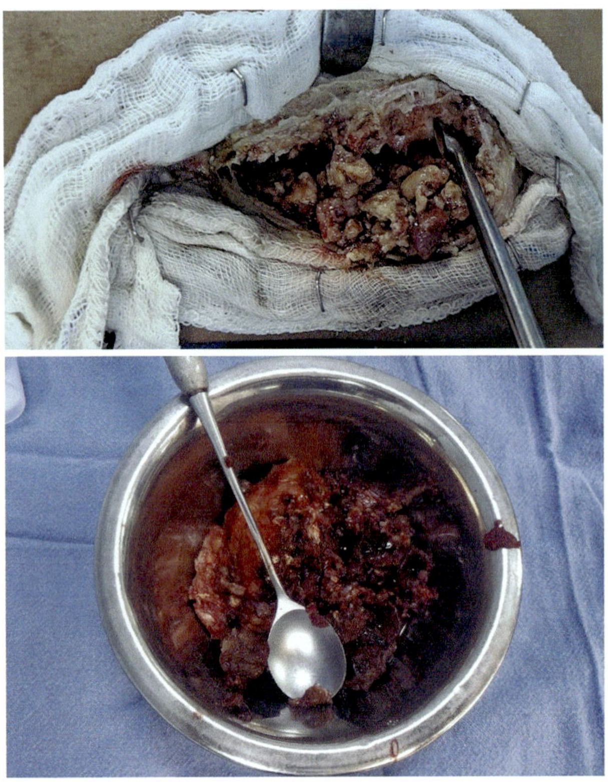

FIGURE 19.4 Gross tumor removal is performed using variable-sized curettes.

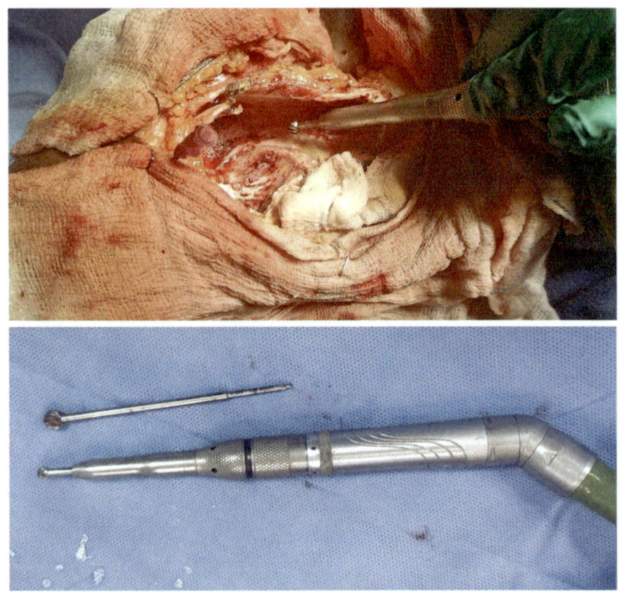

FIGURE 19.5 The walls and edges of the cavity are treated with a high-speed burr to remove residual microscopic tumor and provide access to the trabeculated cavities by smoothing irregular contours within the cavity. Burring effectively "exteriorizes" the cavity, allowing comprehensive debridement that manual curettage alone may not achieve, essential in tumors with trabeculated or septated internal architecture.

Some surgeons repeat curettage and burring after initial lavage ("second pass"), which can yield additional tumor fragments and further reduce recurrence risk. Dental mirrors are useful tools to visualize obscured areas within the cavity (Figure 19.8).

Extending Curettage with Adjuvants

Even with meticulous curettage and burring, the irregular architecture of the tumor cavity may permit residual microscopic disease. Local adjuvants extend the cytotoxic effect intralesionally through chemical, thermal, or physical means. Examples include the following:

- **Chemical agents**: phenol, ethanol, and hydrogen peroxide—cause protein denaturation and membrane disruption (Figure 19.9).
- **Thermal methods**: cryotherapy, cautery—induce cellular apoptosis via extreme temperatures.
- **Physical modalities**: polymethylmethacrylate (PMMA) cementation—provides thermal necrosis during polymerization.

While widely employed, no single adjuvant has demonstrated absolute superiority. The thoroughness of mechanical clearance remains the most critical determinant of local control, with adjuvants serving as complementary, not substitutive, measures.

Rationale and Classification of Adjuvants

The rationale for using local adjuvants in the intralesional management of benign and low-grade malignant bone tumors stems from the goal of eradicating microscopic residual disease that may persist despite meticulous mechanical debridement. While wide resection offers superior oncologic control, it is often associated with disproportionate functional and cosmetic morbidity, particularly in periarticular locations. Adjuvant-enhanced curettage represents a balanced strategy—preserving anatomy while aiming to improve local control rates.

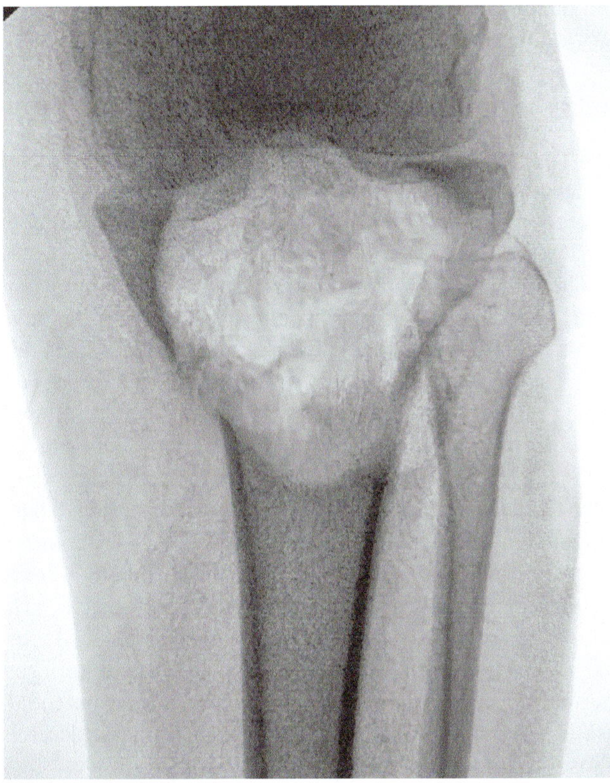

FIGURE 19.6 Intraoperative fluoroscopy may be used to verify the complete spatial reach of curettage.

Classification of Local Adjuvants

Local adjuvants are generally classified into three broad categories:

1. **Thermal agents**—e.g., liquid nitrogen (LN), argon beam coagulation, electrocautery.
2. **Chemical agents**—e.g., phenol, ethanol, hydrogen peroxide (H_2O_2), zinc chloride ($ZnCl_2$).
3. **Mechanical/physical agents**—e.g., high-speed burring (already integral to curettage) and polymethylmethacrylate (PMMA), which functions primarily as a structural filler but also offers limited thermal cytotoxicity.

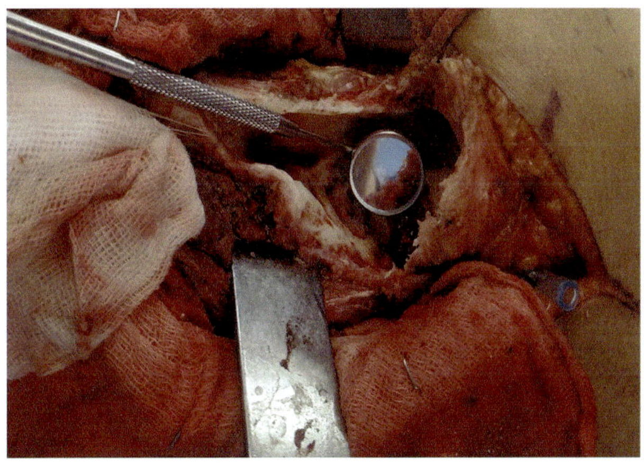

FIGURE 19.8 Dental mirrors are used to visualize obscured areas within the cavity.

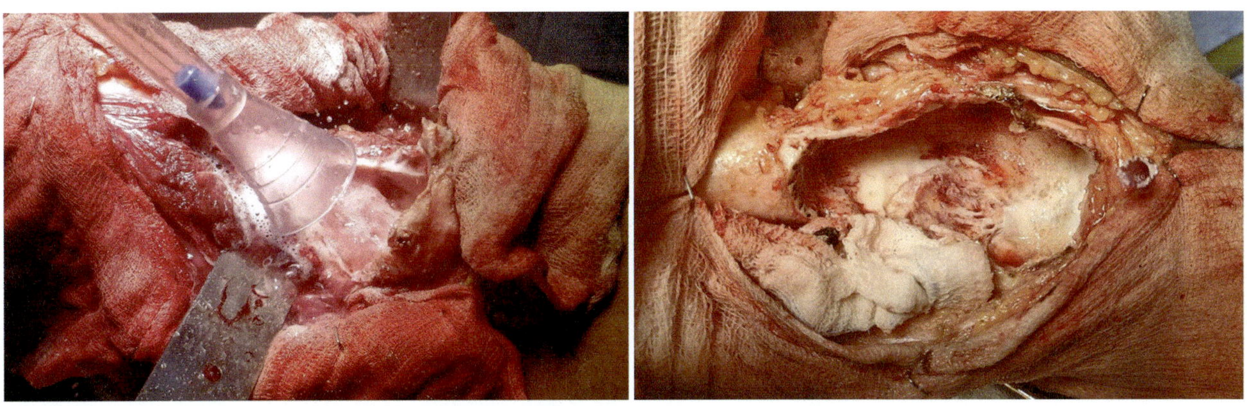

FIGURE 19.7 Pulsatile saline lavage is performed to remove bone dust and necrotic debris from burring, flush microscopic tumor remnants from crevices, and create a clean bed for subsequent adjuvant treatment or grafting.

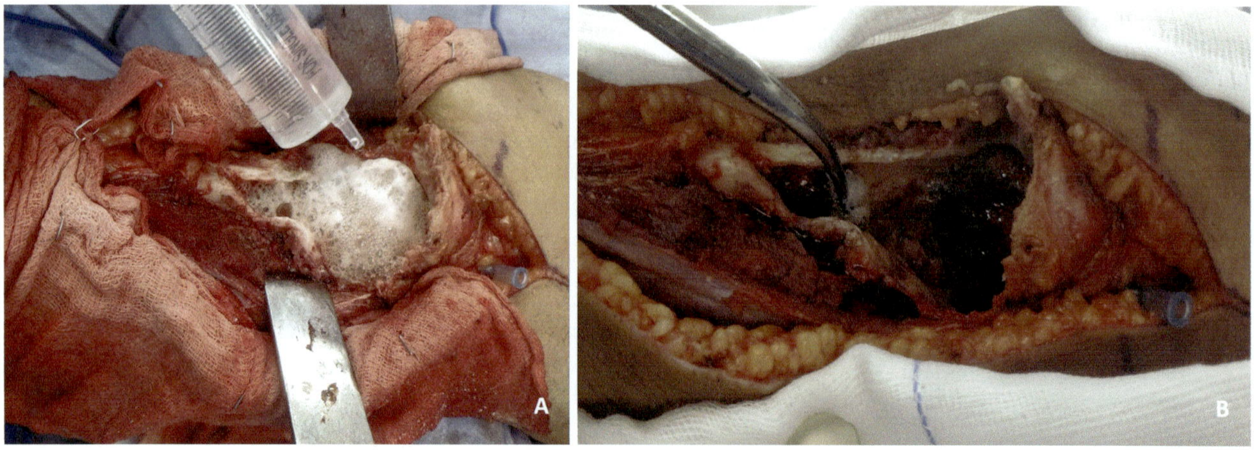

FIGURE 19.9 The cavity is treated with local adjuvants, including hydrogen peroxide (A) and (B) phenol, to extend the margins of the curettage by their cytotoxic effects.

Common Adjuvants and Their Characteristics

Among the various local adjuvants employed in the intralesional management of benign and low-grade malignant bone tumors, **cryoablation** with LN is regarded as one of the most potent. Its mechanism relies on the formation of intracellular ice crystals, disruption of cell membranes, and subsequent vascular stasis, culminating in irreversible cell death. Typically, two to three freeze-thaw cycles are applied directly to the walls of the curetted cavity, achieving bone necrosis to a depth of up to 2 cm [3]. Clinical studies have reported local recurrence rates ranging from 0% to 38%, with a median of approximately 11% [1, 4–7]. Despite its oncological efficacy, cryoablation is associated with notable complications, including pathological fractures in 4.7%–14% of cases, deep infections in 4%–6%, and degenerative joint changes in 2%–16.6% [1]. These complications are primarily related to the extent of thermal injury, particularly in situations where adjacent neurovascular or soft tissue structures are inadequately insulated. The technique is resource-intensive, technically demanding, and is best reserved for aggressive or recurrent lesions where the potential benefit justifies the higher morbidity.

Phenol remains one of the most widely used chemical adjuvants, especially in the treatment of GCTs. Applied in concentrations ranging from 50% to 90%, it induces superficial chemical necrosis through protein coagulation. Following application for approximately two to five minutes, phenol is neutralized with alcohol or saline to prevent collateral tissue injury. Reported recurrence rates after phenol use vary between 0% and 28%, with a median of about 12% [1, 8, 9]. However, its tissue penetration is shallow—approximately 200 microns or 19 cell layers [10, 11]—limiting its cytotoxic effect to superficial residual tumor cells. While phenol is generally safe when handled with appropriate precautions, accidental exposure can cause local tissue damage due to its caustic nature. The evidence supporting its additive benefit remains mixed, with some studies suggesting no significant reduction in recurrence when phenol is used alongside meticulous curettage and high-speed burring [12, 13].

Thermal adjuvants such as **argon beam coagulation** have gained popularity as an alternative to cryotherapy. Argon beam coagulation delivers a unipolar electrical current via a jet of inert argon gas, producing controlled coagulative necrosis of the curetted cavity walls [14]. This allows for uniform treatment of smooth-walled lesions and can be particularly effective in large cavities with accessible geometry. Clinical studies in GCTs treated with argon beam coagulation , high-speed burring, and PMMA have reported recurrence rates of 8.1% [15], while in aneurysmal bone cysts, recurrence rates range between 0% and 7.5% [16, 17]. Limitations of argon beam coagulation include reduced efficacy in irregular or multilobulated cavities where uniform thermal coverage is difficult to achieve and the potential risk of thermal injury to adjacent neurovascular structures if insulation is inadequate.

Polymethylmethacrylate (PMMA), although not strictly classified as an adjuvant, is frequently used for reconstruction after curettage and confers limited tumoricidal benefit through the exothermic polymerization process, which generates heat capable of inducing thermal necrosis up to 1–2 mm from the cement–bone interface. Its primary advantages include immediate mechanical stability, allowing early mobilization, and the facilitation of postoperative surveillance due to its radiopacity. Nevertheless, the thermal effect of PMMA is modest, and its placement near subchondral bone—especially within 1 cm—risks thermal damage to articular cartilage, potentially resulting in degenerative changes [19, 20].

Other chemical agents such as **zinc chloride ($ZnCl_2$), ethanol, and hydrogen peroxide (H_2O_2)** have also been explored. Zinc chloride induces apoptotic cell death while preserving cellular architecture, whereas ethanol and hydrogen peroxide exert cytotoxic effects through membrane disruption, enzyme inactivation, and DNA damage. In vitro studies by Gortzak et al. demonstrated comparable cytotoxicity among these agents and phenol, showing significant reductions in DNA content and metabolic activity in GCT cells at 24 to 120 hours post-exposure [21]. However, despite promising laboratory results, the clinical efficacy of these agents remains uncertain, largely due to their limited tissue penetration, challenges in achieving uniform contact with irregular cavities, and potential local toxicity.

Evidence and Controversy

Despite the widespread use of these adjuvants, no single agent has demonstrated clear superiority in randomized trials. Several comparative studies suggest that the adequacy of curettage—including wide exposure, use of burrs, and pulsatile lavage—is more critical than the specific choice of adjuvant [22, 23]. For instance, van der Heijden et al. found no significant difference in recurrence rates among patients treated with phenol, cryoablation, or PMMA, although complication rates were higher with cryoablation [24]. Similarly, studies by Ghert et al. and Turcotte et al. showed no added benefit of adjuvants over high-speed burring alone [25, 26]. Furthermore, systematic reviews and meta-analyses have concluded that adjuvants may not independently reduce recurrence when curettage and burring are adequately performed [27].

Practical Recommendations

- Phenol remains the most widely used adjuvant due to its ease of application, low cost, and acceptable safety profile.
- Cryoablation may be reserved for aggressive or recurrent lesions, given its higher morbidity and technical demands.
- PMMA is best viewed as a reconstructive filler rather than a tumoricidal agent.
- Adjuvant choice should be individualized based on tumor biology, location, prior treatment, and surgeon experience.

Reconstruction of the Defect Following Curettage

Reconstruction of bone defects after intralesional curettage is an integral component of limb salvage surgery for benign and low-grade malignant bone tumors. The principal objectives are to restore mechanical stability, enable early functional recovery, and reduce the risk of complications such as fracture, joint degeneration, or local recurrence. The choice of reconstructive method is influenced by defect size, anatomical location, subchondral bone involvement, patient age, tumor aggressiveness, and anticipated load-bearing demands.

Small defects that do not compromise bone stability may be left unfilled, allowing spontaneous healing through blood clot organization and ossification. However, larger cavities require structural reconstruction, traditionally achieved with either polymethylmethacrylate (PMMA) cement or bone grafts, each with specific benefits and limitations.

PMMA cement is among the most frequently used reconstructive materials owing to its immediate load-bearing capability, radiopacity for surveillance, and potential tumoricidal effect from exothermic polymerization, which penetrates up to 1–2 mm into adjacent bone [18]. It is especially advantageous in metaphyseal lesions requiring early rehabilitation. Nevertheless, when placed directly beneath subchondral cartilage, PMMA has been associated with degenerative joint changes [19, 20]. To prevent this, the "sandwich technique," interposing cancellous bone graft beneath the subchondral plate and placing cement deeper within the cavity, is recommended (Figure 19.10).

Autologous cancellous bone grafts, commonly harvested from the iliac crest, remain the gold standard for small to moderate-sized defects where biological healing is prioritized. They provide osteoconductive, osteoinductive, and osteogenic properties, enabling complete bone regeneration. Limitations include donor site morbidity, restricted graft volume, and slower consolidation compared to cement. Autografts are preferred in younger patients, epiphyseal lesions, and high-load joint regions, where long-term preservation of joint congruity is essential.

Allografts, either structural or morselized, offer an alternative when autograft volume is inadequate. They act as a scaffold for host bone incorporation without donor site morbidity, though incorporation is generally slower. Potential drawbacks include variable resorption, risk of nonunion, and rare disease transmission.

For complex reconstructions, particularly in weight-bearing bones or juxta-articular locations, composite techniques—combining biological grafts near the joint surface with PMMA in the deeper cavity—allow simultaneous mechanical strength and biological integration, potentially minimizing cartilage degeneration while enabling early mobilization.

Synthetic bone substitutes such as hydroxyapatite, β-tricalcium phosphate, and calcium sulfate provide biocompatible, osteoconductive scaffolds without donor site morbidity. Their ready availability is advantageous, but their mechanical strength is inferior to PMMA, limiting their use to non-weight-bearing applications or as adjuncts in composite constructs. In cases of extensive lesions with substantial cortical thinning, internal fixation may be necessary to prevent pathological fracture and to stabilize the reconstruction.

Key determinants in selecting the reconstruction method include the lesion's proximity to a joint, defect size, patient activity level, and availability of grafting materials or bone bank facilities. When appropriately chosen and executed, reconstruction following curettage achieves high rates of pain relief, functional recovery, and long-term durability without compromising oncological safety. Complications, although infrequent, include fractures when mechanical support is inadequate, joint degeneration following subchondral cementation, graft resorption or nonunion with allografts, and diagnostic challenges in detecting recurrence beneath dense cement.

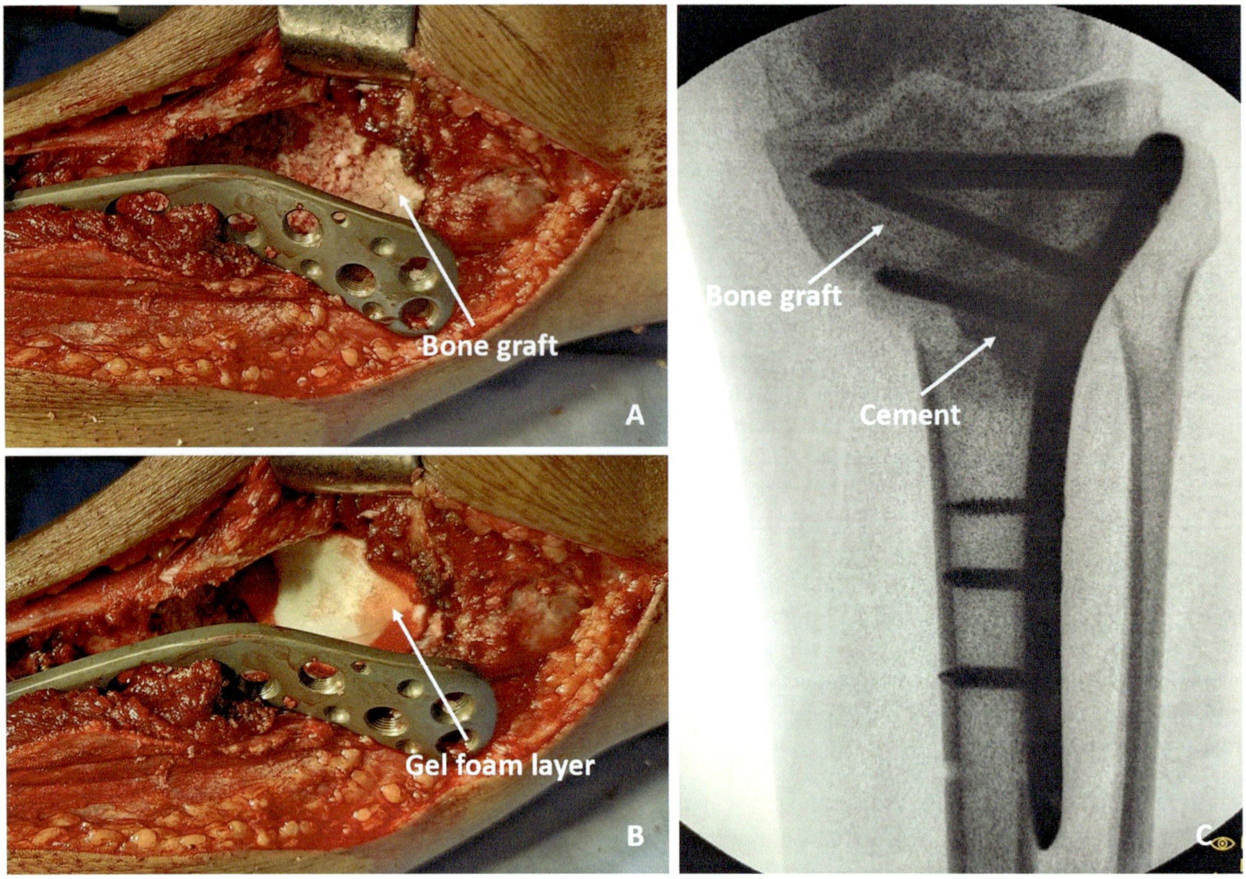

FIGURE 19.10 (A) A layer of morselized allograft juxtaposed beneath the subchondral plate serves as a biological scaffold for host bone incorporation and prevents damage to the articular cartilage by the exothermic polymerization of PMMA cement. (B) A layer of gel foam is positioned between the subchondral bone graft and cement filled within the cavity. (C) Intraoperative fluoroscopic image showing bone graft placed beneath the articular surface and the residual cavity filled with cement, along with plate fixation for structural support.

PERCUTANEOUS TREATMENT OF BENIGN BONE TUMORS

Minimally invasive percutaneous techniques have emerged as effective alternatives or adjuncts to open surgical approaches in the management of benign bone tumors. These image-guided interventions aim to achieve oncologic control while preserving native anatomy, function, and structural integrity. With advances in cross-sectional imaging, needle-based instrumentation, and thermal ablation technology, these techniques allow precise targeting of tumor tissue, minimizing morbidity and expediting recovery. They are particularly valuable in patients with lesions in surgically challenging locations, those unfit for major surgery, or those desiring rapid return to activity with minimal cosmetic impact.

Commonly used percutaneous modalities include thermal ablation methods such as radiofrequency ablation (RFA), cryoablation, and microwave ablation, as well as cementoplasty, curopsy, and sclerotherapy. Procedures are performed under CT, fluoroscopic, or ultrasound guidance, and occasionally under real-time MRI for margin monitoring.

SCLEROTHERAPY IN ANEURYSMAL BONE CYSTS

Aneurysmal bone cysts are benign, expansile, and locally destructive lesions predominantly affecting children and young adults. Once considered reactive in nature, many cases are now recognized to have a neoplastic basis, with USP6 gene rearrangements identified in a significant proportion. While most frequently located in the metaphyseal regions of long bones, aneurysmal bone cysts may also occur in the pelvis, spine, and other skeletal sites. Traditional treatment has been intralesional curettage with or without adjuvants and grafting; however, recurrence rates of 18%–50% and perioperative morbidity have prompted the development of less invasive options.

Sclerotherapy exploits the vascular architecture of aneurysmal bone cysts. Injection of a sclerosant into the cystic spaces induces endothelial damage, thrombosis, and fibrosis, resulting in cavity collapse and eventual ossification. Among various agents, **polidocanol** has gained prominence due to its favorable safety profile and reproducible outcomes. The technique involves aspiration of cyst contents via a Jamshidi or similar needle under fluoroscopic or CT guidance, followed by instillation of 3% polidocanol at approximately 1 ml per cubic centimeter of lesion volume (maximum 6 ml per session; Figure 19.11). Needle tract sealing and saline flushing help prevent extravasation into soft tissues. The procedure is usually outpatient, under local or light general anesthesia, with activity restriction during early healing.

Radiographic and clinical follow-up is conducted every six to eight weeks, with healing indicated by pain resolution, cortical reconstitution, and increasing sclerosis (Figure 19.12). Repeat injections may be given at two to three month intervals if residual cystic spaces persist. Rastogi et al. [28] reported an 84% clinical response and 97% overall healing rate with an average of three injections. Jasper et al. [29] noted an 83% cure rate, though recurrence risk was higher in younger children and in lesions involving the physis or lower limbs. Varshney et al. [30] demonstrated healing in 93.3% of patients treated with sclerotherapy compared with 84.8% after curettage.

Advantages of sclerotherapy include minimal invasiveness, preservation of bone and joint surfaces, avoidance of surgical morbidity, and early return to normal activities—attributes particularly important in skeletally immature patients [31]. Complications are rare but may include skin necrosis, hypopigmentation, and allergic reactions; severe adverse events such as embolic complications have been reported with older agents like Ethibloc, now largely abandoned. Contraindications include lesions with neurological or vascular compression, pathological fracture, and patients with certain comorbidities (e.g., cardiac disease, asthma, pregnancy).

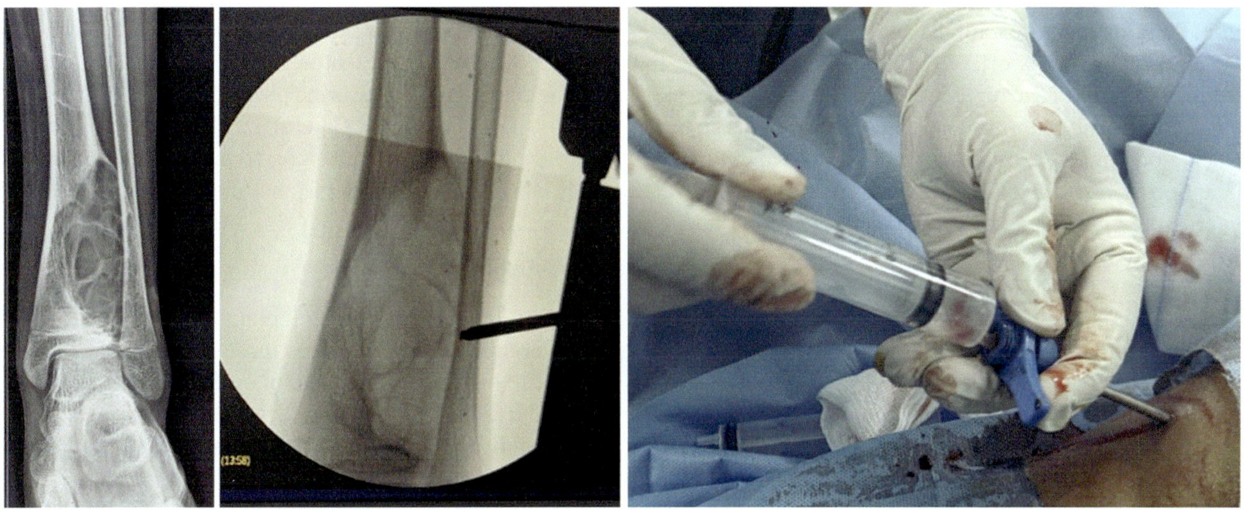

FIGURE 19.11 Percutaneous treatment of aneurysmal bone cysts (ABC) involves aspiration of cyst contents via a Jamshidi needle under fluoroscopic or CT guidance, followed by instillation of 3% polidocanol.

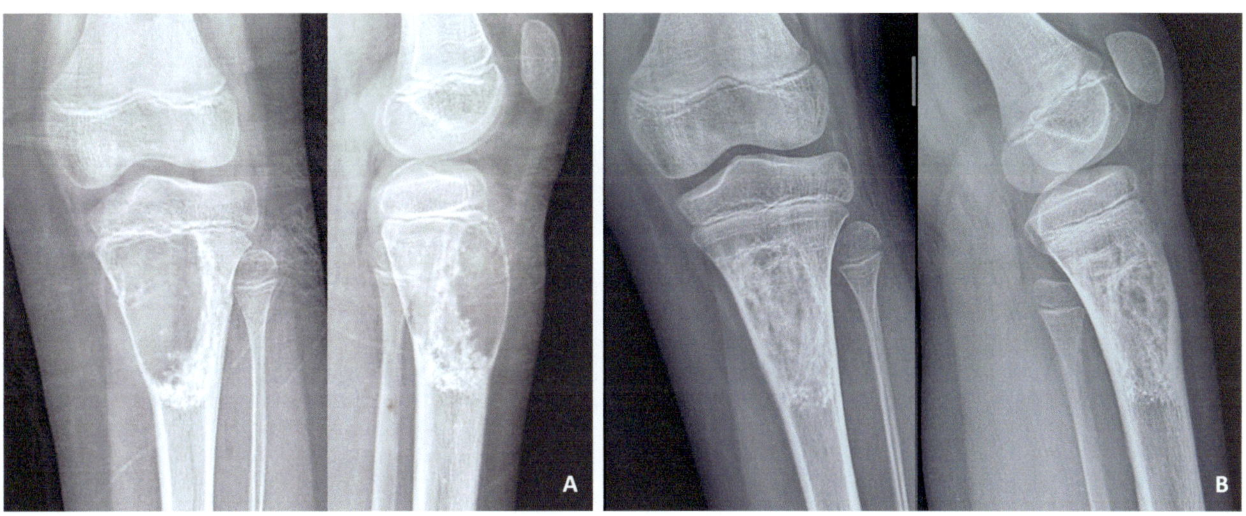

FIGURE 19.12 (A) Plain radiographs of ABC involving the proximal tibia in a 9-year-old female. (B) Radiographs following 2 percutaneous injections of Polidocanol showed a good healing response with cortical reconstitution and sclerosis.

A novel related approach, **curopsy**—percutaneous biopsy combined with limited curettage—has shown spontaneous healing in over 80% of patients in one series [32], suggesting that minimal mechanical disruption may suffice in selected cases. Overall, polidocanol sclerotherapy is now widely regarded as a first-line option for accessible, uncomplicated aneurysmal bone cysts [33].

RADIOFREQUENCY ABLATION (RFA)

RFA is the standard of care for **osteoid osteoma**, offering over 90%–95% success rates with rapid symptom relief and minimal morbidity [34, 35]. It delivers high-frequency alternating current through an electrode positioned in the nidus under CT guidance, heating tissue to approximately 90°C for four to six minutes to induce coagulative necrosis (Figure 19.13).

In larger or more vascular lesions such as **osteoblastoma**, RFA may require multiple applications or electrodes, though cryoablation is often preferred when proximity to neural or vascular structures increases the risk of thermal injury. **Chondroblastomas**, especially those in periarticular locations, may be treated with RFA to avoid surgical disruption of cartilage or growth plates, but caution is warranted in weight-bearing bones due to the risk of chondrolysis or articular collapse [36].

CRYOABLATION

Cryoablation destroys tumor tissue via freeze-thaw cycles that cause membrane rupture, vascular thrombosis, and apoptosis. Argon gas-based probes create an "ice ball" visible under imaging, allowing precise control of ablation margins. This makes it particularly suited for lesions near neurovascular bundles or cartilage, where thermal injury must be avoided. Although widely used for metastatic and malignant bone tumors, its application in benign lesions such as chondroblastomas and aggressive fibrous dysplasia is increasing [37].

RFA for osteoid osteoma achieves durable symptom resolution in over 95% of cases, with recurrence rates below 5% in most series. Cryoablation and microwave ablation have also shown high efficacy, particularly for lesions in anatomically complex or surgically risky locations. Complications, though infrequent, include thermal injury to adjacent structures, post-procedural fractures, and infection; careful ablation planning under image guidance is essential to minimize these risks.

The key benefits of percutaneous therapy include shorter hospital stays, faster recovery, superior cosmetic results, and lower complication rates compared with open surgery. Limitations include reduced ability to histologically assess lesions, potential for incomplete ablation in large or irregular tumors, and the unsuitability of these methods for expansile or structurally destabilizing lesions where reconstruction is required.

In summary, percutaneous treatments—particularly polidocanol sclerotherapy for aneurysmal bone cysts and RFA for osteoid osteoma—represent effective, minimally invasive options that align with the principles of limb preservation and functional optimization. Careful patient selection, precise image-guided technique, and long-term follow-up are critical to achieving optimal oncologic and functional outcomes.

SUMMARY

- Intralesional curettage remains the cornerstone of surgical management for most benign bone tumors, with outcomes improved by extended curettage using adjuvants.
- Adjuvant modalities such as phenol, cryotherapy, argon beam coagulation, and PMMA enhance local control but must be tailored to lesion location and risk profile.
- Defect reconstruction post-curettage requires individualized strategies, balancing biological integration (grafts) and mechanical stability (cement or composites).

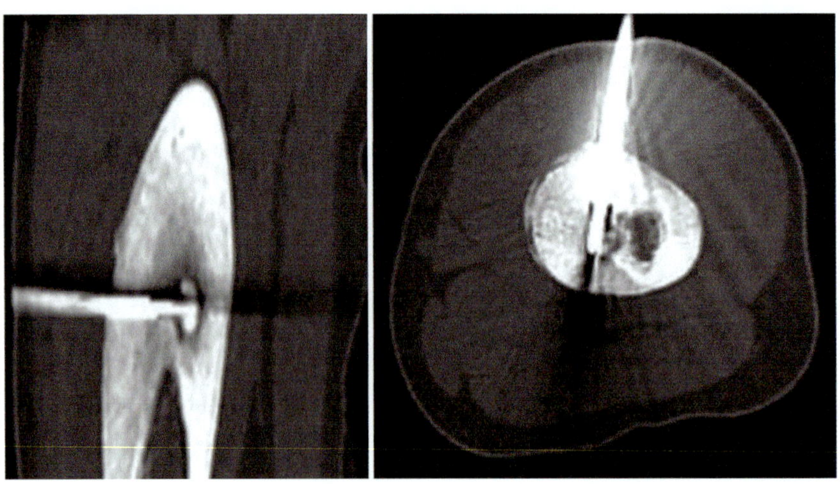

FIGURE 19.13 Radiofrequency ablation of osteoid osteoma of the femur. The figure shows the electrode positioned in the nidus under CT guidance.

- Sclerotherapy, particularly using polidocanol, is an effective and minimally invasive alternative to surgery for aneurysmal bone cysts, offering high cure rates with low morbidity.
- Percutaneous image-guided techniques, including RFA and cryoablation, provide safe and effective management options, especially for osteoid osteomas and deep-seated lesions.

REFERENCES

1. Bickels J, Campanacci DA. Local adjuvant substances following curettage of bone tumors. *J Bone Joint Surg Am.* 2020;102(2):164–174. doi:10.2106/JBJS.19.00470
2. Errani C, Ruggieri P, Asenzio MA, et al. Giant cell tumor of the extremity: a review of 349 cases from a single institution. *Cancer Treat Rev.* 2010;36(1):1–7. doi:10.1016/j.ctrv.2009.09.002
3. Marcove RC, Weis LD, Vaghaiwalla MR, Pearson R, Huvos AG. Cryosurgery in the treatment of giant cell tumors of bone. A report of 52 consecutive cases. *Bull Hosp Joint Dis.* 1978;39(1):12–34.
4. Abdelrahman M, Bassiony AA, Shalaby H, Assal MK. Cryosurgery and impaction subchondral bone graft for the treatment of giant cell tumor around the knee. *HSS J.* 2009;5(2):123–128. doi:10.1007/s11420-009-9125-8
5. Rahman MA, El Masry AM, Azmy SI. Review of 16 cases of aneurysmal bone cyst in the proximal femur treated by extended curettage and cryosurgery with reconstruction using autogenous nonvascularized fibula graft. *J Orthop Surg (Hong Kong).* 2018;26(2):2309499018783905. doi:10.1177/2309499018783905
6. Mohler DG, Chiu R, McCall DA, Avedian RS. Curettage and cryosurgery for low-grade cartilage tumors is associated with low recurrence and high function. *Clin Orthop Relat Res.* 2010;468(10):2765–2773. doi:10.1007/s11999-010-1445-y
7. Meftah M, Schult P, Henshaw RM. Long-term results of intralesional curettage and cryosurgery for treatment of low-grade chondrosarcoma. *J Bone Joint Surg Am.* 2013;95(15):1358–1364. doi:10.2106/JBJS.L.00442
8. Lin WH, Lan TY, Chen CY, Wu K, Yang RS. Similar local control between phenol- and ethanol-treated giant cell tumors of bone. *Clin Orthop Relat Res.* 2011;469(11):3200–3208. doi:10.1007/s11999-011-1962-3
9. Moon MS, Kim SS, Moon JL, Kim SS, Moon H. Treating giant cell tumours with curettage, electrocautery, burring, phenol irrigation, and cementation. *J Orthop Surg (Hong Kong).* 2013;21(2):209–212. doi:10.1177/230949901302100219
10. Mittag F, Leichtle C, Kieckbusch I, et al. Cytotoxic effect and tissue penetration of phenol for adjuvant treatment of giant cell tumours. *Oncol Lett.* 2013;5(5):1595–1598. doi:10.3892/ol.2013.1244
11. Nithyananth M, Priscilla AJ, Boopalan PV, Titus VT, Lee VN. Time required for effective action of phenol against giant cell tumour cells. *J Orthop Surg (Hong Kong).* 2014;22(1):104–107. doi:10.1177/230949901402200126
12. Trieb K, Bitzan P, Lang S, Dominkus M, Kotz R. Recurrence of curetted and bone-grafted giant-cell tumours with and without adjuvant phenol therapy. *Eur J Surg Oncol.* 2001;27(2):200–202. doi:10.1053/ejso.2000.1086
13. O'Donnell RJ, Springfield DS, Motwani HK, Ready JE, Gebhardt MC, Mankin HJ. Recurrence of giant-cell tumors of the long bones after curettage and packing with cement. *J Bone Joint Surg Am.* 1994;76(12):1827–1833. doi:10.2106/00004623-199412000-00009
14. Bickels J, Kollender Y, Merimsky O, Isaakov J, Petyan-Brand R, Meller I. Closed argon-based cryoablation of bone tumours. *J Bone Joint Surg Br.* 2004;86(5):714–718. doi:10.1302/0301-620x.86b5.14416
15. Lewis VO, Wei A, Mendoza T, Primus F, Peabody T, Simon MA. Argon beam coagulation as an adjuvant for local control of giant cell tumor. *Clin Orthop Relat Res.* 2007;454:192–197. doi:10.1097/01.blo.0000238784.98606.d4
16. Cummings JE, Smith RA, Heck RK Jr. Argon beam coagulation as adjuvant treatment after curettage of aneurysmal bone cysts: a preliminary study. *Clin Orthop Relat Res.* 2010;468(1):231–237. doi:10.1007/s11999-009-0914-7
17. Steffner RJ, Liao C, Stacy G, et al. Factors associated with recurrence of primary aneurysmal bone cysts: is argon beam coagulation an effective adjuvant treatment?. *J Bone Joint Surg Am.* 2011;93(21):e1221–e1229. doi:10.2106/JBJS.J.01067
18. Puri A, Agarwal M. Treatment of giant cell tumor of bone: current concepts. *Indian J Orthop.* 2007;41(2):101–108. doi:10.4103/0019-5413.32039
19. van der Heijden L, van de Sande MA, Heineken AC, Fiocco M, Nelissen RG, Dijkstra PD. Mid-term outcome after curettage with polymethylmethacrylate for giant cell tumor around the knee: higher risk of radiographic osteoarthritis?. *J Bone Joint Surg Am.* 2013;95(21):e159. doi:10.2106/JBJS.M.00066
20. Caubère A, Harrosch S, Fioravanti M, Curvale G, Rochwerger A, Mattei JC. Does curettage-cement packing for treating giant cell tumors at the knee lead to osteoarthritis?. *Orthop Traumatol Surg Res.* 2017;103(7):1075–1079. doi:10.1016/j.otsr.2017.06.013
21. Gortzak Y, Kandel R, Deheshi B, et al. The efficacy of chemical adjuvants on giant-cell tumour of bone. An in vitro study. *J Bone Joint Surg Br.* 2010;92(10):1475–1479. doi:10.1302/0301-620x.92b10.23495
22. Prosser GH, Baloch KG, Tillman RM, Carter SR, Grimer RJ. Does curettage without adjuvant therapy provide low recurrence rates in giant-cell tumors of bone?. *Clin Orthop Relat Res.* 2005;(435):211–218. doi:10.1097/01.blo.0000160024.06739.ff
23. Arbeitsgemeinschaft K, Becker WT, Dohle J, et al. Local recurrence of giant cell tumor of bone after intralesional treatment with and without adjuvant therapy. *J Bone Joint Surg Am.* 2008;90(5):1060–1067. doi:10.2106/JBJS.D.02771
24. van der Heijden L, van der Geest IC, Schreuder HW, van de Sande MA, Dijkstra PD. Liquid nitrogen or phenolization for giant cell tumor of bone?: a comparative cohort study of various standard treatments at two tertiary referral centers. *J Bone Joint Surg Am.* 2014;96(5):e35. doi:10.2106/JBJS.M.00516
25. Turcotte RE, Wunder JS, Isler MH, et al. Giant cell tumor of long bone: a Canadian Sarcoma Group study. *Clin Orthop Relat Res.* 2002;(397):248–258. doi:10.1097/00003086-200204000-00029
26. Ghert MA, Rizzo M, Harrelson JM, Scully SP. Giant-cell tumor of the appendicular skeleton. *Clin Orthop Relat Res.* 2002;(400):201–210. doi:10.1097/00003086-200207000-00025
27. Algawahmed H, Turcotte R, Farrokhyar F, Ghert M. High-speed burring with and without the use of surgical adjuvants in the intralesional management of giant cell tumor

of bone: a systematic review and meta-analysis. *Sarcoma.* 2010;2010:586090. doi:10.1155/2010/586090

28. Rastogi S, Varshney MK, Trikha V, Khan SA, Choudhury B, Safaya R. Treatment of aneurysmal bone cysts with percutaneous sclerotherapy using polidocanol. A review of 72 cases with long-term follow-up. *J Bone Joint Surg Br.* 2006;88(9):1212–1216. doi:10.1302/0301-620X.88B9.17829
29. Jasper J, van der Heijden L, van Rijswijk CSP, van de Sande MAJ. Efficacy of sclerotherapy with polidocanol (ethoxysclerol) in primary aneurysmal bone cysts in children and adolescents. *J Pediatr Orthop.* 2021;41(7):e555–e562. doi:10.1097/BPO.0000000000001839
30. Varshney MK, Rastogi S, Khan SA, Trikha V. Is sclerotherapy better than intralesional excision for treating aneurysmal bone cysts?. *Clin Orthop Relat Res.* 2010;468(6):1649–1659. doi:10.1007/s11999-009-1144-8
31. Puthoor D, Francis L, Ismail R. Is sclerotherapy with polidocanol a better treatment option for aneurysmal bone cyst compared to conventional curettage and bone grafting?. *J Orthop.* 2021;25:265–270. Published 2021 May 21. doi:10.1016/j.jor.2021.05.020
32. Reddy KI, Sinnaeve F, Gaston CL, Grimer RJ, Carter SR. Aneurysmal bone cysts: do simple treatments work?. *Clin Orthop Relat Res.* 2014;472(6):1901–1910. doi:10.1007/s11999-014-3513-1
33. Samargandi R, Alkameshki M, Barnawi M, et al. Efficacy of percutaneous treatment of primary aneurysmal bone cysts (ABCs): a systematic review and meta-analysis. *J Clin Med.* 2023;12(23):7213. Published 2023 Nov 21. doi:10.3390/jcm12237213
34. Gangi A, Alizadeh H, Wong L, Buy X, Dietemann JL, Roy C. Osteoid osteoma: percutaneous laser ablation and follow-up in 114 patients. *Radiology.* 2007;242(1):293–301. doi:10.1148/radiol.2421041404
35. Koch G, Cazzato RL, Gilkison A, Caudrelier J, Garnon J, Gangi A. Percutaneous treatments of benign bone tumors. *Semin Intervent Radiol.* 2018;35(4):324–332. doi:10.1055/s-0038-1673640
36. Xie C, Jeys L, James SL. Radiofrequency ablation of chondroblastoma: long-term clinical and imaging outcomes. *Eur Radiol.* 2015;25(4):1127–1134. doi:10.1007/s00330-014-3506-1
37. Callstrom MR, Atwell TD, Charboneau JW, et al. Painful metastases involving bone: percutaneous image-guided cryoablation--prospective trial interim analysis. *Radiology.* 2006;241(2):572–580. doi:10.1148/radiol.2412051247

20 Management of Appendicular Skeletal Metastasis

INTRODUCTION

Skeletal metastases are the most common malignant bone lesions, far exceeding the incidence of primary bone tumors. With improvements in systemic therapies and increased cancer survivorship, the prevalence of metastatic bone disease—particularly in the appendicular skeleton—is rising. Up to 70% of patients with advanced malignancies will develop bone metastases, with the limbs and girdles frequently affected due to their rich vascularity and red marrow content [1, 2]. Breast, prostate, lung, kidney, and thyroid cancers account for the majority of cases, with common metastatic sites including the spine, proximal femur, pelvis, ribs, and proximal humerus.

The management goals for appendicular skeletal metastases are pain relief, preservation or restoration of function, prevention or treatment of pathological fractures, and enhancement of quality of life. Unlike primary bone sarcomas, where curative resection is often attempted, treatment is typically palliative, aiming for rapid recovery with durable solutions that exceed the patient's expected survival [3].

Orthopedic surgeons often play a pivotal role in diagnosis and intervention, requiring close collaboration with medical and radiation oncologists to tailor management. While many lesions respond to systemic therapy and radiation, surgical intervention becomes essential in cases of mechanical instability or high fracture risk. Surgery should provide immediate stability, pain relief, and early mobilization, using mechanically robust and oncologically sound constructs [4].

Recent advances in immunotherapy, targeted agents, and bone-modifying drugs such as bisphosphonates and RANKL inhibitors have extended survival in several cancers [5, 6]. Consequently, orthopedic reconstructions must now meet higher demands for durability, functional restoration, and patient-centered outcomes.

CLINICAL EVALUATION AND DIAGNOSIS

Assessment of suspected appendicular skeletal metastasis begins by distinguishing between patients with a known malignancy and those in whom a bone lesion is the first sign of cancer [7]. In the latter, differential diagnoses include primary bone tumors, benign lesions, and metabolic bone disease. In adults over 40 years, metastasis, multiple myeloma, and lymphoma are the most likely causes of destructive bone lesions unless proven otherwise [3].

HISTORY AND EXAMINATION

A detailed history should document prior or current cancer diagnoses, systemic symptoms (weight loss, fatigue, anorexia), and site-specific complaints. A history of minimal trauma in the setting of a fracture should raise suspicion for pathological fracture. Symptoms pointing to a primary tumor—e.g., chronic cough or hemoptysis (lung), urinary changes (prostate), or breast lumps—should be actively sought.

Physical examination includes systemic and local assessments: neck/chest for lymphadenopathy, breast exam in females, per-rectal exam in males with suspected prostate cancer, and palpation of the affected site for tenderness or masses. Mechanical pain that is activity-related and relieved by rest often suggests structural compromise and impending fracture.

IMAGING

Plain radiographs remain the primary tool for characterizing lesions as lytic, blastic, or mixed. Lytic lesions (renal, thyroid, myeloma) carry a higher risk of fracture than blastic lesions (breast, prostate) (Figure 20.1). CT offers superior cortical detail for surgical planning, while MRI delineates medullary involvement, soft tissue extension, and neurovascular relationships. Whole-body staging with bone scintigraphy, FDG-PET, or PET-CT is crucial to define disease extent; PET-CT provides high sensitivity and specificity for detecting occult metastases and guiding biopsy [7].

LABORATORY WORKUP

Baseline tests include complete blood count, ESR, calcium, alkaline phosphatase, liver function, PSA (men), and serum protein electrophoresis. In selected cases, serum free light chains, and beta-2 microglobulin help diagnose myeloma. Rougraff et al. demonstrated that systematic integration of imaging and laboratory tests identifies the primary tumor in 85%–90% of cases [2].

BIOPSY

Histopathology is the diagnostic gold standard and is essential when the diagnosis is uncertain, particularly in patients without a known primary cancer. Biopsy should follow complete staging to avoid compromising future oncologic resection. Image-guided core needle biopsy of the most

DOI: 10.1201/9780367822002-25

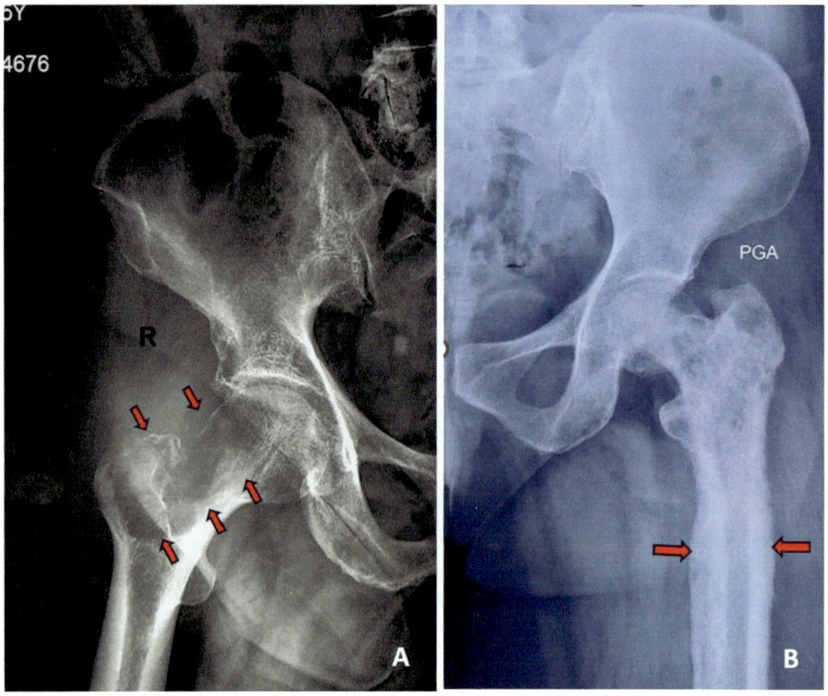

FIGURE 20.1 Plain radiographs showing metastatic involvement of the proximal femur. (A) Lytic metastasis in the proximal femur (red arrows) in a patient with known renal cell carcinoma, demonstrating cortical destruction and loss of trabecular architecture. (B) Sclerotic (blastic) metastatic deposits in the femoral shaft (red arrows) in a patient with breast carcinoma, characterized by diffuse increased bone density and cortical thickening. These radiographic appearances highlight the contrasting patterns of lytic and blastic metastases associated with different primary malignancies.

accessible lesion is preferred. For vascular tumors (renal, thyroid), biopsy should be deferred until after embolization to reduce hemorrhage risk. Careful incision placement and trajectory planning are critical to avoid contamination of uninvolved compartments.

FRACTURE RISK ASSESSMENT

Accurate evaluation of fracture risk is critical in determining the need for prophylactic stabilization of long bones with metastatic lesions. Mirel's scoring system remains the most widely used tool, assessing four parameters—anatomical location, lesion type (lytic, blastic, mixed), lesion size relative to bone diameter, and pain—each graded from 1 to 3, with a total score of 4–12 (Table 20.1) [8]. Scores ≥9 indicate high fracture risk warranting surgical fixation, scores ≤7 suggest conservative management, and a score of 8 lies in a clinical "gray zone," requiring multidisciplinary judgment. Functional pain during activity or weight-bearing is considered the most important predictor, often outweighing radiographic features [9].

While practical, Mirel's system has limitations—particularly low specificity (35%) despite high sensitivity (91%)—leading to potential overtreatment [10]. To improve precision, CT-based structural rigidity analysis (CTRA) quantifies mechanical strength from cross-sectional imaging, achieving 100% sensitivity and 60.6% specificity in femoral lesions, thereby enhancing confidence in borderline cases [11].

Fracture risk assessment should integrate clinical symptoms, lesion morphology, mechanical demands, and imaging findings rather than relying solely on a scoring system [12]. This is especially relevant in equivocal cases, where additional imaging or multidisciplinary discussion can guide management.

A distinct clinical challenge is the presentation with a pathological fracture, often the first manifestation of metastatic disease. Although most are due to metastases, benign bone tumors, metabolic disorders (e.g., hyperparathyroidism), and primary sarcomas must be excluded. Early

TABLE 20.1
Mirel's Scoring System for Predicting Pathologic Fracture Risk

Criteria	Score 1	Score 2	Score 3
1. Site	Upper limb	Lower limb	Peritrochanteric region
2. Pain	Mild	Moderate	Functional
3. Lesion Type	Blastic	Mixed	Lytic
4. Size (Cortical Involvement)	< 1/3	1/3 to 2/3	> 2/3

orthopedic–oncology–radiology collaboration is essential to ensure accurate diagnosis and appropriate treatment planning.

CLINICAL DECISION-MAKING FOR PATIENTS WITH METASTATIC BONE DISEASE

The decision to undertake surgical intervention for appendicular skeletal metastasis must be guided by a multidisciplinary evaluation that balances the goals of palliation, mechanical stability, functional restoration, and, in selected cases, disease control. The primary objective of surgery in the metastatic setting is not oncologic cure, but rather maximization of quality of life through restoration of function and relief of pain.

Surgical treatment is generally indicated in the following scenarios:

- **Impending or actual pathological fractures**, especially in weight-bearing bones.
- **Intractable pain** not responsive to medical or radiation therapy.
- **Failure of nonoperative measures**, including radiotherapy or pharmacologic interventions.
- **Solitary or oligometastatic lesions**, particularly in long-term survivors, where definitive control may be beneficial.
- **Mechanical instability**, threatening mobility and independence.

The **selection of surgical candidates** must be individualized, considering several factors:

- The **nature of the primary malignancy**, including responsiveness to systemic therapies.
- The **number and anatomical location of metastases**.
- **Patient's life expectancy**, which can be estimated using prognostic models such as PATHFx.
- **Performance status and comorbidities**.
- The **extent of local bone destruction**.
- **Patient's activity level and expectations**.

Patients with generalized metastatic disease, surgically inaccessible lesions, or extensive locoregional tumor extension with a poor prognosis are typically best managed with palliative modalities, including limited surgical interventions (e.g., cement augmentation), low-dose radiation, or systemic therapies [3].

SURVIVAL PREDICTION AND IMPLICATIONS

Accurate estimation of survival is central to planning treatment for appendicular skeletal metastases. As management is largely palliative, surgical interventions must balance expected life expectancy, anticipated functional benefit, and quality of life; both undertreatment of patients likely to live longer and overtreatment of those with limited survival risk offer suboptimal results. Survival prediction models are therefore increasingly integrated into surgical planning to optimize intervention type, implant choice, and rehabilitation strategy.

DETERMINANTS OF SURVIVAL

Several variables influence survival in skeletal metastases:

- **Primary tumor type**: Breast, prostate, and thyroid cancers often have longer survival, particularly with modern targeted therapies, while lung cancer and melanoma carry a poorer prognosis [3, 13]. Average life expectancy with bone metastasis is ~48 months for thyroid, 40 months for prostate, 24 months for breast, 6 months–4–5 years for renal (type dependent), and 6–7 months for lung cancer.
- **Visceral metastases**: Spread to liver, lung, or brain markedly reduces survival.
- **Number and location of bone lesions**: Solitary or oligometastatic disease confers a better prognosis and may justify aggressive surgery [14].
- **Functional status and comorbidities**: Higher performance scores (Karnofsky, ECOG) and fewer comorbidities correlate with prolonged survival.
- **Response to systemic therapy**: Effective chemotherapy, hormonal therapy, or immunotherapy, especially in renal, breast, or myeloma metastases, can extend survival.

PROGNOSTIC TOOLS

The **PATHFx** Bayesian machine-learning algorithm incorporates demographic, oncologic, clinical, and laboratory parameters to predict individualized 3- and 12-month survival probabilities [6]. It has demonstrated good external validation and assists in stratifying patients for durable versus limited interventions [6, 15]. Other prognostic models include the **Bauer Score**, **Katagiri Score**, and **Tokuhashi Score** (more spinal-specific), which provide quick bedside estimations but are less precise than PATHFx.

IMPLICATIONS FOR SURGICAL PLANNING

Survival prediction directly informs surgical decision-making:

- **<3 months survival** → Prioritize nonoperative or minimally invasive palliation (e.g., PMMA (Poly methyl methacrylate) augmentation, intralesional curettage, radiotherapy).
- **3–12 months survival** → Opt for prophylactic fixation with or without cement augmentation, or simpler reconstructions aimed at immediate stability and minimal morbidity.

- **>12 months survival** → Consider durable reconstructions (segmental resection, modular endoprosthesis, biological reconstruction) to avoid revision and accommodate longer postoperative function.

Implant selection should match the mechanical demand for the patient's projected lifespan. Overengineering in short-survival patients can increase operative burden without benefit, whereas underestimating survival risks early implant failure, reoperation, and functional decline. Integrating robust prognostic tools into multidisciplinary planning ensures individualized, durable, and goal-directed care.

PREOPERATIVE CONSIDERATIONS

Preoperative multidisciplinary evaluation is essential to assess surgical candidacy, oncologic control, and optimal timing. Tyrosine kinase inhibitors should be discontinued approximately seven days prior to surgery to minimize bleeding risk and restarted only after satisfactory wound healing. Anti-angiogenic agents such as bevacizumab should be withheld for at least 28 days pre- and postoperatively to reduce wound complications [3].

Highly vascular tumors, particularly renal cell carcinoma, and thyroid carcinoma, benefit from preoperative arterial embolization within 24–48 hours of surgery, which can markedly reduce intraoperative blood loss. Anticipation of significant bleeding warrants cross-matched blood availability, arterial pressure monitoring, and central venous access if necessary. Given that many patients are immunocompromised or have treatment-related comorbidities, optimization of nutrition, coagulation status, renal function, and cardiopulmonary reserve is critical [3].

TREATMENT OF COMPLETE AND/OR IMPENDING FRACTURES IN METASTATIC BONE DISEASE

The primary aim in managing pathological fractures from metastatic disease is to provide immediate mechanical stability, pain relief, and functional restoration rather than fracture healing. Management begins with full staging and diagnostic workup. Radiographs of pathological fractures through metastatic lesions typically reveal destructive lytic lesions, often in the metaphyseal or diaphyseal regions, with minimal periosteal reaction, limited soft tissue swelling, and short fracture lines—features distinguishing them from primary sarcomas (Figure 20.2).

A critical oncologic pitfall is misdiagnosing a primary malignant bone tumor as metastasis. Performing intramedullary nailing without biopsy in such cases can lead to catastrophic tumor contamination of the medullary canal—a "rodded sarcoma" scenario (Figure 20.3). This not only compromises future limb salvage but also increases recurrence and metastasis risk. Inappropriately placed fixation incisions can violate oncologic principles, rendering definitive resection more difficult.

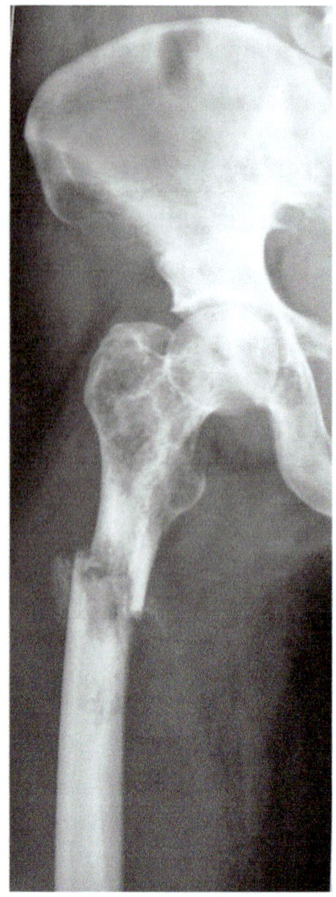

FIGURE 20.2 Plain radiograph of the proximal femur showing a pathological fracture through a metastatic lesion. The destructive lytic focus at the epicenter demonstrates cortical erosion with a short fracture line, minimal periosteal reaction, and limited soft tissue involvement—typical features of metastatic bone disease.

Therefore, in any case where the diagnosis is uncertain, a biopsy planned along future resection lines must precede fixation. This ensures oncologic safety, preserves surgical options, and prevents inadvertent dissemination of a potentially curable primary malignancy.

SURGICAL PRINCIPLES AND IMPLANT SELECTION

The management of complete pathological fractures and impending fractures in metastatic bone disease is guided by similar surgical principles, with the distinction that impending fractures are addressed prophylactically to prevent fracture-related complications, whereas complete fractures require urgent stabilization.

Key oncologic and biomechanical considerations include:

1. **Extent of disease** – differentiating solitary from disseminated lesions.
2. **Primary tumor biology** – accounting for variable healing potential and treatment response (e.g., breast, thyroid vs. lung, renal).

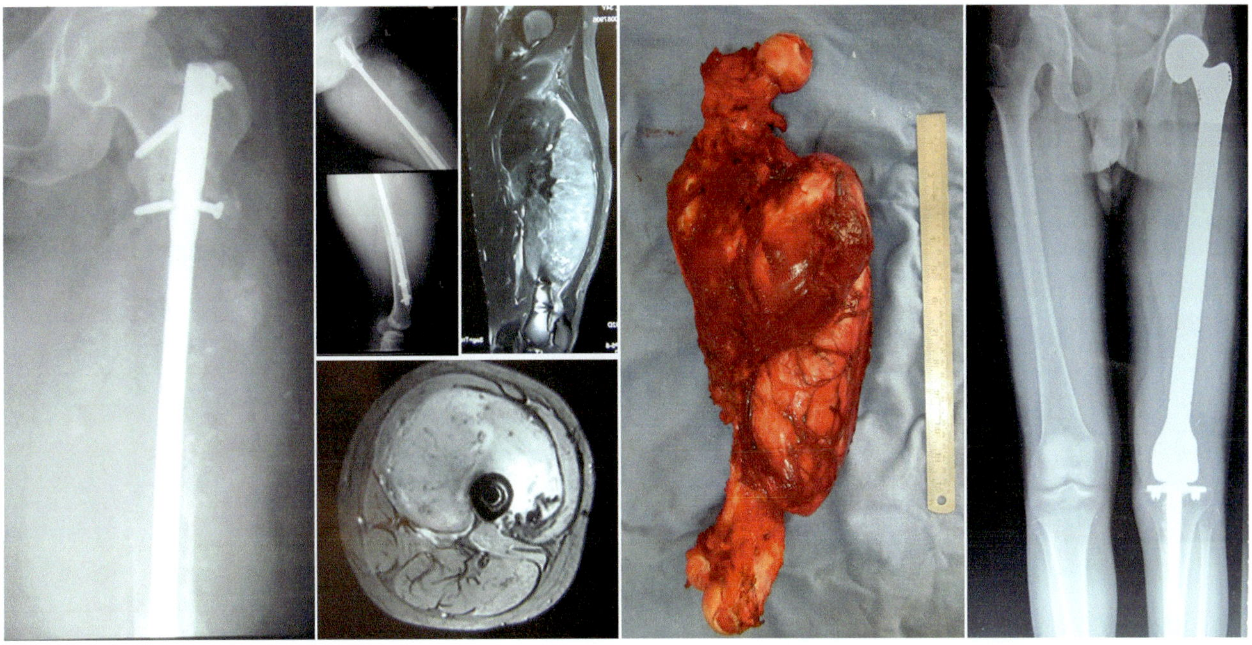

FIGURE 20.3 A 52-year-old male with a presumed pathological fracture of the femur in a known case of prostate cancer. Radiographs showing intramedullary nail fixation performed without biopsy. MRI demonstrating an aggressive lesion with intramedullary and soft tissue involvement surrounding the implant. The unplanned surgical intervention necessitated a wide total femur resection and replacement. Gross specimen of the excised femur with extensive tumor mass following wide total femur resection. Postoperative radiograph showing reconstruction with a total femur megaprosthesis. This case highlights the importance of mandatory biopsy before fixation in suspected pathological fractures to avoid compromising oncological outcomes.

3. **Implant durability** – selecting constructs that withstand high stress without failure.
4. **Prognosis and activity level** – tailoring reconstruction longevity to patient survival and function.

The surgical objective is to create a load-bearing construct that allows immediate mobilization and remains functional for the patient's lifetime. Standard load-sharing devices, such as non-augmented plates, are prone to failure in poorly healing metastatic bone. Instead, **load-bearing implants**—including intramedullary nails (Figures 20.4 and 20.5), modular endoprostheses, and cement-augmented locking plates—are preferred (Table 20.2). In non-healing pathological fractures, cemented fixation or prosthetic replacement should be prioritized. For patients with good prognosis and high activity demands, durable reconstructions such as endoprosthetic replacement or arthroplasty reduce the risk of mechanical failure and the need for revision surgery.

MANAGEMENT OF IMPENDING FRACTURES

Prophylactic fixation of impending fractures is associated with better functional outcomes, lower complication rates, and shorter hospital stays than surgery after fracture occurrence. Prophylactic surgery enables immediate mobilization and mitigates the risk of emergent fracture and complex revision procedures [4].

Indicators for surgical prophylaxis include:

- Pain with functional loading (the most predictive clinical sign)
- Cortical destruction >50% or lesion >2.5 cm (Harrington criteria) [16]
- Mirel's score ≥9 strongly predicts fracture risk and typically warrants surgical stabilization

In the prophylactic management of metastatic bone lesions, diaphyseal involvement is typically addressed using intramedullary fixation (Figures 20.6 and 20.7). In contrast, metaphyseal or periarticular lesions, particularly those sparing the joint, may benefit from cement augmentation with locking plate constructs. When extensive bone lysis is present or systemic therapy is unlikely to be effective, reinforcement with polymethylmethacrylate (PMMA) enhances both initial stability and the longevity of the construct. For lesions with severe structural compromise or when metastectomy offers a survival advantage, segmental resection followed by reconstruction may be the optimal choice to ensure a single-stage, definitive solution.

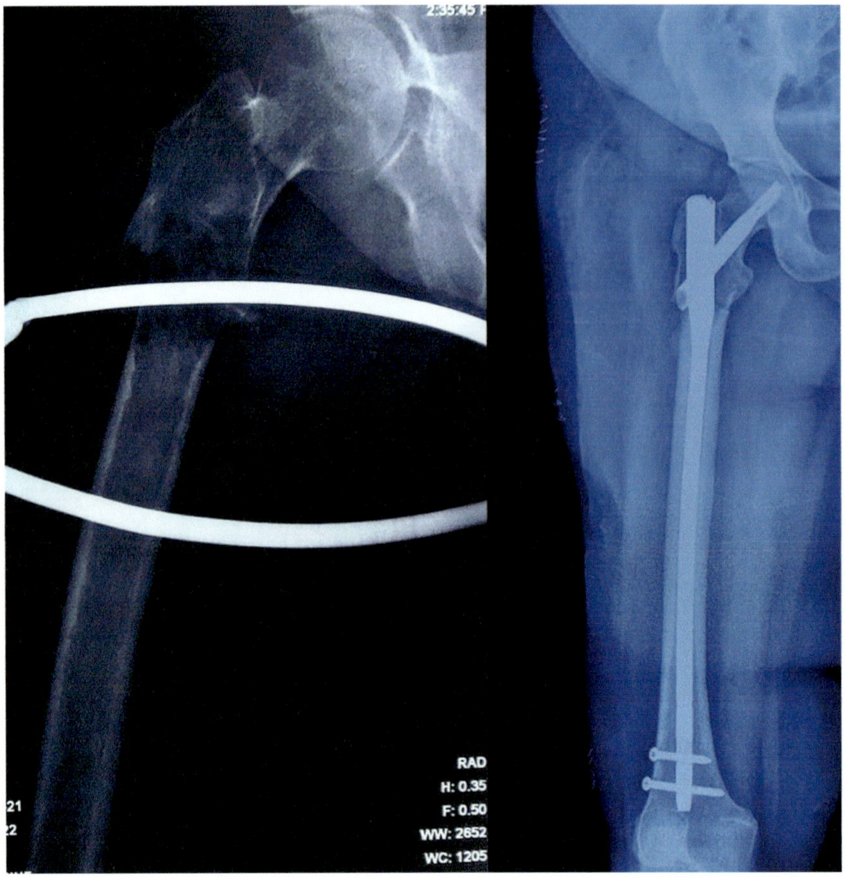

FIGURE 20.4 Intramedullary fixation of a pathological fracture in the subtrochanteric femur secondary to disseminated thyroid cancer. The left image shows a preoperative radiograph with a destructive lytic lesion and pathological fracture through the subtrochanteric region. The right image demonstrates postoperative radiographs following intramedullary fixation with a proximal femoral nail, achieving stable reconstruction and functional restoration.

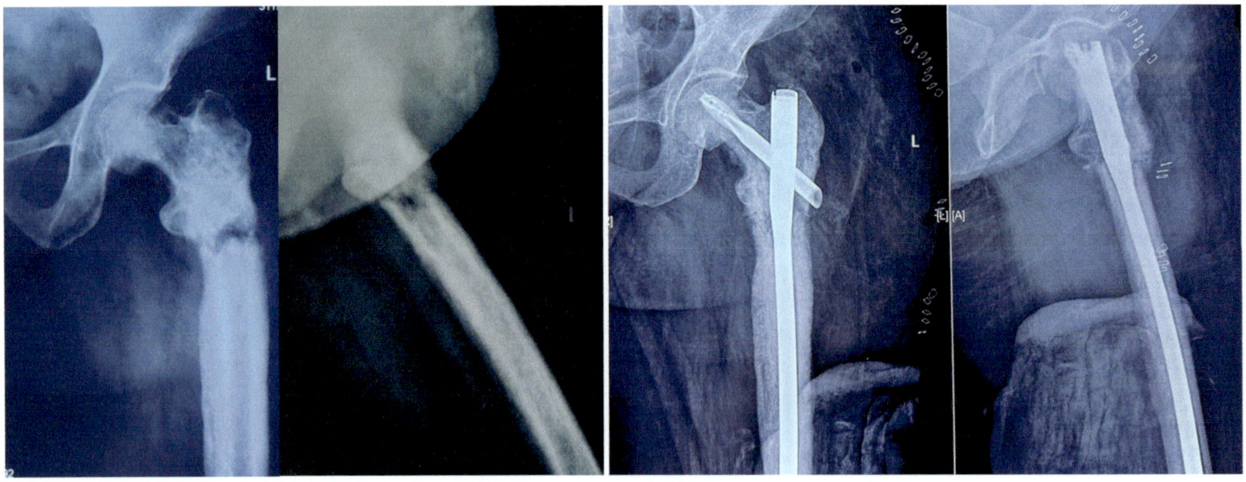

FIGURE 20.5 Intramedullary fixation of a pathological fracture through a metastatic subtrochanteric femoral lesion in a 58-year-old female with disseminated breast cancer. The left image shows a pathological fracture with underlying lytic destruction. The right image demonstrates intramedullary nail fixation with distal locking, offering structural stability and facilitating early mobilization.

TABLE 20.2
Fixation Options Based on Location

Location	Preferred Fixation Options
Diaphyseal fractures	Cement-augmented intramedullary nails or intercalary prostheses
Proximal femur	Cemented hemiarthroplasty, cephalomedullary nails, or total hip arthroplasty
Periarticular or metaphyseal regions	Endoprosthetic replacement for durable reconstruction
Long bone shaft fractures with major destruction	Segmental resection and modular megaprosthesis

RESECTION & ENDOPROSTHETIC REPLACEMENT/ARTHROPLASTY IN METASTATIC BONE DISEASE

Endoprosthetic replacement combined with tumor resection is a definitive and highly effective option for managing appendicular skeletal metastases, particularly in cases where joint involvement or extensive bone destruction preclude reliable fixation. It provides immediate structural stability, enables early full weight-bearing, and offers rapid pain relief with durable functional restoration—critical in patients with limited healing potential. Compared with internal fixation, it is especially advantageous in periarticular and metaphyseal lesions.

INDICATIONS

Endoprosthetic reconstruction is preferred in:

- Extensive metaphyseal or periarticular bone loss
- Articular fractures not amenable to fixation
- Solitary/oligometastatic lesions with longer survival prognosis
- Failed fixation or unstable implants
- High functional demand requiring early mobilization

Commonly reconstructed sites include the proximal humerus, distal femur, and proximal femur (Figure 20.8). Modular prosthetic systems allow precise adaptation to the extent of resection, restoring limb length, alignment,

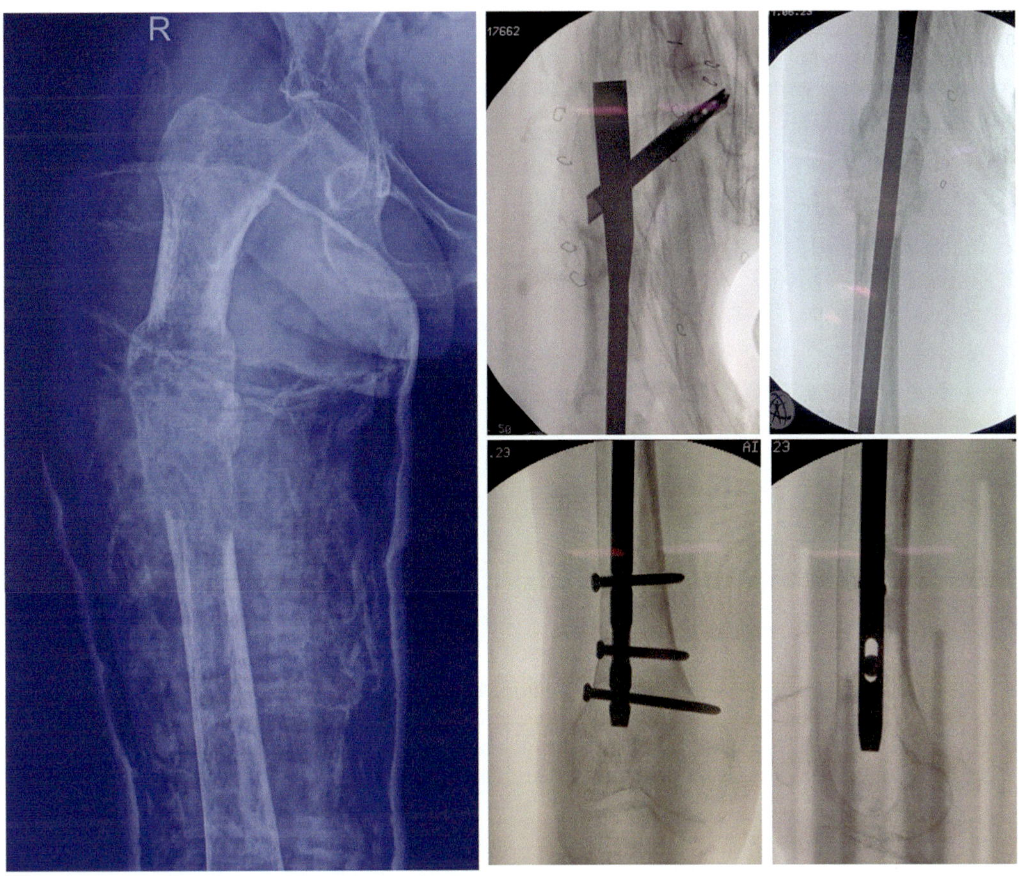

FIGURE 20.6 Prophylactic intramedullary fixation of the femur in disseminated metastatic lung carcinoma. The left image shows a preoperative radiograph demonstrating diffuse metastatic involvement of the femur with an impending subtrochanteric fracture. The right images depict intraoperative fluoroscopy following intramedullary nail placement spanning the full length of the femur, with proximal and distal interlocking screws ensuring stable fixation and fracture prevention.

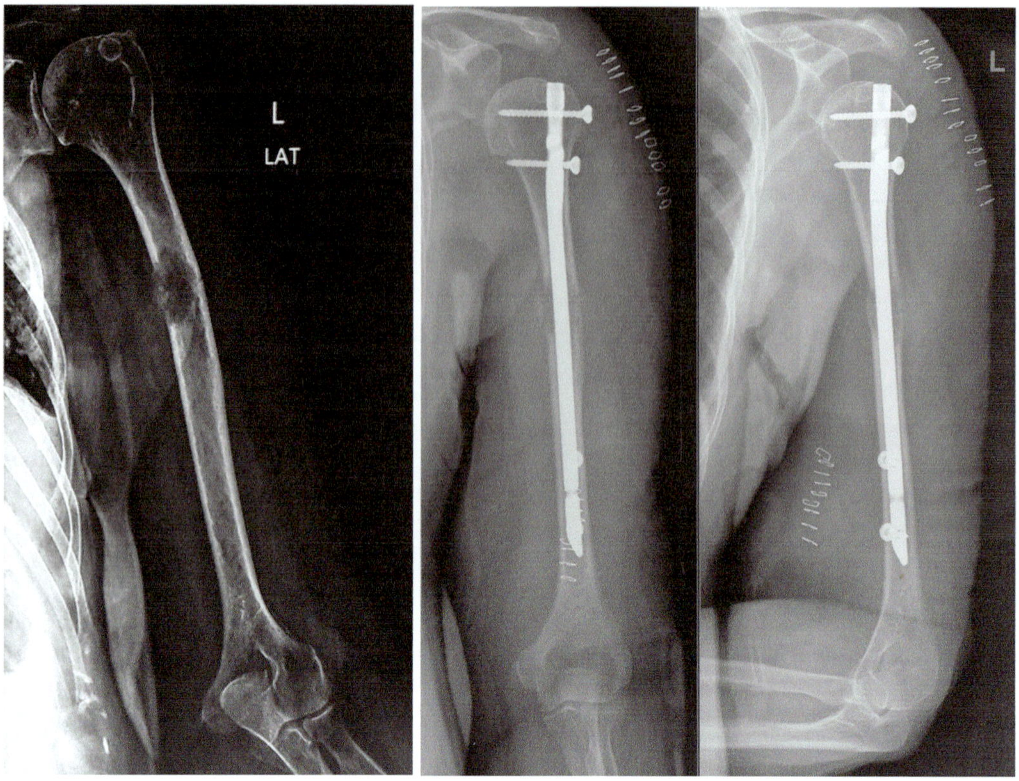

FIGURE 20.7 Prophylactic intramedullary fixation of the humerus in disseminated metastatic breast carcinoma. The left image shows a preoperative radiograph demonstrating a lytic metastatic lesion in the humeral diaphysis with impending fracture. The right images depict postoperative radiographs showing intramedullary nail fixation with proximal and distal interlocking screws, providing stability and preventing pathological fracture.

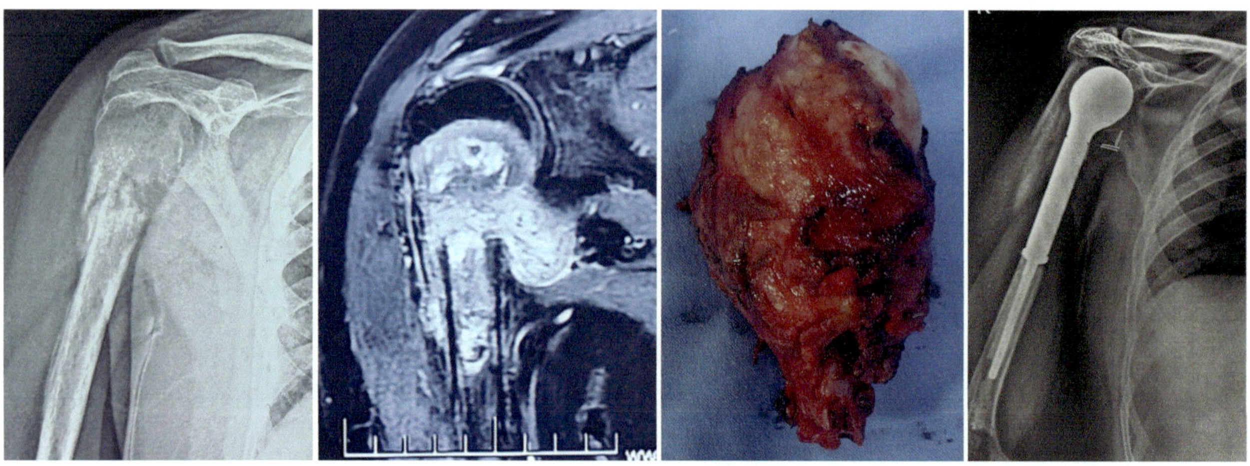

FIGURE 20.8 Metastatic thyroid carcinoma involving the proximal humerus. Preoperative radiograph (left) and MRI (second from left) show a destructive metaphyseal and peri-articular lesion with cortical breach and soft tissue extension. The excised specimen (second from right) demonstrates the tumor-involved proximal humerus following wide resection. Postoperative radiograph (right) depicts endoprosthetic replacement, achieving stable reconstruction and restoration of proximal humeral anatomy.

and function. Intercalary or segmental reconstructions are indicated for diaphyseal lesions, offering definitive, single-stage treatment.

In femoral neck metastases, arthroplasty is favored over intramedullary fixation due to high implant failure rates (Figure 20.9). Cemented fixation is recommended in pathologic or irradiated bone, where biological ongrowth is unlikely. Periacetabular reconstructions follow similar principles, with early studies supporting porous tantalum components for durable fixation.

While long-stem cemented implants have been traditional to span diseased bone and prevent future fractures,

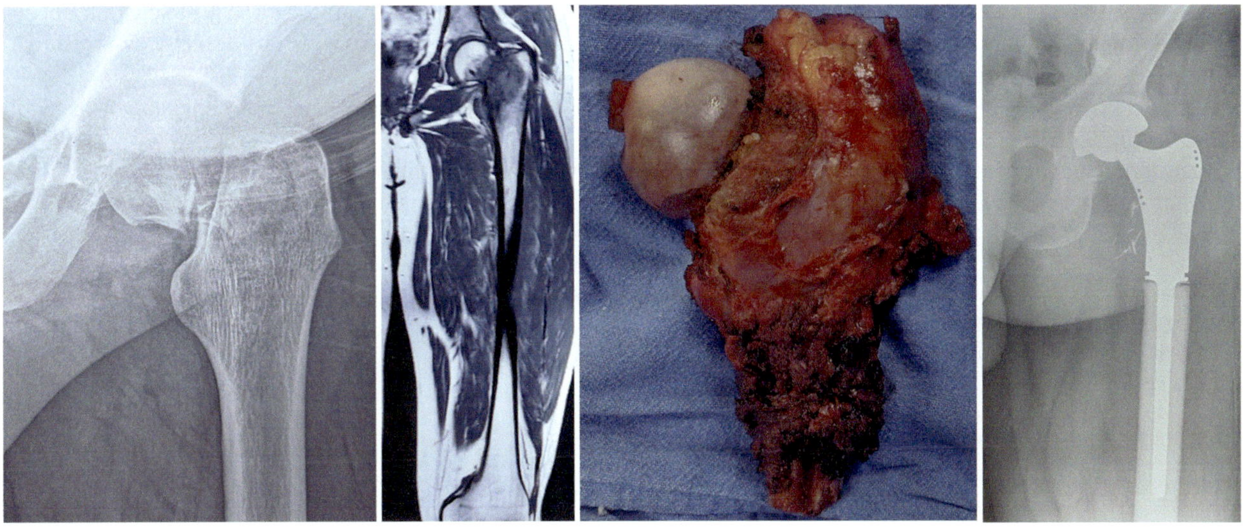

FIGURE 20.9 Metastatic renal cell carcinoma involving the proximal femur. Preoperative radiograph (left) demonstrates a lytic lesion with cortical destruction and pathological fracture. MRI (second from left) confirms a solitary metastatic lesion with soft tissue extension. The excised specimen (second from right) shows the tumor-involved proximal femur after wide resection. Postoperative radiograph (right) illustrates endoprosthetic replacement providing stable reconstruction and restoration of hip anatomy.

selective segmental replacement may suffice in certain patients—except in myeloma or renal cell carcinoma, where skip lesions are more likely [17].

Bone Cement Implantation Syndrome (BCIS) is a recognized intraoperative hazard during cementation, particularly in proximal femoral metastases and in patients with cardiopulmonary disease. It presents with hypoxia, hypotension, arrhythmias, or cardiac arrest. Risk mitigation includes pre-oxygenation, invasive hemodynamic monitoring, adequate volume resuscitation, femoral canal venting, and minimizing cement pressurization [17, 18].

When applied to appropriately selected patients, endoprosthetic and arthroplasty reconstructions achieve predictable results, with Musculoskeletal Tumor Society (MSTS) functional scores typically exceeding 60%–80%. Even in patients with limited life expectancy, over half experience meaningful pain relief, restored mobility, and improved independence. For those with longer survival, durable implants minimize the risk of mechanical failure and reoperation, aligning surgical goals with oncologic prognosis.

By integrating oncologic resection principles with robust mechanical reconstruction, endoprosthetic replacement offers a single, definitive intervention that can maintain patient mobility, optimize function, and preserve dignity in the palliative setting of metastatic bone disease.

PERIACETABULAR METASTASIS

Metastatic involvement of the acetabulum, although less common than other skeletal sites, presents a formidable surgical challenge due to its central role in hip biomechanics and weight transmission. Such lesions can cause acetabular insufficiency or pathological fractures, leading to severe pain, instability, and marked functional loss.

A widely accepted surgical method for reconstruction in this setting is the **Harrington technique**, later refined for improved longevity. This involves retrograde placement of threaded pins through the acetabular dome into the iliac wing to reinforce the weakened bone (Figure 20.10). The pins are embedded within **polymethylmethacrylate (PMMA) cement**, which secures an acetabular support ring, into which a cemented polyethylene liner is inserted. This construct provides strong mechanical stability, enabling early mobilization, effective pain relief, and restoration of hip function. It remains particularly valuable in

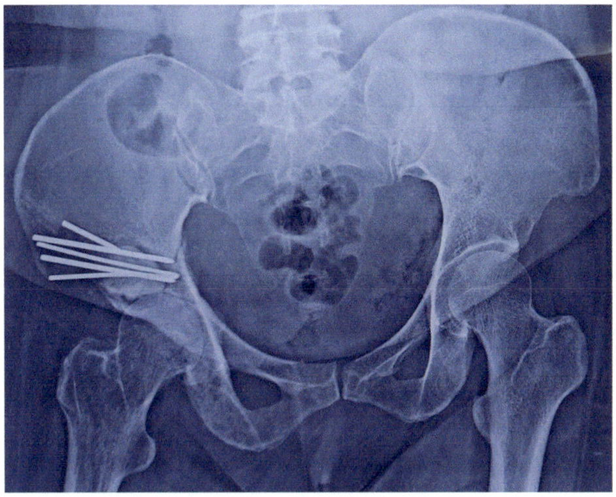

FIGURE 20.10 Harrington technique for peri-acetabular metastasis. Radiograph shows retrograde placement of threaded pins through the acetabular dome into the iliac wing, reinforced with polymethylmethacrylate (PMMA) cement to secure an acetabular support ring, thereby providing structural stability for reconstruction in metastatic acetabular involvement.

patients with limited life expectancy, offering a cost-effective and durable solution.

In cases of extensive periacetabular bone loss, **cemented total hip arthroplasty** is the mainstay of treatment. For patients with longer anticipated survival and adequate residual bone stock, **porous tantalum components** show promising early results by enabling potential biologic fixation and enhanced long-term stability [19].

RESECTION ARTHRODESIS USING INTRAMEDULLARY NAILS AND PMMA CEMENT

In selected cases—particularly young patients with metastatic disease involving the distal femur or proximal tibia—**resection arthrodesis** with intramedullary nailing and PMMA cement provides a stable, durable joint fusion. It can serve as a definitive salvage option or as a temporary reconstruction until prognosis allows for joint-preserving procedures. Limitations include complete loss of knee motion, lower functional scores, and risks of infection, implant failure, and peri-implant fracture. Despite these drawbacks, it remains a viable option when mobility and stability take precedence over joint motion.

POSTOPERATIVE CONSIDERATIONS

Patients undergoing surgery for metastatic bone disease face a higher risk of venous thromboembolism, with reported rates of 7.1% overall, 3.9% for pulmonary embolism, and 3.3% for deep vein thrombosis [20]. Initiation of chemoprophylaxis—unless contraindicated—is essential, with ongoing research needed to define the most effective anticoagulation regimens.

Postoperative radiation therapy is routinely advised to control residual disease, reduce recurrence, and relieve pain, except in patients with very limited life expectancy or prior maximum radiation exposure. The entire implant should be included in the radiation field, typically commencing 2–4 weeks after surgery once wounds have healed.

Systemic cancer therapies—including chemotherapy, targeted agents, and hormonal therapy—should be resumed after adequate wound healing and hematologic recovery. Tyrosine kinase inhibitors and immunotherapies are generally withheld for at least seven days pre- and postoperatively to minimize bleeding and infection risk. Close coordination with oncology ensures optimal, individualized postoperative care.

COMMON COMPLICATIONS AND FAILURE PATTERNS IN METASTATIC BONE DISEASE

Treatment failures may arise due to:

- Inappropriate implant selection (e.g., using load-sharing instead of load-bearing implants).
- Misjudgment of pathology (e.g., using intramedullary nails for solitary lesions wrongly assumed to be metastatic).
- Inadequate fixation length or cementation in highly lytic bones.
- Implant failure or peri-implant fractures due to insufficient mechanical support.
- Non-union and pseudarthrosis, which are frequent due to poor healing capacity of metastatic bone.
- Infection and wound dehiscence, exacerbated by immunosuppression and prior radiotherapy.
- Mechanical loosening of prosthetic components, particularly in the setting of extensive tumor or poor host bone.

KEY TECHNICAL RECOMMENDATIONS

- Rule out a primary tumor of the bone before surgical intervention by biopsy of the lesion.
- Always favor **load-bearing constructs** over load-sharing ones in metastatic fractures.
- Avoid **short segment fixation**; aim to **span the entire diseased bone**.
- Consider **adjuvant bone cement** in cases with poor bone stock or severe osteolysis.
- Ensure that the chosen construct **outlives the patient's survival expectancy**.
- **Cemented constructs** offer immediate mechanical fixation and do not rely on bone ingrowth, making them advantageous in irradiated or lytic bone.

NONOPERATIVE MANAGEMENT OF APPENDICULAR BONE METASTASIS

Nonoperative management plays a pivotal role in patients with appendicular skeletal metastases who have limited life expectancy, poor performance status, or are unsuitable for surgery. The primary aims are fracture prevention, pain palliation, and preservation of function and quality of life.

Pharmacologic options include bisphosphonates, which inhibit osteoclast-mediated bone resorption, reducing skeletal-related events (SREs) and hypercalcemia [20]. Denosumab, a RANKL monoclonal antibody, offers equal or superior efficacy, fewer renal effects, and better compliance [5].

External beam radiotherapy (EBRT) remains the mainstay for painful lesions, achieving pain relief in up to 90% of patients, with complete relief in 50%. Single-fraction (8 Gy) and multi-fraction (20–30 Gy) schedules are effective; however, higher doses carry an increased fracture risk [21].

Radiopharmaceuticals such as Strontium-89, Samarium-153, Rhenium-186, and Radium-223 can provide systemic pain relief and reduce SREs, especially in bone-dominant disease.

Minimally invasive interventions include radiofrequency ablation, CT-guided cryoablation, MR-guided focused ultrasound (rapid pain relief), and electrochemotherapy (bleomycin via electroporation) for refractory pain [22, 23].

Transarterial embolization offers effective palliation in hypervascular metastases, though post-embolization syndrome should be anticipated.

SUMMARY

- **Multidisciplinary evaluation and individualized surgical planning** are paramount to ensure optimal outcomes in skeletal metastasis.
- The principles of orthopedic treatment of metastatic bone disease are to rule out a primary tumor of the bone, to provide adequate stability, and, consequently, to allow early mobilization.
- **Survival prediction and life expectancy** are critical in guiding surgical decision-making.
- **Endoprosthetic replacement and arthroplasty** offer durable reconstruction, especially in periarticular or extensively lytic lesions.
- **Prophylactic fixation** of impending fractures reduces morbidity and enhances postoperative recovery.

REFERENCES

1. American Cancer Society. *Cancer facts & figures 2017*. Atlanta: American Cancer Society; 2017.
2. Rougraff BT, Kneisl JS, Simon MA. Skeletal metastases of unknown origin. A prospective study of a diagnostic strategy. *J Bone Joint Surg Am.* 1993;75(9):1276–1281. doi:10.2106/00004623-199309000-00003
3. Johnson CN, Gurich RW Jr, Pavey GJ, Thompson MJ. Contemporary management of appendicular skeletal metastasis by primary tumor type. *J Am Acad Orthop Surg.* 2019;27(10):345–355. doi:10.5435/JAAOS-D-17-00749
4. Talbot M, Turcotte RE, Isler M, Normandin D, Iannuzzi D, Downer P. Function and health status in surgically treated bone metastases. *Clin Orthop Relat Res.* 2005;438: 215–220. doi:10.1097/01.blo.0000170721.07088.2e
5. Wang X, Yang KH, Wanyan P, Tian JH. Comparison of the efficacy and safety of denosumab versus bisphosphonates in breast cancer and bone metastases treatment: a meta-analysis of randomized controlled trials. *Oncol Lett.* 2014;7(6):1997–2002. doi:10.3892/ol.2014.1982
6. Forsberg JA, Wedin R, Bauer HC, et al. External validation of the bayesian estimated tools for survival (BETS) models in patients with surgically treated skeletal metastases. *BMC Cancer.* 2012;12:493. Published 2012 Oct 25. doi:10.1186/1471-2407-12-493
7. Cirstoiu C, Cretu B, Iordache S, Popa M, Serban B, Cursaru A. Surgical management options for long-bone metastasis. *EFORT Open Rev.* 2022;7(3):206–213. Published 2022 Mar 17. doi:10.1530/EOR-21-0119
8. Mirels H. Metastatic disease in long bones. A proposed scoring system for diagnosing impending pathologic fractures. *Clin Orthop Relat Res.* 1989;249:256–264.
9. Healey JH, Brown HK. Complications of bone metastases: surgical management. *Cancer.* 2000;88(12 Suppl):2940–2951. doi:10.1002/1097-0142(20000615)88:12+<2940::aid-cncr10>3.0.co;2-w
10. Damron TA, Morgan H, Prakash D, Grant W, Aronowitz J, Heiner J. Critical evaluation of Mirels' rating system for impending pathologic fractures. *Clin Orthop Relat Res.* 2003;415:S201–S207. doi:10.1097/01.blo.0000093842.72468.73
11. Nazarian A, Entezari V, Zurakowski D, et al. Treatment planning and fracture prediction in patients with skeletal metastasis with CT-based rigidity analysis. *Clin Cancer Res.* 2015;21(11):2514–2519. doi:10.1158/1078-0432.CCR-14-2668
12. Damron TA, Mann KA. Fracture risk assessment and clinical decision making for patients with metastatic bone disease. *J Orthop Res.* 2020;38(6):1175–1190. doi:10.1002/jor.24660
13. Sugiura H, Yamada K, Sugiura T, Hida T, Mitsudomi T. Predictors of survival in patients with bone metastasis of lung cancer. *Clin Orthop Relat Res.* 2008;466(3):729–736. doi:10.1007/s11999-007-0051-0
14. Lin PP, Mirza AN, Lewis VO, et al. Patient survival after surgery for osseous metastases from renal cell carcinoma. *J Bone Joint Surg Am.* 2007;89(8):1794–1801. doi:10.2106/JBJS.F.00603
15. Kirkinis MN, Lyne CJ, Wilson MD, Choong PF. Metastatic bone disease: a review of survival, prognostic factors and outcomes following surgical treatment of the appendicular skeleton. *Eur J Surg Oncol.* 2016;42(12):1787–1797. doi:10.1016/j.ejso.2016.03.036
16. Harrington KD. New trends in the management of lower extremity metastases. *Clin Orthop Relat Res.* 1982;(169):53–61.
17. Terek RM. CORR Insights®: complications of cemented long-stem hip arthroplasties in metastatic bone disease revisited. *Clin Orthop Relat Res.* 2013;471(10):3308–3309. doi:10.1007/s11999-013-3177-2
18. Donaldson AJ, Thomson HE, Harper NJ, Kenny NW. Bone cement implantation syndrome. *Br J Anaesth.* 2009;102(1):12–22. doi:10.1093/bja/aen328
19. Khan FA, Rose PS, Yanagisawa M, Lewallen DG, Sim FH. Surgical technique: porous tantalum reconstruction for destructive nonprimary periacetabular tumors. *Clin Orthop Relat Res.* 2012;470(2):594–601. doi:10.1007/s11999-011-2117-2
20. Shallop B, Starks A, Greenbaum S, et al. Thromboembolism after intramedullary nailing for metastatic bone lesions. *J Bone Joint Surg Am.* 2015;97(18):1503–1511. doi:10.2106/JBJS.N.01067
21. Lutz S, Balboni T, Jones J, et al. Palliative radiation therapy for bone metastases: update of an ASTRO evidence-based guideline. *Pract Radiat Oncol.* 2017;7(1):4–12. doi:10.1016/j.prro.2016.08.001
22. Lee HL, Kuo CC, Tsai JT, Chen CY, Wu MH, Chiou JF. Magnetic resonance-guided focused ultrasound versus conventional radiation therapy for painful bone metastasis: a matched-pair study. *J Bone Joint Surg Am.* 2017;99(18):1572–1578. doi:10.2106/JBJS.16.01248
23. Bianchi G, Campanacci L, Ronchetti M, Donati D. Electrochemotherapy in the treatment of bone metastases: a phase II trial. *World J Surg.* 2016;40(12):3088–3094. doi:10.1007/s00268-016-3627-6

21 Bone Grafting, Allograft, and Tissue Processing

INTRODUCTION

Bone grafting remains a foundational aspect of orthopedic reconstruction, employed to address skeletal deficits arising from trauma, oncologic resections, infections, congenital anomalies, and degenerative conditions. Since the late 19th century, the field has progressed from experimental grafting techniques to biologically and mechanically sophisticated interventions.

The primary goals of bone grafting include achieving fusion between osseous segments, promoting union in delayed or nonunion cases, and reconstructing structural defects that compromise mechanical integrity. These objectives must be pursued with careful attention to the unique biological and biomechanical demands of each clinical scenario—ranging from small defects to large segmental reconstructions following tumor excision.

Graft incorporation is governed by a triad of interdependent factors: recipient site vascularity, mechanical stability, and the biological properties of the graft itself. Autografts, allografts, and synthetic alternatives vary widely in their regenerative potential and structural contribution. This chapter provides a comprehensive examination of bone grafting principles, focusing on the biological mechanisms of graft incorporation, the clinical applications of autografts and allografts, modern tissue banking practices, and emerging alternatives such as osteoinductive growth factors and synthetic scaffolds.

BIOLOGY OF BONE GRAFTS

The Triad of Bone Graft Function

Bone regeneration following grafting is orchestrated by three primary biological processes: **osteogenesis**, **osteoinduction**, and **osteoconduction** [1]. Although overlapping in effect, these mechanisms are biologically distinct and critical in selecting graft materials.

Osteogenesis

Osteogenesis refers to the direct formation of bone by viable osteoprogenitor cells transplanted within the graft. These cells, including osteoblasts and mesenchymal stem cells, are capable of surviving transplantation, proliferating, and synthesizing osteoid. This mechanism is exclusive to fresh autografts, particularly those harvested with bone marrow, and initiates bone formation even in avascular environments.

Factors influencing osteogenic capacity include

- **cell viability**, which is preserved through atraumatic harvesting techniques;
- **the local microenvironment**, rich in oxygen and biochemical cues; and
- **recipient site vascularity**, enhancing survival and proliferation.

While crucial in early healing, osteogenesis is typically supplemented and eventually overtaken by host-derived osteoinductive and osteoconductive responses.

Osteoinduction

Osteoinduction involves recruitment of host mesenchymal stem cells and their differentiation into osteoblasts under the influence of signaling molecules such as bone morphogenetic proteins (BMPs), TGF-β, FGFs, and platelet-derived growth factors (PDGFs). This multistep cascade—chemotaxis, proliferation, differentiation, and matrix formation—is key to bone regeneration in avascular or poorly cellular environments.

Preclinical models, particularly ectopic implantation in athymic mice, demonstrate the potential for bone formation even in non-osseous tissues. However, clinical translation is tempered by

- patient variability (age, comorbidities),
- regulatory limits on growth factor concentrations, and
- mechanical complexity of clinical sites compared to controlled experimental settings.

Osteoconduction

Osteoconduction refers to the role of the graft as a scaffold that facilitates host cell migration, vascular ingrowth, and subsequent bone formation. Osteoconductive efficacy depends on physical and chemical attributes, including

- **porosity** (100–500 μm) for vascular and cellular infiltration;
- **surface topography** influencing protein adsorption and cell adhesion;
- **resorption kinetics**, balancing degradation, and new bone formation; and
- **mechanical strength**, supporting load transmission.

DOI: 10.1201/9780367822002-26

Materials such as hydroxyapatite, calcium phosphate ceramics, processed allografts, and collagen-based matrices serve as effective osteoconductive scaffolds. Their function may be augmented through combination with cells or osteoinductive agents to form composite grafts.

The Ideal Bone Graft

The theoretical ideal graft combines osteogenic cells, osteoinductive signals, and an osteoconductive matrix. Fresh cancellous autografts most closely approximate this standard, but limitations in availability and donor-site morbidity drive the pursuit of engineered alternatives.

AUTOGRAFTS: BIOLOGICAL PERFORMANCE AND CLINICAL APPLICATION

Autografts, derived from the patient, offer the advantage of histocompatibility and no risk of disease transmission. Their intrinsic osteogenic, osteoinductive, and osteoconductive properties make them the reference standard.

Cancellous Autografts

Cancellous bone, with its trabecular structure and cellular richness, enables rapid incorporation. Healing progresses through three overlapping phases:

1. **Inflammatory Phase (Days 0–7)**: Hematoma forms; host immune cells infiltrate; graft-resident osteoprogenitor cells initiate osteoid production.
2. **Reparative Phase (Weeks 1–8)**: Capillary ingrowth and osteoblast proliferation result in new bone formation on necrotic trabeculae (creeping substitution).
3. **Remodeling Phase (Months 2–12)**: Woven bone matures into lamellar bone through osteoclastic resorption and mechanoadaptive remodeling [2, 3].

Complete biological incorporation typically occurs within 6–12 months. Cancellous grafts are ideal for

- metaphyseal defect filling,
- spinal fusions,
- nonunion repair in stable mechanical environments, and
- joint arthrodesis enhancement.

The iliac crest remains the preferred harvest site due to its cellular richness and accessibility, although alternative sites like the proximal tibia and distal femur may be used.

Cortical Autografts

Cortical grafts provide superior mechanical strength but incorporate slowly due to their density and limited vascular access. Integration involves the following:

1. **Revascularization (Weeks 1–4)**: Host capillaries penetrate haversian canals; limited cell survival occurs via diffusion.
2. **Resorptive Phase (Months 1–6)**: Osteoclastic resorption reduces structural integrity.
3. **Reparative Phase (Months 6–24)**: New bone forms in remodeled haversian spaces; mechanical properties gradually return.
4. **Remodeling (Years 1–3)**: Composite structure forms; central graft regions may remain avascular [4].

Used in diaphyseal reconstructions and structural support post-tumor resection, nonvascularized cortical grafts offer immediate load-bearing capacity. The fibula is commonly used due to its straight geometry, sufficient length, and low morbidity.

However, during the resorptive phase, cortical grafts are susceptible to fatigue fractures. Supplemental fixation is often necessary in weight-bearing applications.

Vascularized Bone Grafts

Vascularized autografts, harvested with their nutrient blood supply and reanastomosed microsurgically, maintain cell viability and offer distinct advantages:

- Immediate biologic activity without relying on creeping substitution
- Maintained mechanical strength
- Enhanced infection resistance via intrinsic perfusion
- Accelerated interface healing

Common indications include the following:

- Segmental defects >6 cm
- Refractory nonunions in compromised beds
- Mandibular or maxillofacial reconstructions
- Osteonecrosis
- Complex composite tissue loss

The fibula is the most widely used vascularized graft due to its reliable vasculature, osteocutaneous harvest capability, and acceptable donor morbidity. Other options include vascularized iliac crest, scapula, or medial femoral condyle.

Despite their advantages, vascularized grafts require microsurgical expertise, longer operative time, and carry risks of flap failure and donor morbidity. Their use must be carefully weighed against case complexity and resource availability.

Allografts

Allografts are harvested from human donors and transplanted into recipients of the same species. These may be fresh, fresh-frozen, or freeze-dried. Fresh allografts are seldom used due to logistical challenges, immunologic rejection, and high cost. Fresh-frozen allografts, stored at –80°C, are the most commonly used in clinical practice. They retain much of the biomechanical integrity of cortical bone but are devitalized and have diminished biological activity [5, 6].

During transplantation, any remaining donor cells that attempt to proliferate may elicit an immune response, leading to inflammatory reactions, inhibition of osteoblast function, and destruction of neovascular connections. As such, fresh-frozen allografts are processed to reduce immunogenicity by removing marrow elements and destroying cell-surface antigens. Antigens present on the collagen matrix of cortical bone are weakly antigenic and generally do not trigger strong immune reactions.

Allograft incorporation is less robust than autografts. While periosteal and endosteal callus can bridge the graft-host junction, internal remodeling is limited. The incorporation occurs predominantly at the graft-host interface, with poor central graft remodeling. This limited repair capability, coupled with mechanical fatigue over time, leads to higher rates of nonunion and stress fractures, particularly in large segmental reconstructions [6].

BONE BANKING AND TISSUE PROCESSING

Bone grafts are often recovered from deceased donors, making bone banking a critical step in ensuring graft safety and efficacy. Ethical considerations are paramount; grafts are viewed as donated tissues rather than commodities. Bone banks must follow stringent guidelines for tissue recovery, processing, and distribution [7].

Donor screening involves a detailed medical history, lifestyle risk assessment, and laboratory testing for transmissible diseases, including HIV, hepatitis B and C, and syphilis. The advent of nucleic acid testing (NAT) has significantly improved detection sensitivity, shortening the window period for viral identification to seven days for both HIV and hepatitis C [8].

Tissue procurement may be aseptic, conducted in sterile operating room environments, or performed in clean rooms within 24 hours of death and 12 hours of refrigeration. Post-harvest processing includes lavage, ultrasonic cleaning, ethanol treatment, and antibiotic exposure to eliminate residual marrow, fat, and pathogens. In some cases, tendon insertions are preserved for specific applications.

Demineralized bone matrix (DBM) is prepared from cortical bone after acid extraction. This process retains BMPs and growth factors, endowing DBM with osteoinductive potential. However, variations in donor characteristics and processing methods lead to inconsistent BMP content and variable clinical efficacy.

STERILIZATION TECHNIQUES AND BIOMECHANICAL CONSIDERATIONS

Terminal sterilization is crucial to ensure safety but must preserve the biological and mechanical properties of the graft. Gamma irradiation is widely used, typically delivered in doses of 10–25 kGy. Doses above 25 kGy effectively eliminate pathogens but significantly degrade mechanical strength and osteoinductive proteins in a dose-dependent fashion [9]. Lower doses (<17 kGy) strike a balance between sterility and functional preservation but may not guarantee complete inactivation of viruses like HIV [10].

Freeze-drying, or lyophilization, allows storage at room temperature by removing >94% of water content. While this extends shelf life, it also reduces graft strength and biological activity. Fresh-frozen grafts, though logistically demanding, retain superior mechanical properties and are preferred for load-bearing reconstructions.

Sterility testing is performed as per United States Pharmacopeia (USP) <71> standards, seeking to ensure the absence of viable microbes. Aseptic allografts are processed with minimal irradiation and retain more native structure, whereas sterile-labeled grafts undergo terminal irradiation with contamination probabilities of <1 in 1 million.

BONE GRAFT SUBSTITUTES

Bone graft substitutes encompass a wide variety of biologic and synthetic materials intended to replicate the structural and functional properties of autografts. They can be broadly classified into allograft-derived, synthetic, and biologic-enhanced substitutes. The development and utilization of these alternatives are particularly valuable in scenarios where autograft availability is limited or when donor-site morbidity must be avoided.

DBM is derived from cortical bone after undergoing acid extraction to remove its mineral content. This process exposes growth factors, including BMPs, which are responsible for its osteoinductive properties [11]. However, DBM lacks inherent structural strength and must often be combined with carriers such as glycerol or hyaluronic acid for handling and implantation. The variability in BMP content due to differences in donor tissue and processing techniques leads to inconsistency in osteoinductive potential and clinical outcomes.

Despite the theoretical advantages, proving the clinical superiority of one DBM product over another remains challenging due to the heterogeneity of products, processing methods, and study designs. Several studies have demonstrated fusion and healing potential in preclinical models, but their translation to consistent clinical success is limited [11].

Synthetic Substitutes: Synthetic materials include ceramics like calcium sulfate, calcium phosphate ceramics (hydroxyapatite, tricalcium phosphate), and composite materials. Calcium sulfate is resorbable and biocompatible, with dissolution occurring within 6–17 weeks, making it useful for temporary scaffolding [12]. However, it lacks long-term structural support.

Calcium phosphate ceramics are more robust and porous, promoting osteoconduction by supporting cellular attachment, migration, and proliferation. Pore size between 300 to 500 µm is considered optimal for vascular and bone ingrowth [12]. Hydroxyapatite, due to its close resemblance to natural bone mineral, has excellent biocompatibility and is slowly resorbed, offering long-term stability in defect reconstruction.

Calcium phosphate ceramics provide good compressive strength and moldability, making them suitable for metaphyseal defects. They set in situ and can be drilled or tapped for screw fixation. Newer formulations have improved resistance to shear forces and show promise in weight-bearing applications. However, these materials are primarily osteoconductive and lack intrinsic osteoinductive or osteogenic properties.

Growth Factor–Based and Cell-Based Substitutes: Among biologically active substitutes, recombinant human BMPs (rhBMP-2 and rhBMP-7) have shown the ability to induce bone formation through direct osteoinductive activity. These proteins, produced via recombinant DNA technology, are applied with carriers to sites of bone loss or nonunion. Clinical trials have demonstrated efficacy in spinal fusion and tibial nonunion, with fusion rates comparable to autografts [13].

Nevertheless, concerns remain regarding the supraphysiologic doses required, off-label usage, cost, and potential adverse effects including local inflammatory reactions and cancer risk. As a result, BMP use is typically reserved for complex cases where standard treatments have failed.

A newer category of graft substitutes includes cell-containing grafts, incorporating mesenchymal stem cells (MSCs) into scaffolds. These cellular constructs aim to provide both osteogenic and osteoinductive capacities, bridging the gap between biologically inert materials and living bone. Early in vitro and preclinical studies suggest potential efficacy, but larger clinical trials are needed to establish safety and effectiveness.

Commercial Products Several commercially available bone graft substitutes combine various features:

- Ceramics: Vitoss (Stryker), Norian SRS (Synthes), BoneSource (Stryker)
- Plaster-based: Osteoset (Wright Medical)
- DBM products: Grafton (Medtronic), AlloFuse (AlloSource), DBX (MTF)
- Cell-based: Trinity Evolution (MTF), NuVasive (AlloSource)
- BMP-based: Infuse (Medtronic)

The choice among these products should be guided by defect size, mechanical requirements, biological environment, and patient-specific factors. While many options are available, no single product has proven universally superior. Comparative studies remain limited, and product selection often relies on surgeon preference and institutional availability.

BIOLOGICS AND FUTURE DIRECTIONS

Biologic agents such as recombinant human BMPs (rhBMP-2 and rhBMP-7) have demonstrated efficacy in promoting bone healing in difficult cases such as tibial nonunions. Randomized controlled trials have shown fusion rates comparable to autografts. Nevertheless, supraphysiologic doses, high costs, and emerging safety concerns, including cancer risk, have limited their widespread adoption [13]. Meta-analyses have questioned long-term outcomes and identified complications associated with off-label use.

Emerging therapies include stem cell-enriched grafts and tissue-engineered constructs that combine scaffolds with cellular and molecular components. Early studies suggest potential for these constructs to offer osteoinductive and osteogenic benefits without relying on carriers. Regulatory classification as human cell and tissue products (HCT/P) by the Food and Drug Administration (FDA) requires stringent quality control.

CONCLUSION

Bone grafting continues to evolve as a fundamental component of orthopedic reconstruction. While autografts remain the gold standard due to their unmatched biological properties, limitations in availability and donor-site morbidity necessitate alternatives. Allografts provide structural support and have expanded indications due to advances in tissue processing and sterilization. Synthetic and biologically enhanced substitutes are gaining ground, though variability in clinical efficacy remains a challenge.

Surgeons must consider graft size, mechanical demands, recipient site vascularity, and infection risk when selecting the appropriate graft. A comprehensive understanding of the biology, processing, and limitations of each graft type will enable clinicians to tailor solutions to individual patient needs and improve reconstructive outcomes.

SUMMARY

- Bone grafting relies on three key biological mechanisms—osteogenesis, osteoinduction, and osteoconduction—which collectively determine graft incorporation and guide the selection of autografts, allografts, or substitutes.
- Autografts remain the gold standard due to their superior biological activity, offering viable cells, inductive signals, and a natural scaffold; vascularized grafts provide additional advantages in large or biologically compromised defects.
- Allografts serve as essential structural options in orthopedic oncology, with their safety and mechanical performance shaped by modern tissue banking practices, including donor screening, processing, and sterilization techniques.

- Bone graft substitutes—including DBM, ceramics, growth factor–based products, and emerging cell-based constructs—expand reconstructive options, though variability in biological potency and clinical outcomes necessitates careful, indication-specific use.

REFERENCES

1. Blokhuis TJ, Arts JJ. Bioactive and osteoinductive bone graft substitutes: definitions, facts and myths. *Injury.* 2011;42(Suppl 2):S26–S29.
2. Chase SW, Herndon CH. The fate of autogenous and homogenous bone grafts. *J Bone Joint Surg Am.* 1955;37(4):809–841.
3. Phemister DB. The fate of transplanted bone and regenerative power of its various constituents. *Surg Gynecol Obstet.* 1914;19:303–333.
4. Enneking WF, Burchardt H, Puhl JJ, Piotrowski G. Physical and biological aspects of repair in dog cortical-bone transplants. *J Bone Joint Surg Am.* 1975;57(2):237–252.
5. Tomford WW. Bone allografts: past, present and future. *Cell Tissue Bank.* 2000;1(2):105–109.
6. Enneking WF, Campanacci DA. Retrieved human allografts: a clinicopathological study. *J Bone Joint Surg Am.* 2001;83(7):971–986.
7. American Association of Tissue Banks. Available at: http://www.aatb.org. Accessed August 12, 2012.
8. Tomford WW. Transmission of disease through transplantation of musculoskeletal allografts. *J Bone Joint Surg Am.* 1995;77(11):1742–1754.
9. Nguyen H, Morgan DA, Forwood MR. Sterilization of allograft bone: effects of gamma irradiation on allograft biology and biomechanics. *Cell Tissue Bank.* 2007;8(2):93–105.
10. Hernigou P, Gras G, Marinello G, Dormont D. Inactivation of HIV by application of heat and radiation: implication in bone banking with irradiated allograft bone. *Acta Orthop Scand.* 2000;71(5):508–512.
11. Bae HW, Zhao L, Kanim LE, et al. Intervariability and intravariability of bone morphogenetic proteins in commercially available demineralized bone matrix products. *Spine (Phila Pa 1976).* 2006;31(12):1299–1306.
12. LeGeros RZ. Properties of osteoconductive biomaterials: calcium phosphates. *Clin Orthop Relat Res.* 2002;395:81–98.
13. Carragee EJ, Chu G, Rohatgi R, et al. Cancer risk after use of recombinant bone morphogenetic protein-2 for spinal arthrodesis. *J Bone Joint Surg Am.* 2013;95(17):1537–1545.

22 Recent Advances in Limb Salvage Surgery

INTRODUCTION

The field of musculoskeletal oncology continues to pose substantial challenges for orthopedic oncologists. Despite these hurdles, ongoing research into tumors affecting the musculoskeletal system has generated valuable data that aids in guiding clinical decisions. Given the rarity and diverse nature of these conditions, much of the existing literature comprises retrospective studies. This chapter aims to highlight recent advancements, summarize the current body of evidence, and underscore the importance of ongoing and future collaborative research initiatives.

ADVANCES IN ENDOPROSTHESIS

Reconstruction of the femur and tibia following tumor resection remains a focal point in orthopedic oncology, especially with growing interest in the long-term outcomes of endoprosthetic reconstructions. Over the years, these reconstructions have evolved to include diverse implant options such as rotating-hinge prostheses for the distal femur, cementless stemmed nonextendable endoprostheses, and innovative compressive osseointegration devices [1–5].

While the fixed-hinge knee prosthesis has demonstrated generally favorable outcomes after distal femoral resection [6], long-term follow-up raises concerns. In a study by Grimer et al., only a 10% implant survival rate was observed at 20 years in a cohort of 102 patients who underwent fixed-hinge distal femoral replacement, highlighting the importance of vigilant, extended monitoring and the likelihood of reoperation [7]. To address these limitations, rotating-hinge prostheses were introduced to enhance implant longevity (Figure 22.1). Ogura et al. evaluated outcomes in 214 patients treated over 26 years at Memorial Sloan Kettering Cancer Center using the Finn/Orthopedic Salvage System (OSS) rotating-hinge knee prosthesis (Zimmer Biomet), documenting 312 reoperations and a 10-year cumulative incidence of 30.1% for implant removal or revision, with a steady annual failure rate of 1.24% [1].

A broader analysis involving 209 patients treated between 1991 and 2016 identified specific risk factors for prosthetic failure, including the extent of femoral and quadriceps resection. Additionally, infection risk correlated with the type of joint resected, while a bone-to-stem ratio exceeding 2.5 was predictive of aseptic loosening [2].

In skeletally immature patients, stemmed cementless nonextendable endoprostheses have been employed with mixed outcomes. El Ghoneimy et al. analyzed 328 such cases in individuals under 18 years and reported a substantial early revision rate. Complications included aseptic loosening, hinge, and stem breakage, periprosthetic fractures, and cortical stress shielding. The overall cumulative revision incidence at eight years reached 32% [3].

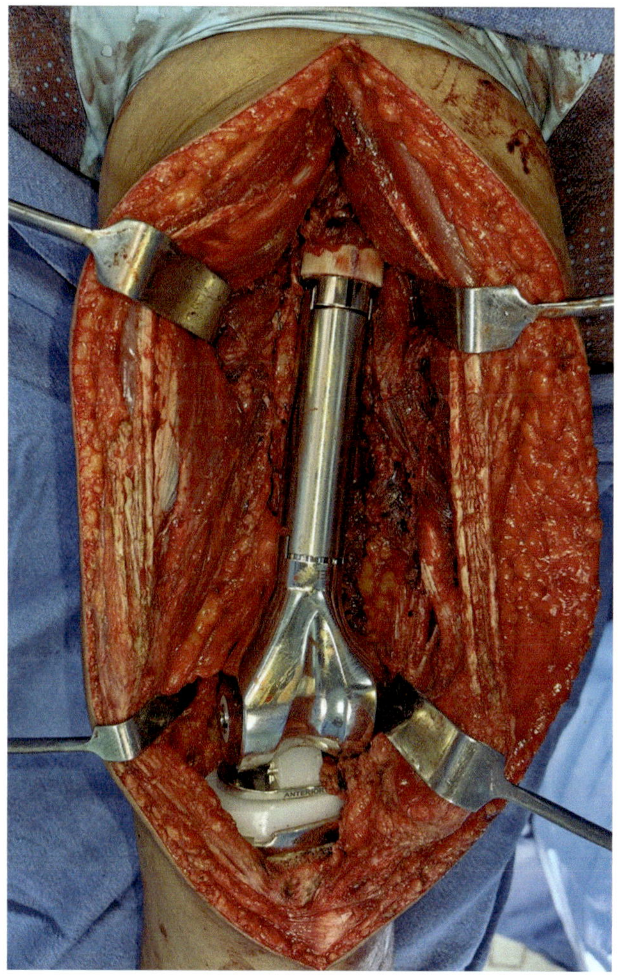

FIGURE 22.1 Intraoperative photograph showing implantation of a rotating hinge distal femur endoprosthesis following wide resection of a distal femoral tumor. The rotating hinge design provides stability while allowing controlled axial rotation, thereby reducing torsional stresses at the bone–implant interface. This biomechanical advantage helps in enhancing implant longevity, minimizing aseptic loosening, and improving long-term functional outcomes in limb salvage surgery.

DOI: 10.1201/9780367822002-27

Achieving robust fixation between the prosthesis and residual host bone remains a critical factor in endoprosthetic success. Compressive osseointegration has emerged as a viable alternative to traditional stemmed implants, particularly in challenging anatomical locations. A single-center retrospective review of 25 patients with primary sarcomas in the proximal or distal femur treated with compressive osseointegration prostheses reported only three cases of spindle loosening or fracture. The reoperation rate stood at 12% over a ten-year follow-up. Radiographs showed cortical hypertrophy in over half the cohort and no evidence of interface atrophy or narrowing, indicating promising long-term implant-host integration [4].

Compliant compression fixation systems aim to promote biological osteointegration while preserving bone stock (Figure 22.2). In the distal femur, this method has been associated with durable outcomes and consistent cortical remodeling near the implant. A retrospective series of 12 patients undergoing proximal femoral reconstruction with this technology found limited bone formation at the interface, yet survivorship remained favorable in patients younger than 65 years with localized tumors and nonirradiated bone [5].

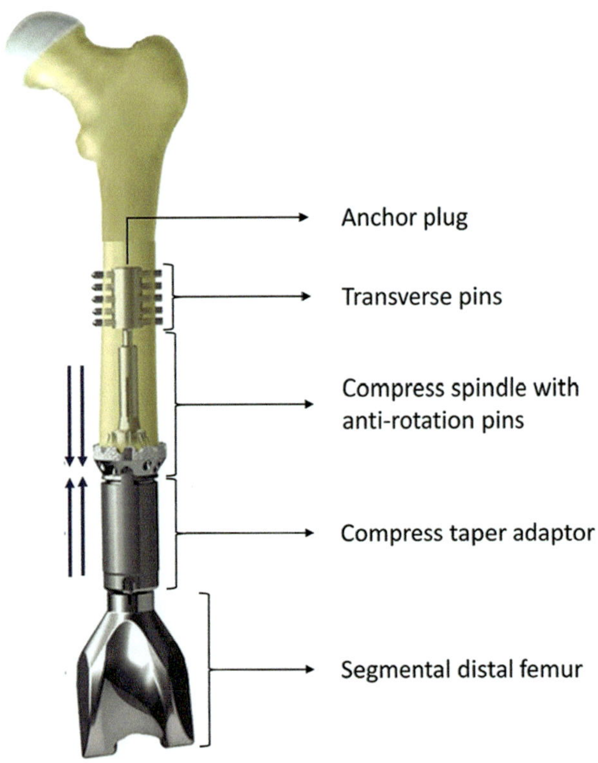

FIGURE 22.2 Diagram illustrating the components of a compliant compression fixation system used in limb salvage surgery. The system consists of an anchor plug, transverse pins, a compress spindle with anti-rotation pins, a compress taper adaptor, and a segmental distal femur replacement. These devices provide continuous axial compression at the bone–implant interface, thereby promoting biological osteointegration, reducing stress shielding, and preserving host bone stock. This principle offers enhanced long-term fixation and durability compared to conventional cemented or press-fit stems.

Across various studies, patient cohorts have ranged from 12 to over 300 individuals, with follow-up durations extending up to several decades. Reported revision rates commonly approximate 30% over long-term observation. It is noteworthy that complications associated with compressive osseointegration, which facilitates fixation even in short residual segments, tend to occur early. Nonetheless, as these systems are relatively recent, definitive conclusions on their long-term performance are still pending.

When dealing with massive tumors or complex revisions, surgeons are often faced with extremely short residual bone segments, rendering standard intramedullary stem fixation unfeasible. To address this, multiple strategies have been explored, including compressive osseointegration, custom short medullary stems, cross-fixation pin constructs, and extracortical plates [8, 9]. However, these approaches do not enhance the remaining bone length. To bridge this gap, the telescoping allograft technique was introduced, which involves inserting an allograft into the short native bone to effectively augment its length. Initially proposed by Healey et al., this method aims to recreate diaphyseal continuity in limb salvage procedures [10]. Hindiskere et al. reported on its application in augmenting residual femoral segments, demonstrating an implant survivorship of 80% at seven years [11]. Another promising development is the use of custom-made 3D-printed short stems with a porous structure, which allow secure fixation of massive endoprostheses in short segments, offering favorable limb function, implant stability, and low complication rates [12].

Reconstruction of the proximal humerus poses unique challenges, largely due to the extensive soft tissue and muscle detachments required, making implant-related complications—particularly instability—a major concern [13]. To mitigate this, reverse total shoulder arthroplasty with a constrained design is increasingly used (Figure 22.3). While such implants can offer improved stability compared to unconstrained options, which may compromise elbow and hand function due to instability, they are also prone to early aseptic loosening of the glenoid component due to increased stress at the bone-implant interface.

In a study assessing the short-term functional results of reverse total shoulder prostheses in 18 patients, the revision rate was higher than that reported for other types of proximal humerus prostheses. The authors attributed this to the greater stress transmitted through the constrained design, potentially accelerating loosening at the humeral interface [14]. To address this issue, a novel constrained implant consisting of two serially connected constrained joints via a dumbbell link has been developed. This system is particularly suited for extra-articular resections of the proximal humerus involving loss of deltoid and rotator cuff function, and has shown encouraging early outcomes [15].

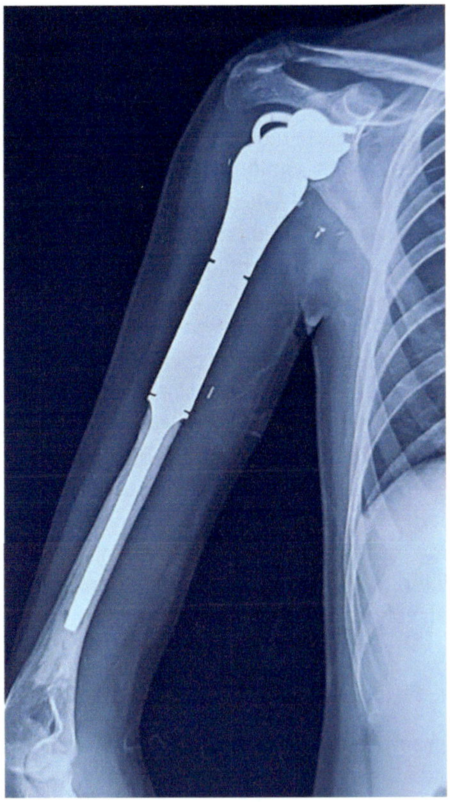

FIGURE 22.3 Postoperative radiograph demonstrating a reverse total shoulder arthroplasty performed following proximal humeral resection for tumor. The reverse prosthesis design medializes and lowers the center of rotation, thereby allowing the deltoid muscle to compensate for rotator cuff deficiency and restore functional range of motion. This reconstruction option is particularly valuable in oncological resections of the proximal humerus, where soft-tissue preservation is limited.

3D BIOPRINTING IN LIMB SALVAGE SURGERY

Limb salvage surgery has evolved significantly over the last few decades, shifting from a domain primarily dominated by amputation to a reconstructive approach driven by technological advances in microsurgery, imaging, and biomaterials. In this continuum, three-dimensional (3D) bioprinting has emerged as a disruptive innovation, offering the potential to replicate complex anatomical and functional structures using customized, biologically active constructs. recent advances in three-dimensional (3D) technologies, including 3D printing (3DP) and surgical navigation systems, have emerged as transformative tools in musculoskeletal oncology. These innovations facilitate not only anatomical reconstruction but also biological integration, enhancing outcomes in oncological and traumatic reconstructions [16].

Unlike traditional subtractive manufacturing methods, 3DP constructs objects layer by layer using high-resolution imaging data such as CT or MRI to generate precise and detailed structures. Several 3DP techniques have been adopted in orthopedic surgery, including powder-based printing, vat polymerization, and droplet-based methods [16, 17].

THE RATIONALE FOR 3D BIOPRINTING IN LIMB SALVAGE SURGERY

Conventional limb salvage often relies on metallic endoprostheses, structural allografts, or arthrodesis. These techniques, while functionally effective, are often associated with complications such as poor implant-host integration, stress shielding, infection, and mechanical failure [16]. Moreover, these approaches lack the bioactivity required for remodeling, vascularization, and innervation—critical components of tissue homeostasis and long-term success.

3D bioprinting, by combining viable cells (in bioinks) with structural biomaterials, seeks to recreate living tissues that not only provide mechanical stability but also actively participate in biological processes such as osteogenesis and angiogenesis. This paradigm shift enables the fabrication of constructs that closely mimic the structural, functional, and biological attributes of native tissues, thus offering a potential solution to the unmet needs in limb salvage surgery [16].

A key advantage of 3DP lies in its capacity for customization—allowing material properties such as pore size, porosity, and elastic modulus to be tailored to replicate native bone architecture. This personalization promotes biomechanical compatibility, enhances osseointegration, and potentially improves implant survival [17].

Moreover, the utility of 3DP spans both preoperative and intraoperative phases. Preoperatively, 3D-printed anatomical models offer a precise and concise visualization of tumor margins and adjacent critical structures. These are valuable not only for surgical planning but also as educational tools. Patient-specific instruments (PSIs), derived from 3D-printed data, enable accurate translation of preoperative planning into real-time surgical execution—especially in anatomically complex tumors, where standard implants may be insufficient [18].

Intraoperatively, navigation-assisted surgery utilizes preoperative imaging to provide real-time guidance during tumor resections, thereby improving the precision of osteotomies and enhancing the likelihood of achieving clear surgical margins. This contributes significantly to local disease control and functional preservation [19].

These technologies should be viewed not in isolation but as interlinked components of an integrated treatment strategy. 3D planning, PSIs, and navigation systems must be selected based on tumor location, anatomical constraints, and surgical objectives, to yield optimal clinical outcomes [20].

BIOPRINTING TECHNOLOGIES AND BIOMATERIALS

Multiple printing techniques are now adapted for orthopedic use, including extrusion-based, inkjet, stereolithography, and laser-assisted bioprinting. The selection of technology is dictated by the resolution, biocompatibility of the material, and the complexity of the construct required.

Bioinks commonly consist of combinations of polymers (natural or synthetic), ceramics, and viable cells. Natural materials such as silk fibroin and alginates are favored for their biocompatibility, biodegradability, and ability to promote cellular proliferation and differentiation [21, 22]. For instance, silk fibroin has demonstrated osteoinductive potential and has been used to promote vascular endothelial growth factor (VEGF) synthesis and mesenchymal stem cell (MSC) differentiation [23]. Synthetic biopolymers like polycaprolactone (PCL), polylactic acid (PLA), and polyetheretherketone (PEEK) offer structural integrity and have been used in hybrid constructs that combine mechanical and biological functions [24].

Ceramic components such as hydroxyapatite (HA) and β-tricalcium phosphate (β-TCP) are often integrated for their osteoconductive properties, enhancing bone-implant integration. More recent innovations include smart materials with "4D" functionalities—materials that respond to environmental cues such as pH or temperature, enabling controlled release of growth factors or antibiotics over time [16, 25].

PRECLINICAL APPLICATIONS

In vitro and animal model studies have provided encouraging evidence for the efficacy of 3D-bioprinted constructs. Various biocompatible scaffolds have successfully demonstrated the promotion of osteogenesis and angiogenesis. For example, β-TCP scaffolds coated with dipyridamole significantly enhanced bone formation in rabbit models. Similarly, PCL-based scaffolds integrated with osteogenic agents like BMP-2 or Wnt3a have shown successful bone regeneration in long bone defects [16, 26].

The bioactivity of scaffolds has also been enhanced through the use of functional coatings, including collagen, alginate-catechol, and antimicrobial agents. In animal studies, these combinations have led to improved cell attachment, differentiation, and resistance to infection—laying the foundation for future clinical translation [27].

CLINICAL APPLICATIONS IN UPPER AND LOWER LIMB SALVAGE

Although most clinical applications currently utilize metal-based 3D-printed implants, bioprinted constructs are beginning to make their way into clinical practice. Titanium and tantalum prostheses have been employed in patients with upper limb malignancies, including scapular and clavicular resections. These implants often incorporate porous structures and bioactive coatings to facilitate osseointegration and soft tissue attachment [16, 28].

In lower limb reconstruction, 3D-printed titanium implants have been used to reconstruct diaphyseal defects of the femur and tibia caused by osteomyelitis or tumor resections [29]. These constructs can be further enhanced by incorporating β-TCP (β-Tricalcium Phosphate) granules or stem cell-seeded hydrogels to promote osteogenesis and vascularization [16, 30].

FIXATION STRATEGIES AND HYBRID APPROACHES

A key challenge in 3D bioprinting remains the mechanical fixation and biological integration of the implant. Several strategies have been explored, including designing constructs with pre-drilled holes for soft tissue reattachment, using porous zones for enhanced tissue in-growth, and hybrid builds combining metal cores with biologically active coatings. For example, porous tantalum implants with peripheral anchoring holes have been used successfully in phalangeal replacements, enabling both functional restoration and biological integration [16, 31].

The development of hybrid constructs—combining rigid load-bearing structures with 3D-bioprinted cell-laden hydrogels—is increasingly being viewed as a future direction for large bone defect reconstructions. These hybrids can provide mechanical support while simultaneously promoting biological healing, effectively bridging the gap between structural and biological requirements [32].

FUTURE DIRECTIONS AND CHALLENGES

Despite promising results, several challenges hinder the widespread adoption of 3D bioprinting in limb salvage surgery. These include the following:

- **Cell viability and scalability**: Maintaining cell viability during printing, and scaling up constructs for large defects remains technically complex.
- **Regulatory hurdles**: Clinical translation of bioprinted tissues is hindered by stringent regulatory frameworks, especially concerning the use of viable cells.
- **Biomechanical limitations**: Most bioprinted constructs are yet to match the long-term mechanical performance of traditional prostheses.
- **Cost and accessibility**: High production costs and limited availability of certified bioprinters pose barriers, particularly in low-resource settings.

Nevertheless, ongoing research in bioinks, vascularized constructs, and in situ bioprinting holds promise. Techniques such as bioprinting tendon–bone interfaces, incorporating neural elements for proprioception, and using AI-based anatomical modeling may further refine the outcomes of limb salvage surgery.

3D bioprinting has the potential to redefine the landscape of limb salvage surgery by offering personalized, biologically active, and mechanically competent constructs. While still in its nascent stage, this technology promises to address many of the limitations of conventional reconstructive techniques. With continued interdisciplinary collaboration among surgeons, materials scientists, and bioengineers, 3D bioprinting could soon become a cornerstone in the reconstructive armamentarium of orthopedic oncologists and trauma surgeons alike.

THE PARITY TRIAL AND OTHER COLLABORATIVE STUDIES

The *Prophylactic Antibiotic Regimens in Tumor Surgery (PARITY)* trial, published on January 6, 2022, represents a major milestone in collaborative musculoskeletal oncology research [33]. This multicenter, parallel, blinded randomized controlled trial was conducted between January 2013 and October 2019 across 55 institutions in 12 countries. It focused on patients undergoing femoral or tibial tumor resections followed by endoprosthetic reconstruction. Participants were randomized to receive either a one-day or a five-day course of postoperative intravenous cephalosporin, with the primary endpoint being the incidence of surgical site infection. Secondary outcomes included antibiotic-associated adverse events, need for unplanned reoperations, functional and oncologic outcomes, and overall survival.

Of the 604 patients analyzed, 311 received the 1-day regimen and 293 received the 5-day regimen. Surgical site infections occurred in 16.7% of the one-day group and 15.0% of the five-day group. The hazard ratio for infection was 0.93 (95% CI, 0.62–1.40; $p = 0.73$), indicating no statistically significant difference. However, antibiotic-related complications were significantly more common in the five-day group (5.1%) compared to the one-day group (1.6%), with a hazard ratio of 3.24 (95% CI, 1.17–8.98; $p = 0.02$). These findings emphasize that extending antibiotic prophylaxis beyond 24 hours may increase the risk of complications without reducing infection rates. Importantly, the PARITY trial generated a high-quality prospective dataset that provides a platform for further analysis and secondary research in orthopedic oncology.

In a complementary development, Gazendam et al. established minimally important differences (MIDs) for key outcome measures, including the Musculoskeletal Tumor Society Rating Scale-93 (MSTS-93) and the Toronto Extremity Salvage Score (TESS-79), facilitating the interpretation of treatment effects. These thresholds help clinicians and patients discern whether observed changes in scores after treatment are not only statistically but also clinically meaningful [34].

Two notable prospective collaborative studies are currently underway. The Musculoskeletal Tumor Registry (MsTR), initiated by the American Academy of Orthopedic Surgeons (AAOS) in collaboration with the Musculoskeletal Tumor Society (MSTS), began as a pilot project in 2018 and expanded into a full registry in 2019 [35]. As one of the subspecialty registries within the AAOS network, MsTR enables aggregation of patient data related to rare musculoskeletal tumors across participating centers, supporting long-term evaluation of functional outcomes, complications, and oncologic control.

Another prominent initiative is the *Surveillance After Extremity Tumor Surgery (SAFETY)* trial, a randomized controlled study that has recruited over 150 patients with soft tissue sarcomas from 25 sites in 10 countries [36]. In this trial, participants are randomized to undergo either intensive or less intensive surveillance post-surgery, with outcomes tracked for oncologic recurrence and quality of life. The SAFETY trial is preparing to enter its definitive phase as of 2023, aiming to provide evidence-based guidelines on optimal post-treatment follow-up strategies.

PREDICTIVE MODELING

Efforts to better predict surgical and oncologic outcomes in patients with musculoskeletal tumors continue to evolve, particularly in resource-constrained environments. Ganguly et al. developed and validated a baseline prognostic scoring system for osteosarcoma patients treated with a uniform, non-high-dose methotrexate-based protocol in a lower middle-income health-care setting [37]. Their analysis identified tumor size, presence of metastases at diagnosis, and elevated serum alkaline phosphatase levels as independent predictors of poor event-free survival. These factors were integrated into a composite prognostic score.

In a similar vein, the same group proposed a baseline prognostic score for Ewing sarcoma. Their model included tumor diameter >5 cm, baseline metastatic disease, and total leukocyte count >11,000/mm^3 as significant indicators of poor overall survival. These parameters were used to construct a risk stratification tool to guide treatment planning and prognostication [38].

SUMMARY

- Advances in endoprostheses, including rotating-hinge designs and compressive osseointegration, have enhanced reconstruction options but require long-term follow-up.
- 3D printing and navigation technologies enable personalized, precise tumor resections and reconstructions.
- The PARITY trial supports limiting postoperative antibiotics to 24 hours to reduce complications without increasing infection risk.
- Multicenter collaborations like MsTR and the SAFETY trial are driving evidence-based improvements in sarcoma care.
- Prognostic models using clinical and laboratory parameters aid in risk stratification and treatment planning for osteosarcoma and Ewing sarcoma.

REFERENCES

1. Ogura K, Yakoub MA, Boland PJ, Healey JH. Finn/orthopaedic salvage system distal femoral rotating-hinge megaprostheses in oncologic patients: long-term complications, reoperations, and amputations. *J Bone Joint Surg Am.* 2021 Apr 21;103(8):705–714. doi:10.2106/JBJS.20.00696
2. Ogura K, Fujiwara T, Morris CD, Boland PJ, Healey JH. Long-term competing risks for overall and cause-specific failure of rotating-hinge distal femoral arthroplasty for tumour reconstruction. *Bone Joint J.* 2021 Aug;103-B(8):1405–1413. doi:10.1302/0301-620X.103B8.BJJ-2020-2323.R1

3. El Ghoneimy AM, Shehab AM, Farid N. What is the cumulative incidence of revision surgery and what are the complications associated with stemmed cementless nonextendable endoprostheses in patients 18 years or younger with primary bone sarcomas about the knee. *Clin Orthop Relat Res.* 2022 Jul 1;480(7):1329–1338. doi:10.1097/CORR.0000000000002150
4. Groundland J, Brown JM, Monument M, Bernthal N, Jones KB, Randall RL. What are the long-term surgical outcomes of compressive endoprosthetic osseointegration of the femur with a minimum 10-year follow-up period? *Clin Orthop Relat Res.* 2022 Mar 1;480(3):539–548. doi:10.1097/CORR.0000000000001979
5. Christ AB, Fujiwara T, Fabbri N, Healey JH. Compliant compression reconstruction of the proximal femur is durable despite minimal bone formation in the compression segment. *Clin Orthop Relat Res.* 2021 Jul 1;479(7):1577–1585. doi:10.1097/CORR.0000000000001663
6. Myers GJ, Abudu AT, Carter SR, Tillman RM, Grimer RJ. Endoprosthetic replacement of the distal femur for bone tumours: long-term results. *J Bone Joint Surg Br.* 2007 Apr;89(4):521–526. doi:10.1302/0301-620X.89B4.18631. Erratum in: J Bone Joint Surg Br. 2007 May;89(5):706.
7. Grimer RJ, Aydin BK, Wafa H, Carter SR, Jeys L, Abudu A, Parry M. Very long-term outcomes after endoprosthetic replacement for malignant tumours of bone. *Bone Joint J.* 2016 Jun;98-B(6):857–864. doi:10.1302/0301-620X.98B6.37417
8. Stevenson JD, Wigley C, Burton H, Ghezelayagh S, Morris G, Evans S, Parry M, Jeys L. Minimising aseptic loosening in extreme bone resections: custom-made tumour endoprostheses with short medullary stems and extra-cortical plates. *Bone Joint J.* 2017 Dec;99-B(12):1689–1695. doi:10.1302/0301-620X.99B12.BJJ-2017-0213.R1
9. Calvert GT, Cummings JE, Bowles AJ, Jones KB, Wurtz LD, Randall RL. A dual-center review of compressive osseointegration for fixation of massive endoprosthetics: 2- to 9-year followup. *Clin Orthop Relat Res.* 2014 Mar;472(3):822–829. doi:10.1007/s11999-013-2885-y. Erratum in: Clin Orthop Relat Res. 2013 Jun;471(6):2041.
10. Healey JH, Abdeen A, Morris CD, Athanasian EA, Boland PJ. Telescope allograft method to reconstitute the diaphysis in limb salvage surgery. *Clin Orthop Relat Res.* 2009 Jul;467(7):1813–1819. doi:10.1007/s11999-008-0548-1
11. Hindiskere S, Staals E, Donati DM, Manfrini M. What is the survival of the telescope allograft technique to augment a short proximal femur segment in children after resection and distal femur endoprosthesis reconstruction for a bone sarcoma? *Clin Orthop Relat Res.* 2021 Aug 1;479(8):1780–1790. doi:10.1097/CORR.0000000000001686
12. Li Z, Lu M, Zhang Y, Gong T, Min L, Zhou Y, Luo Y, Tu C. 3D-printed custom-made short stem with porous structure for fixation of massive endoprosthesis in joint-preserving reconstruction after tumor resection. *J Orthop Surg Res.* 2023 Jun 29;18(1):468. doi:10.1186/s13018-023-03954-8
13. Denissen JJPM, Koenders N, van Hinte G, Groen F, van der Wees PJ, van der Geest ICM, Dierselhuis EF. Functional outcomes after reverse shoulder megaprosthesis following resection of malignant bone tumor in the proximal humerus: a systematic review and meta-analysis. *JSES Int.* 2023 Mar 31;7(4):592–600. doi:10.1016/j.jseint.2023.02.018
14. Ayvaz M, Cetik RM, Bakircioglu S, Tokgozoglu AM. Proximal humerus tumors: higher-than-expected risk of revision with constrained reverse shoulder arthroplasty. *Clin Orthop Relat Res.* 2020 Nov;478(11):2585–2595. doi:10.1097/CORR.0000000000001245
15. Lesensky J, Belzarena AC, Daniel M. Reconstruction with a double-constrained implant design after complex shoulder extra-articular resection. *World J Surg Oncol.* 2023 Sep 18;21(1):295. doi:10.1186/s12957-023-03173-9
16. Timofticiuc IA, Dragosloveanu S, Caruntu A, et al. 3D bioprinting in limb salvage surgery. *J Funct Biomater.* 2024;15(12):383. Published 2024 Dec 19. doi:10.3390/jfb15120383
17. Kotrych D, Angelini A, Bohatyrewicz A, Ruggieri P. 3D printing for patient-specific implants in musculoskeletal oncology. *EFORT Open Rev.* 2023 May 9;8(5):331–339. doi:10.1530/EOR-23-0066
18. Thadani VN, Riaz MJ, Singh G. The evolution of three-dimensional technology in musculoskeletal oncology. *J Clin Orthop Trauma.* Jul–Sep 2018;9(3):269–274. doi: 10.1016/j.jcot.2018.07.020. Epub 2018 Jul 25.
19. Kim Y. Three-dimensional printing technolgy in orthopedic oncology. *Clin Exp Pediatr.* 2022 Oct;65(10):496–497. doi:10.3345/cep.2022.00080
20. Zhang Z, Shi Y, Fu J, Liu D, Zhu D, Liu X, Dang J, Fan H. Customized three dimensional printed prosthesis as a novel intercalary reconstruction for resection of extremity bone tumours: a retrospective cohort study. *Int Orthop.* 2022 Dec;46(12):2971–2981. doi:10.1007/s00264-022-05559-y
21. Gungor-Ozkerim PS, Inci I, Zhang YS, Khademhosseini A, Dokmeci MR. Bioinks for 3D bioprinting: an overview. *Biomater Sci.* 2018;6(5):915–946. doi:10.1039/c7bm00765e
22. Kong Z, Wang X. Bioprinting technologies and bioinks for vascular model establishment. *Int J Mol Sci.* 2023;24(1):891. Published 2023 Jan 3. doi:10.3390/ijms24010891
23. Agostinacchio F, Mu X, Dirè S, Motta A, Kaplan DL. In situ 3D printing: opportunities with silk inks. *Trends Biotechnol.* 2021;39(7):719–730. doi: 10.1016/j.tibtech.2020.11.003
24. Roseti L, Parisi V, Petretta M, et al. Scaffolds for bone tissue engineering: state of the art and new perspectives. *Mater Sci Eng C Mater Biol Appl.* 2017;78:1246–1262. doi:10.1016/j.msec.2017.05.017
25. Fang Y. Guo Y, Liu T, Xu R, Mao S, Mo X, Zhang T, Ouyang L, Xiong Z, Sun W. Advances in 3D bioprinting. *Chin. J. Mech. Eng. Addit. Manuf. Front.* 2022, 1, 100011.
26. Wang W, Yeung KWK. Bone grafts and biomaterials substitutes for bone defect repair: A review. *Bioact Mater.* 2017;2(4):224–247. Published 2017 Jun 7. doi:10.1016/j.bioactmat.2017.05.007
27. Kang HW, Lee SJ, Ko IK, Kengla C, Yoo JJ, Atala A. A 3D bioprinting system to produce human-scale tissue constructs with structural integrity. *Nat Biotechnol.* 2016;34(3): 312–319. doi:10.1038/nbt.3413
28. Li J, Chen M, Fan X, Zhou H. Recent advances in bioprinting techniques: approaches, applications and future prospects. *J Transl Med.* 2016;14:271. Published 2016 Sep 20. doi:10.1186/s12967-016-1028-0
29. Lu Y, Chen G, Long Z, et al. Novel 3D-printed prosthetic composite for reconstruction of massive bone defects in lower extremities after malignant tumor resection. *J Bone Oncol.* 2019;16:100220. Published 2019 Jan 25. doi:10.1016/j.jbo.2019.100220
30. Wang W, Liu P, Zhang B, et al. Fused deposition modeling printed PLA/nano β-TCP composite bone tissue engineering scaffolds for promoting osteogenic induction function. *Int J Nanomedicine.* 2023;18:5815–5830. Published 2023 Oct 17. doi:10.2147/IJN.S416098
31. Moroni L, de Wijn JR, van Blitterswijk CA. 3D fiber-deposited scaffolds for tissue engineering: influence of pore distribution and architecture on mechanical properties. *Biomaterials.* 2006;27(7):974–985.

32. Daly AC, Critchley SE, Rencsok EM, Kelly DJ. A comparison of different bioinks for 3D bioprinting of fibrocartilage and hyaline cartilage. *Biofabrication.* 2016;8(4):045002. Published 2016 Oct 7. doi:10.1088/1758-5090/8/4/045002
33. Ghert M, Schneider P, Guyatt G, Thabane L, Vélez R, O'Shea T, Randall RL, Turcotte R, Wilson D, Wunder JS, Baptista AM, Cheng EY, Doung YC, Ferguson PC, Giglio V, Hayden J, Heels-Ansdell D, Khan SA, Sampath Kumar V, McKay P, Miller B, van de Sande M, Zumárraga JP, Bhandari M. Comparison of prophylactic intravenous antibiotic regimens after endoprosthetic reconstruction for lower extremity bone tumors: a randomized clinical trial. *JAMA Oncol.* 2022 Mar 1;8(3):345–353. doi:10.1001/jamaoncol.2021.6628
34. Gazendam AM, Schneider P, Bhandari M, Busse JW, Ghert M; on behalf of the PARITY Investigators. Defining minimally important differences in functional outcomes in musculoskeletal oncology. *J Bone Joint Surg Am.* 2022 Sep 21;104(18):1659–1666. doi:10.2106/JBJS.21.01539
35. Musculoskeletal Tumor Society. MSTS. Accessed Aug 4, 2022. www.msts.org/index.php/registry
36. Surveillance After Extremity Tumor Surgery. What is the SAFETY trial? Accessed 2023 Oct 24. https://safetyrct.com/
37. Ganguly S, Sasi A, Khan SA, Kumar VS, Kapoor L, Sharma MC, Mridha A, Barwad A, Thulkar S, Pushpam D, Bakhshi S. Formulation and validation of a baseline prognostic score for osteosarcoma treated uniformly with a non-high dose methotrexate-based protocol from a low middle income healthcare setting: a single centre analysis of 594 patients. *Front Oncol.* 2023 Apr 28;13:1148480. doi:10.3389/fonc.2023.1148480
38. Sasi A, Ganguly S, Biswas B, Pushpam D, Kumar A, Agarwala S, Khan SA, Kumar VS, Deo S, Sharma DN, Biswas A, Mridha A, Barwad A, Thulkar S, Bakhshi S. Development and validation of a prognostic score at baseline diagnosis for Ewing sarcoma family of tumors: a retrospective single institution analysis of 860 patients. *Am J Transl Res.* 2022 Feb 15;14(2):927–941.

Index

Pages in *italics* refer to figures and pages in **bold** refer to tables.

A

abductor lever arm, 88
above-knee amputation, 93
acetabular considerations, 89
acetabular wear, 91
Adams–Berger tendon graft technique, 76
advanced imaging, 10–15
allograft-prosthesis composite (APC) reconstruction, 36–38, 91, 170; *see also* autograft-prosthesis composites
  advantages, 69–70
  distal humerus, 69–70
  technique, 51
allografts, 201, 219–220
  intercalary resection, 177–178, **178**
  pelvic bone tumors, 145–148
  reconstruction, 50, 78, 170
  reconstructions, 120–121
American Joint Committee on Cancer (AJCC) staging system, 4
  for bone sarcoma, **6**
anatomical endoprosthesis, 48
anesthesia, 26
aneurysmal bone cysts (ABC), 8, 202–204, *203*
angiography; *see also* CT angiography
  distal femur resection, 94
ankle mortise, 118
anterior approach, 84–85
anterior dissection, 120
anterior intraperitoneal approach, 155–156
anterior skin incision, *96*
anterior spinal column fixation (ASCF), 159
antibiotics, 191
appendicular skeletal metastases, 207–217
argon beam coagulation, 200
arithmetic method, 166
arthroplasty in metastatic bone disease, 213
aseptic allografts, 220
aseptic loosening, 68
autoclaving, 179
autograft-prosthesis composites (AuPCs), 91–92
autografts, 201, 219–220
  pelvic bone tumors, 145–148
  reconstructions, 50
axillary nerve, 55–56

B

barrier
  effect, 32
  types, **33**
baseline tests, 207
baseplate positioning, 49
benign bone tumors, 4, **4**, 11, *11*
  aneurysmal bone cysts, 202–204
  cryoablation, 204
  Enneking staging system for, **6**
  limb salvage in, 196–205
  and malignant bone tumors, **4**, **10**
  percutaneous treatment of, 202
  radiofrequency ablation (RFA), 204
  reconstruction of, 201
  surgical technique of curettage, 196–202
benign lesions, 3
biceps femoris tendon, 76, 128–130, *129*
biceps muscle, 63, *65*
biologic agents, 221
biological reconstruction, 170
  distraction osteogenesis, 124
  nonvascularized fibular autografts, 35–36
  proximal humerus, 50–51
  recycled tumor-bearing autografts, 36
  structural or osteoarticular allografts, 35
  techniques, 35, 176
  vascularized fibular autografts, 35–36
biomaterials, 225–226
bioprinting technologies, 225–226
biopsy, 22–30, 44, 207–208
  common pitfalls in, **29**
  execution of, 26–29
  incisions misplacement, 23
  misplacement, *23*
  percutaneous core needle biopsy (CNB), 25–29
  principles, 22–23
  technique types, 23–25
    core needle (Trocar) biopsy, 24
    fine-needle aspiration (FNA) biopsy, 23–24
    incisional (open) biopsy, 25
  transverse, *24*
  types, **24**
bone banking, 220
Bone Cement Implantation Syndrome (BCIS), 215
bone cement spacer, 185
bone edema, 170
bone grafting
  allografts, 219–220
  autografts, 219–220
  biology of, 218–219
  cancellous autografts, 219
  cortical autografts, 219
  function, 218
  ideal, 219
  osteoconduction, 218–219
  osteogenesis, 218
  osteoinduction, 218
  substitutes, 220–221
  vascularized bone grafts, 219
bone integration, 131
bone resection, 66
bone scan, 20
bone scintigraphy, 63
bone tumors
  AJCC Staging System for, 6
  biopsy of, *see* biopsy
  classification, 4
  clinical evaluation of, 3
  clinical presentation of, 3
  computed tomography in, 15
  diagnoses by age, **3**
  en bloc resection of, **74**
  history, 3
  imaging of, 8–21
  matrix types in, *9*
  pelvic, 137–150
  physical examination, 3–4
  radiographic evaluation of, 8–10
  scapular resection for, *see* scapular resection
  staging, 4–7
  surgical management of, 31–40
  WHO classification of, **5**
bony and articular anatomy, 43
brachialis muscle, 65, *66*

C

calcium phosphate, 220–221
cancellous autografts, 219
capsule and ligamentum teres, 83
carpal-ulnar junction, 77
cavity, walls and edges of, *198*
cement augmentation, 181
cemented APC, 37
cemented fixation, 214
cemented stems, 101
cemented total hip arthroplasty, 216
chemical agents, 198
chemotherapeutic agents, 166
chest wall assessment, 57
chondroid matrix, 8–9
chondroid tumors, 15
chondrosarcoma, *18*, *147*
  of sacrum, *156*
  scapula, *57*
  Type III pelvic resection in, *143*
clavicula pro humero (CPH), 50
complications
  aseptic loosening, 102
  hardware failure, 101
  infection, 101
  of limb salvage surgery, 39, **39**
  neurovascular injury, 102
  patellar complications, 102
  periprosthetic fracture, 102
component failure or fracture, 68
compressive osseointegration, 224
computed tomography (CT) scan, 15–19, 63
  chest for pulmonary metastasis, 20
  chondrosarcoma, *18*
  CT angiography (CTA), 15–19, *19*, 63, *107*
  distal femur resection, 94–95
  giant cell tumor, *17*
  osteochondroma, 19
  "rings-and-arcs" pattern, *19*
continuous passive motion (CPM) devices, 102
contrast-enhanced MRI, 10, 154
conventional radiography, 8
conventional reconstruction techniques, 188
core biopsy needle, *28*
core needle (Trocar) biopsy, 24, 44
  image-guided, 22, 207–208
cortical autografts, 219
cryoablation, 200, 204
CT angiography (CTA), 15–19, *19*, 63, *107*
curettage, surgical technique of, 196–202
curopsy, 204
custom-made prostheses, 145
custom stem, 89

D

definitive implantation, 89
delayed functional recovery, 70
deltopectoral approach, 45–46
dental mirrors, *199*
digital rectal examination (DRE), 154
distal femoral osteosarcoma, *13*
distal femur resection, 93–103, *94–95*
angiography, 94
closure, 101
computed tomography, 94–95
endoprosthesis, *101–102*
femoral osteotomy and margin assessment, 96–97
final assembly and assessment, 100–101
haemostasis and field preparation, 97
infection, 101–102
knee joint, 93
limb-sparing procedures, 95
local recurrence, 93
magnetic resonance imaging, 94
nuclear scintigraphy, 95
plain radiographs, 94
pop+liteal vesse+l+s+ and nerves, 93–94
prosthetic reconstruction, 102–103
sartorial (adductor) canal, 93
skeletal defect–endoprosthesis reconstruction, 97–99
surgical resection, 96
trial placement and adjustments, 99–100
distal fibula resection, 126
fibular resections, 131
distal humerus tumor, *68*, *70*
allograft-prosthetic composite reconstruction, 69–70
endoprosthetic reconstruction, 66
implant survival, 68
infection, 68–70
osteoarticular allograft reconstruction, 68–69
preoperative planning, 62–63
preparation for reconstruction, 66–67
soft tissue dissection, 64–66
soft tissue reconstruction, 67–68
surgical anatomy, 62
surgical technique, 63–64
distal radioulnar joint (DRUJ), 76–77
distal radius, 71
distal tibia resection, 118–124
bone resection, 120
distraction osteogenesis, 124
endoprosthetic reconstruction, *123*, 123–124
implant survival, 123
incision and approach, 120
osteosarcoma, *122*
patient positioning, 120
soft tissue dissection, 120
surgical anatomy and preoperative planning, 118–119
surgical margin planning, 119
surgical technique, 119
distal ulna, 76
distraction osteogenesis, 124
documentation, 29
double-barrel fibula, 178–179
dual tendon stabilization, 77
DWI, 14
dynamic contrast–enhanced MRI (DCE-MRI), 14, 20
dynamic humeral suspension, 59
dynamic radioulnar convergence, 76

E

elbow and hand function, 55
elbow joint capsule, 66
emerging imaging techniques, 8
en bloc tumor resection, **76**, 151, 177
endoprosthesis, 223–225; *see also* endoprosthetic reconstruction; prosthetic reconstruction
expandable prosthesis, 167–169
hemipelvic endoprosthesis, 145
intercalary endoprostheses, 181–185
endoprosthetic reconstruction, *33*, *34*, 33–35
distal humerus, 66
distal tibia resection, 123–124
scapular resection, 59–60
technique of, 67
Enneking staging system, 4, **6**, *32*
classification of surgical margins, **32**, *32*
epiphyseal lesions, 9
Ewing sarcoma, 8, 10, 44, 93, *183*
distal humerus, *63–64*, *70*
femur, *12*
humerus, *193*
ilium, *142*
magnetic resonance imaging (MRI) of, *46*, *127*
pathological fracture in, *11*
planned skin incision, *182*
of proximal femur, *16*, *85–86*
proximal humerus, 45, *46*
radiological images of, *146*
tibia, *10*
trans-acetabular resection, *147*
Excisional biopsy, 25
expandable prosthesis, 167–169
extensive extremity sarcomas, 188–195
extensor mechanism reconstruction techniques, 115
extensor musculature, 65
external beam radiotherapy (EBRT), 216
external fixation index (EFI), 124
extra-articular resection (Malawer type V/VI), 47
extracorporeal irradiation (ECRT), 36, *37*, 122–123, 179, 185; *see also* recycled autograft reconstructions

F

fatigue fractures, 179
Fédération Nationale des Centres de Lutte Contre le Cancer (FNCLCC), 4
femoral component cementation, 100
femoral nerve, 85
femoral osteotomy, 96–97
femoral preparation, 99, *99*
femoral stem fractures, 101
F-18 fluorodeoxyglucose (18F-FDG), 20
fibular autograft reconstructions, 121
fibular diaphysis, 126
resection, 131
fibular head autograft arthroplasty, 73, 75
fibular resections, 126–133, *127*
distal fibula, 126
distal fibula resection, 131
fibular diaphysis resection, 131–132
plain radiographs of, *127*
postoperative rehabilitation protocol, 131–133
proximal fibula, 126
proximal fibula resections, 126–128
Type I resection, 128
Type II resection, 128–130, *129*
final implantation and assembly, *100*
fine-needle aspiration (FNA) biopsy, 23–24
flexorplasty, 67
flexor-pronator muscles, 65
fracture risk assessment, 208–209
free fibular autografts (FFAs), 170–171, 178–179
free vascularized fibula graft (FVFG), 50
fresh-frozen allografts, 220
functional outcomes, 31, 39, 48, 50, 59, 72, **74**, 93, 103, 105, 121, 123, 130, 144–148, 154, 160, 169, 191–192, 204, 211
functional preservation, 31
function testing, 99
fungating synovial sarcoma, *194*

G

gamma irradiation, 220
gastrocnemius muscle, 130
genetic syndromes, 3
Giant cell tumor of bone (GCTB), *73–74*, 76; *see also* giant cell tumors (GCT)
giant cell tumors (GCT), 14, 71, *71*, *121*
computed tomography (CT) scan, *17*
computed tomography (CT) scan for, *17*
glenohumeral involvement, 43
glenoid component placement, 49
gluteus maximus, 84
gold standard, 25
graft fracture, 59, 69
graft-host fixation, 51
graft incorporation, 218

H

haemostasis, 97
hematologic malignancies, 55
hematoma, 29
heterogeneous tumors, 24
high-field MRI, 15
high-grade tumors, 33
hip joint capsule, 83
hip rotationplasty (Type B), 189–190
hip transposition, 146
humeral component placement, 49
humeral suspension, 59

I

ice-cream cone prosthesis, 144
ideal bone graft, 219
iliofemoral arthrodesis, 144
ilioinguinal extension, 84, 141
ilium, 141, *142*
image-guided core needle biopsy, 22, 207–208
imaging, of bone tumors, 8–21
advanced, 10–15
assessment, 8–10
CT angiography in, 15–19
evaluation of systemic extent, 19–20
surveillance imaging, 21
therapeutic response, assessment of, 20–21
impending fractures, 210–213
implant selection, 88–89
incisional (open) biopsy, 25
induced membrane technique, 185
intercalary allograft, 131
intercalary reconstruction, 185

intercalary resection, 176–185
allograft reconstruction, 177–178, **178**
bone quality and defect, 176–177, *177*
Capanna technique, 179
implant survival, 183
local recurrence, 177
oncological safety, 177
reconstruction methods, 176
tumor location and extent, 176
intra-articular resection (Malawer type I), 47, *98*
intralesional margin, 32
intramedullary nails, 216
intraoperative fluoroscopy, *199*
intraosseous bone lesions, 29
ipsilateral nonvascularized fibular autograft (fibular centralization), 121–122
ischiofemoral arthrodesis, 144

J

joint cartilage, 32
joint degeneration, 191
joint resection, 57

K

Karnofsky Performance Score, 145
knee disarticulation, 96–97
knee joint, 93
knee rotationplasty (Type A), 189–190

L

lateral femoral cutaneous nerve (LFCN), 84
LCL reconstruction, 130
lesion, in long bones, **8**, *9*
Ligament Augmentation and Reconstruction System (LARS), 59
limb-length discrepancies (LLD), 166, 174
limb salvage surgery, 31, 165
allograft-prosthesis composite (APC) reconstruction, 36–38; *see also* autograft-prosthesis composite; limb sparing surgery
barrier effect, 32
in benign bone tumors, 196–205
bioprinting technologies and biomaterials, 225–226
complications of, 39, **39**
compression fixation system used in, *224*
endoprosthesis, 223–225
goals of, 31
Henderson classification, 39
implant survival, 223, 225
local recurrence, 31–32
margin selection in practice, 33
principles, 31
recent advances in, 223–227
reconstruction strategies in, 33–35
site-specific approaches, 38
in skeletally immature patients, 167
soft tissue reconstruction in, 38–39
surgical margins, concept of, 31–32
techniques, 3
3D bioprinting, 225–226
limb sparing surgery, 95
liquid nitrogen–treated autograft, 123
local adjuvants, 199
local recurrence, 31–32, 93, 105, 137, 145, 177, 191
long-term follow-up, 60
low-grade tumors, 33
lyophilization, 220

M

magnetic resonance angiography (MRA), 15
magnetic resonance imaging (MRI), 10–15, 62–63, 126
contrast-enhanced, 154
diffusion-weighted imaging, 8
dynamic contrast–enhanced MRI (DCE-MRI), 14, 20
of Ewing sarcoma, *46*, *127*
high-field MRI, 15
of osteosarcoma, *15*, *119*, *168*, *179*
pelvis and lumbosacral spine, *155*
malignant bone tumors, 4, **4**, **10**
malignant tumors, 3–4, 71
marginal margin, 32
margin assessment, 96–97
Masquelet (induced-membrane) technique, 185; *see also* induced membrane technique
massive allografts, 71
reconstruction, 120
massive bone allografts, 59
medial gastrocnemius muscle, *111*
medial malleolus, 118
mesh-based static suspension, 60, *60*
mesh suspension techniques, 59
metaphyseal lesions, 9
metastatic disease, 55
metastatic renal cell carcinoma, *215*
metastatic thyroid carcinoma, *214*
meticulous hemostasis, 22
minimally invasive percutaneous techniques, 202
modular hemipelvic endoprosthesis, 145
modular intercalary endoprostheses, 181–185
multidisciplinary planning, 44
multimodal analgesia, 160
musculocutaneous nerve, 56
musculoskeletal neoplasms, 22
musculoskeletal oncology, 32
Musculoskeletal Tumor Registry (MsTR), 227
musculoskeletal tumors, 4
musculoskeletal tumor society (MSTS) score, 48, 59, 91, 123–124, 146
myocutaneous flaps, 159–160
myositis ossificans, 15

N

nail-cement spacer reconstruction, 52–53
navigation-assisted surgery, 225
neoadjuvant chemotherapy, 44
neurovascular bundle, 57
neurovascular examination, 3
neurovascular injury, 102
neurovascular management, 85–88
nonabsorbable sutures, 66
nonbiological reconstruction techniques, 176
nonreconstructive soft tissue closure, 60
nonvascularized fibular autografts, 72
nonvascularized fibular grafts, 36, 131, 178
nuclear scintigraphy, 95
nutritional optimization, 63

O

occupational therapy, 160
oncological control, 31
on-site evaluation, 29
operative time, 121
osseous anatomy, 83
osteoarticular allograft
arthroplasty, 73–75
reconstruction, 50, 68–69
osteoconduction, 218–219
osteogenesis, 218
osteoid matrix, 8–9, *9*
osteoid osteoma, 15, *204*
osteoinduction, 218
osteosarcoma, 8, 93, *165*, *179*, 188
CT angiography of, *19*, *95*
distal femur in, *95*
distal tibia, *122*
magnetic resonance imaging (MRI) of, *15*, *119*, *168*, *179*
patient with, *44*
plain radiographs of, *45*
proximal humerus, *45*
proximal tibia, *106–107*, *110*
osteotomies, 120

P

pain, 3
pain management, 191
partial limb salvage, 188–195
classification, 189
growth prediction and limb length considerations, 189
hip rotationplasty (Type B), 190
knee rotationplasty (Type A), 190
local recurrence, 191, 196
neurovascular assessment, 189
oncologic staging and imaging, 189
pain management and antibiotics, 191
preoperative evaluation and planning, 189
prerequisites, 188
prosthetic consultation, 190
psychosocial counseling, 189
psychosocial support, 191
quality of life, 192
rehabilitation and prosthetic planning, 191
rotationplasty, 188
surgical phocomelia, 192–194
surgical technique, 190
vascular and limb monitoring, 190
partial wrist arthrodesis, 72–73
patient positioning, 26
pedestal cup prostheses, 144
pelvic resections, 137–150
allografts and autografts, 145–148
anatomical considerations, 138
biopsy planning, 139–140
Enneking/Dunham classification, 137–138
general surgical principles, 140
hip joint, 138
implant survival, 145
inguinal and anterior pelvic region, 139
key decision factors, 142
local recurrence, 137, 145
navigation in, 149
osseous framework, 138
postoperative care and rehabilitation, 148–149

reconstruction, 141
reconstructive options, 142
sacrum and sacroiliac joint, 138
sciatic notch region, 138–139
surgical techniques and resection planning, 140
Type I pelvic resections, 142–143
Type II pelvic resections, 143–145
Type III pelvic resections, 148
utilitarian pelvic incision, 140–141
visceral relationships, 139
pelvis, 38
percutaneous core needle biopsy (CNB), 25–29, *27*
percutaneous image-guided techniques, 205
percutaneous therapy, 204
periacetabular metastasis, 215–216
Harrington technique for, 215, *215*
periacetabular replacement (PAR) Endoprosthesis, 144–145
periprosthetic infection, 68
peroneal nerve injury, 133
phenol, 200
physeal sacrifice, 165
physical examination, 207
physical modalities, 198
plain radiographs, 84
polidocanol, 202
polidocanol sclerotherapy, 204–205
polymethylmethacrylate (PMMA), 185, 200–201
polymethylmethacrylate (PMMA) cement, 215–216
polypropylene mesh, 59, 146
popliteal artery, **106**
popliteus muscle, *110*
porous tantalum components, 216
positron emission tomography–CT (PET–CT), 20–21, 84
post-chemotherapy MRI, 11
posterior approach, 156–157
posterior pelvic ring fixation, 159
postoperative management, 160
postoperative rehabilitation, 53, 60
protocol, 131–133
post-scapulectomy reconstruction, 57
preoperative angiography, 83
preoperative planning, 56
primary bone malignancies, 31, 93, 137
profunda femoris artery, 85
prolene mesh, 48, *49*, 52, *114*
Prophylactic Antibiotic Regimens in Tumor Surgery (PARITY) trial, 227
proposed algorithmic approach, 167
prosthesis
reconstruction, 48
templating, 84
types of, 48
prosthetic reconstructions, 53
distal femur resection, 102–103
prosthetic replacement, 78
prosthetic wrist replacement, 75–76
proximal femur, *210*
proximal femur endoprosthesis, 88, *90*
proximal femur resection, 83–92
allograft-prosthesis composite, 91
anterior approach, 84–85
autograft-prosthesis composite (AuPC), 91–92
capsule and ligamentum teres, 83
clinical considerations, 91
implant survival, 91
infection, 91, 101
muscular attachments and function, 83
neurovascular anatomy, 83
neurovascular management, 85–88
osseous anatomy, 83
preoperative planning, 84
reconstruction options, 88–90
resection level and osteotomy, 88
soft tissue dissection, 85–88
surgical anatomy, 83
surgical technique of, 84
proximal fibula, 126
proximal humerus, 43–53, *45–46*
anatomic considerations, 43
biological reconstruction techniques, 50–51
bony and articular anatomy, 43
clinical assessment, 44
extra-articular resection (Malawer type V/VI), 47
imaging and staging, 44
implant survival, 49
infection, 51, 59–60
intra-articular resection (Malawer type I), 47
muscular attachments, 43
nail-cement spacer reconstruction, 52–53
neurovascular structures, 43
postoperative rehabilitation, 53
prosthetic reconstruction, 48
soft tissue reconstruction, 48
surgical implications, 43–44
surgical management, 44–46
surgical technique, 51
proximal polymethylmethacrylate (PMMA) cement, 52
proximal tibia, 105–117
endoprosthesis, *112*
local recurrence, 105
psoas tendon, 85
psychosocial implications, 166
pulsatile saline lavage, 197–198, *199*

Q

quality of life, 192; *see also* functional outcomes

R

radial/ulnar nerve palsy, 68
radiation therapy, 166
radiofrequency ablation (RFA), 204
radionuclide bone scan (99mTc-MDP), 20
randomized controlled trials, 221
RANKL inhibitors, 207
rapid on-site evaluation (ROSE), 29
reconstruction techniques, 38
reconstructive strategies, 131
rectum, 155
rectus femoris, 84, *87*, 96
recurrence, *see* local recurrence, tumor recurrence
recurrent tumors, 33
recycled autograft reconstructions, 122
extracorporeal irradiation (ECRT), 36, *37*, 122–123, 179, 185
liquid nitrogen freezing, 180
recycled tumor-bearing autografts, 36, **184**
rehabilitation
postoperative management, 160
and prosthetic planning, 191
renal cell carcinoma, *208*
resected tumor specimen, *66*
resection arthrodesis, 216
resurfaced APC, 37
reverse total shoulder arthroplasty (RTSA), 48–49
rhabdomyosarcoma, *58*
rotational alignment, 89
rotationplasty, 188; *see also* partial limb salvage
hip (Type B), 189–190
knee (Type A), 189–190
surgical technique, 190
rotator cuff, 43, 52

S

sacral tumors, 151–161
anatomical overview, 151
anterior intraperitoneal approach, 155–156
biomechanical considerations, 151–152
biomechanical studies, 160
classification and levels, 153
local recurrence, 151
lumbosacropelvic junction, 151
operative techniques of spinopelvic reconstruction, 157
posterior approach, 156–157
postoperative management and rehabilitation, 160
preoperative evaluation and planning, 153–155
sacral neural anatomy, 153
soft tissue coverage and myocutaneous flaps, 159–160
spinopelvic fixation (SPF) techniques, 159
surgical approaches to, 155
vascular anatomy of, 152–153
sacrectomy; *see also* sacral tumors
complications, **161**
levels of, *154*
reconstruction techniques, 160
sacroiliac joint (SIJ), 151
sacrum, 151
chondrosarcoma of, *156*
chordoma of, *158*
saddle prosthesis, 144
sampling error, 25
sandwich technique, 201
sartorial (adductor) canal, 93
sartorius, 84
Sauvé–Kapandji (S-K) procedure, 72, 76
scapular pillar graft, 50
scapular resection, 55–60
classification, 56
dissection and exposure, 57
dynamic humeral suspension, 59
endoprosthetic reconstruction, 59–60
humeral suspension, 59
local recurrence, 55
massive bone allografts, 59
mesh-based static suspension, 60
nonreconstructive soft tissue closure, 60
patient positioning, 56
postoperative rehabilitation, 60
preoperative planning, 56
reconstruction options, 57–59
rhabdomyosarcoma of, *58*

surgical anatomy of, 55–56
surgical approaches, 56
surgical technique and, 56
sciatic nerve, 189
sclerotherapy, 202–204
segmental transport, 185
shoulder girdle resections, **56**
single fibula, 178
size-matched allograft, 51
skeletal defect–endoprosthesis reconstruction, 97–99
skeletal defect, reconstruction of, 48
skeletally immature patients, 165–174
expandable prosthesis, 167–169
growth prosthesis, 166
limb-length discrepancy, 166
limb salvage and reconstruction strategies, 167
implant survival, 169
local recurrence, 170
patterns and timing, 166
physeal sacrifice and growth disturbance, 165
proposed algorithmic approach, 167
psychosocial implications, 166
surgical strategy, 166–167
technical constraints, 166
transepiphyseal resection (TER), 169
skeletal metastases, 207–217
bone disease, 209
clinical decision-making, 209
complete and/ or impending fractures in, 210
fracture risk assessment, 208–209
impending fractures, 211–213
nonoperative management of, 216
periacetabular metastasis, 215–216
postoperative radiation therapy, 216
preoperative multidisciplinary, 210
prognostic tools, 209
resection & endoprosthetic replacement/ arthroplasty in, 213
surgical planning, 209–210
surgical principles and implant selection, 210–211
survival in, 209
survival prediction and implications, 209
small longitudinal skin incision, 29
soft tissue coverage, 159–160
soft tissue dissection, 85–88, 120
bone resection, 66
distal humerus, 64–66
elbow joint resection, 66
muscular dissection, 65
neurovascular dissection, 64–65
soft tissue exposure, 45
soft tissue management, 120
soft tissue reconstruction, 38–39, 48, 66, 67–68, 89, 141
proximal humerus, 48
soft tissue tumors, 8
spermatic cord/round ligament, 141
spinal and pelvic tumors, 6, **6**
spinopelvic fixation (SPF) techniques, 159
spinopelvic reconstruction, 157, 160; *see also* sacrectomy
Stanmore design, 167
sterile preparation, 26
sterility testing, 220
structural iliac crest bone grafting, 72
structural/osteoarticular allografts, 35
structured physiotherapy program, 148
strut grafts, 143
suprascapular nerve, 56
surgical management
of bone tumors, 31–40
deltopectoral approach, 45–46
implant survival, 35, 38
infection, 35, 38
patient positioning, 44
principles, 44
proximal humerus, 44–46
surgical margins
concept of, 31–33
curative, 32
intralesional, 32
marginal, 32
wide, 32
surgical phocomelia, 192–194
Surveillance After Extremity Tumor Surgery (SAFETY) trial, 227
surveillance imaging, 21
suture anchor fixation, 130
systemic extent evaluation, 19–20
systemic symptoms, 3

T

Telengiectatic Osteosarcoma, *52*
therapeutic response, assessment of, 20–21
3D bioprinting, 225–226
3D-printed implants, 60
tibia cortical strut autografts (TCSA), 72
tibia, of Ewing sarcoma, *10*
tibiotalar arthrodesis, 131
Tikhoff–Linberg resection, *58*
tissue processing, 220
tissue sampling, 22
total wrist arthrodesis, 71–72
transarterial embolization, 217
transepiphyseal resection (TER), 169–170
transverse biopsy scars, 24, *24*
transverse incisions, 119
trendelenburg gait, 83
trial assembly, 89
trial placement and adjustments, 99–100, *100*
triangular fibrocartilage complex (TFCC), 76
triceps muscle, 65
trochanteric osteotomy, 84
tumor-devitalized autografts, 171–173
tumor recurrence, 188
tumor resection, 131
Type I fibula resections, **128**, 128–130, *129*
Type II fibula resections, **128**, 128–130, *129*
Type I pelvic resections, *142*, 142–143
Type II pelvic resections, 143–145
Type III pelvic resections, 148

U

ulnar buttress arthroplasty, 77
ulnar centralization techniques, 72
ulnar translocation techniques, 72
uncemented APC, 37
uncemented porous-coated/fluted stems, 89
utilitarian fibular incision, 126
utilitarian pelvic incision, 140–141, *141*

V

vascular and limb monitoring, 190
vascular endothelial growth factor (VEGF), 20
vascular imaging, 94
vascularized bone grafts, 219
vascularized fibular autograft, 122
vascularized fibular grafts (VFGs), 35, 170–171, 178–179, **181**; *see also* free vascularized fibula
vastus intermedius, 96
vastus lateralis, 84

W

wet sponges, *198*
whole-body imaging MRI, 20–21
wound closure, 90–91
wrist
alternative reconstruction techniques, 78
arthrodesis, **74**
arthroplasty, 73, **75–76**
distal radius, 71
distal ulna, 76
fibular head autograft arthroplasty, 75
osteoarticular allograft arthroplasty, 73–75
partial wrist arthrodesis, 72–73
prosthetic wrist replacement, 75–76
reconstruction, stabilization strategies in, 76
total wrist arthrodesis, 71–72
ulnar buttress arthroplasty, 77
ulnar stump, 77

Z

zinc chloride, 200

For Product Safety Concerns and Information please contact our
EU representative GPSR@taylorandfrancis.com Taylor & Francis
Verlag GmbH, Kaufingerstraße 24, 80331 München, Germany